WILDERNESS EMERGENCY CARE
Third Edition, Revised

Steve Donelan

With special chapters on:

Solar Radiation and Eye Protection *by Stephen R. Chun, OD, FAAO*
Herbal First Aid *by Charles Garcia*

Supporting courses in:
- Basic Wilderness First Aid
- Wilderness First Aid
- Wilderness First Responder
- Wilderness EMT Upgrade

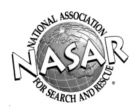

i

ISBN 978-0-9864440-6-7 (Paperback Edition)

Editing by Steve Donelan and Emily E. James

Cover design and drawings by Evelyn Sinclair, www.gangof1.com

Front cover art adapted from *The Domes of Yosemite* by Albert Bierstadt

Back cover inset photos by Ben Schifrin, MD, FACEP

Photographs by Ben Schifrin, MD, FACEP; Joanne Clapp Fullager; Ruth McConnell; Mike Cardwell; Oleg Grachev; Linda Garcia; and other sources as credited

Printed and bound in the United States of America

First Printing, 2018

Published by The National Association For Search And Rescue, Inc.

PO Box 232020

Centreville, VA 20120-2020

Visit www.NASAR.org

To my students,
Who are also my teachers

Steve

Contents

Biological hazards

Medical problems

Evacuation and survival

Introduction

Wilderness Emergency Care can be used as a textbook in emergency care courses or by autodidacts who want to learn and practice on their own. I hope that you will find this book interesting and enjoyable to read, and that it will help you avoid, prevent and prepare for emergencies by guiding you through mental rehearsals of what can happen and what you can do. I also hope that you will find the book to be a useful reference.

In wilderness or disaster situations, where resources are limited and medical care is not available, you need to know more and have a much larger repertory of skills to cope with emergencies than you would when an ambulance is 10 minutes away. But as a teacher, I have seen that people learn and remember best if they know the reasons for what they learn, rather than just memorizing signs, symptoms and procedures. My experience is supported by many studies of skills learning and retention. So I always explain topics, rather than just describing problems and treatments, and I encourage you to make logical and causal connections.

For example, what damage does an injury do, and how does the body react? How does that reaction produce the signs and symptoms that we find when we assess the patient? Similarly, how do the body and brain react to the stress of heat, cold or altitude? Once you've thought through these questions, you should be able to figure out what is going on in an emergency and what to do about it, even if you can't remember exactly what I or another writer recommended.

Medical terms are descriptive and sometimes humorous, but they come from Latin or Greek. So I demystify terms by breaking them down and showing their literal sense. I put ideas into historical and cultural context because that helps us to understand them. It also reminds us that some ideas may turn out to be wrong, as so many of their predecessors were. So the same process of inquiry and analysis that gives us some confidence in current ideas about emergency care should prevent us from getting too dogmatic.

Most of the chapters in this book started as lesson plans and handouts for my classes and articles that I published in various journals. These chapters have been updated and expanded for the Third Edition. Sources used for each chapter are in the Bibliography. In Recommended Reading, you will find an annotated list of the books and journals that I find most useful and interesting. The *Wilderness Medical Society Practice Guidelines for Wilderness Emergency Care* (of which I am a contributor and peer reviewer) provides a consensus of wilderness medical experts and educators on how to deal with medical problems and injuries in the wilderness. For resuscitation, the *2015 American Heart Association Guidelines for CPR and ECC* explains the current standards.

In the chapters on injuries, you will find illustrated guides to bandaging and splinting methods, including improvised techniques. You will not find many of these in other books. Urban rescuers use standard equipment, and their bandages and splints only need to stay on for a short ambulance ride to the hospital. But wilderness rescuers need to improvise with what is available. Also, their bandages and splints need to stay in place while the patient walks, skis, or scrambles out, or is evacuated.

Even more important than physical skills are the mental and social skills of emergency care: figuring out what the problems are and what is causing them; setting priorities and making a plan; organizing and leading a rescue or working in a team; communicating with the patient and other people on the scene; and coping with the psychological stress of an emergency in yourself and others. I describe these skills in the first chapter and refer to them throughout the book. You can develop the mental and social skills of emergency care by practicing techniques realistically and doing role-playing scenarios.

A supplementary chapter on herbal first aid by Charles Garcia will introduce you to beneficial plants that you can find in the wilderness. But to learn how to identify and use these plants, you should take a course from an herbalist.

However you use this book, I hope that it will make your wilderness activities safer and more enjoyable. I also hope that it will prepare you to help yourself and other people in a wilderness emergency or an urban disaster.

Chapter 1. Training for wilderness emergencies

Urban rescuers face many challenges – technical, physical and psychological. Unless they are involved in a major disaster, however, urban rescuers usually have quick access to medical care, transportation, shelter, supplies and reinforcements. And although they may go into hazardous situations to perform emergency care, these rescuers can usually retreat to safe surroundings.

In the wilderness or a disaster situation, you can count on none of these advantages. You may have to care for patients for many hours during bivouacs or strenuous evacuations. Your shelter and supplies will be what you have with you or can improvise, and reinforcements may be long in coming. With limited resources, you must protect your patients and yourself against weather and other environmental hazards. What kind of training prepares you for wilderness emergencies or major disasters?

Before you can take care of others, you must first learn the survival skills needed to take care of yourself in the wilderness. These skills include knowing what to carry and to wear to survive the worst possible conditions. You should learn how the body interacts with environmental stresses such as heat, cold and altitude; and how clothing and shelter can control this interaction. You should also practice first aid skills, such as bandaging and splinting, on yourself as well as on others because you may have to treat your own injuries.

Throughout training, you must play an active learning role. Passive learning conditions people to absorb information and regurgitate it onto exam papers. TV and other passive recreations condition people to be spectators, and so do instructors who talk at length without student interaction.

Instructors who teach interactively and ask frequent questions, however, put you in an active learning mode. They guide you through the process of making the connections between cause and effect, mechanisms of injury and damage, signs and symptoms and what is going on in the body. Once you have made these connections in the classroom, you are more likely to be able to figure out what is going on and what to do in a real emergency.

Skills demonstrations and practice should be role-playing. You should always get into the role during skills practice by talking to the patient and saying only what you would say in a real emergency. By doing that, you will train yourself to provide good patient care, which is more important than any single mechanical skill; and you will develop mental as well as physical reflexes to carry you through an emergency.

Psychological aspects of first aid

Any serious emergency can make rescuers as well as victims feel that they are losing control of events. In the wilderness, the strange surroundings, exposure, and insidious effects of environmental stress on the brain all can combine to induce fear, despair or apathy. You can begin training yourself to cope with these stresses by understanding them.

Everyone is susceptible to stress. Behavior that denies or evades the reality of an unpleasant situation is common. This behavior may range from unrealistic assessments or plans to apathy or withdrawal. Some may react by blaming themselves or others in the group. Others may have sensory disturbances like tunnel vision or muffled hearing.

By recognizing these behavioral problems as signs of emergency stress, you can avoid being pulled into unproductive emotional responses. When causes of the stress are physical, simple physical measures, such as rehydration, energy food, and protection from the elements, can have major psychological benefits. Productive action also gives people a sense of regaining control. Reasoning with the unrealistic and reassuring the fearful may help, but tactful redirection to useful tasks is often more effective therapy.

Every serious injury or illness has psychological effects. Patients may be locked into an internal conversation about pain or fear. As a rescuer, you need to join in this conversation and redirect it to what you and the patient can do, together, to help. Those who are seriously ill or injured are often in a highly suggestible state, so what you say and how you say it can influence autonomic nervous system functions, positively or negatively. These functions include pulse, blood pressure, respiration, and the inflammatory response to an injury. Even in a positive context, scare words like "die" or "bleeding" can have a negative effect. Instead, use only positive or neutral words (and never describe the injuries) when a patient can hear; but always tell the truth.

If a patient asks about his or her injuries, acknowledge the problem in neutral terms, then redirect the conversation to what you can do to help. For example, if a patient asks "Is my leg broken?" you can say "There is an injury, but let's put a splint on it, and tell me if that makes it more comfortable." Give a patient choices whenever possible, and set it up as a win-win situation. For example, "Would you be more comfortable in this position or that position?"

Recognizing problems and understanding their causes, however, are not enough. You must train yourself to respond as a rescuer to behavioral problems. Behavioral emergencies can be acted out in class. You can take turns trying to talk down someone playing the role of a suicidal victim, for instance. Clues to organic causes of behavioral problems, often overlooked, can be scattered about. Realistic role-playing, along with discussion, teaches you how to talk to a disturbed patient and when to back off or seek reinforcements.

Communication and teamwork

Communication is not by voice alone. Short team exercises done in complete silence train you to become more aware of body language and of what others on the team are doing. For example, each team can be challenged to do as many splints as possible in five minutes on one victim. Teams should be given a few moments to make a plan, but once the clock starts, every word spoken costs a point. This exercise also helps cure the habit of unnecessary chatter, which can turn emergency responses into chaos.

Injury or illness can suppress or alter body language and facial expression as well as speech. While rescuers usually understand this in theory, the absent or altered signals can still make it hard for them to communicate with patients. Realistic role-playing in scenarios trains you to respond to the victim's condition, not to the distortions of communication caused by the condition. Too often, specific skills are practiced out of context. Practicing a splint on a partner

who is joking and moving the supposedly injured limb about freely does not prepare you to treat someone with a real fracture.

One of the hardest lessons to learn in emergency care is that democracy does not work at an accident scene. Group efforts like backboarding and extrication train you in scene leadership and teamwork. When acting as leader, you learn to plan ahead and give unambiguous directions. As a member of the team, you learn to listen to the leader, talk as little as possible, and address questions or suggestions to the leader. Cross discussions cut the lines of leadership. It is also important that only one rescuer talk to each patient. When you play the role of patient in class, you learn how disorienting it is to have several voices competing for your already distracted attention.

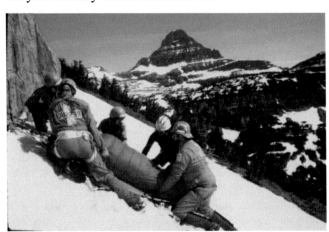

Photo courtesy of Ben Schifrin, MD

Legal and ethical aspects

Before providing emergency care, you need the **consent** of the patient. You should also explain what you want to do so that the patient understands the **risks** (if any) – that makes it **informed consent**. If the patient is (or becomes) unresponsive, that is **implied consent**. The law presumes that anyone who cannot respond needs help. When treating a **minor**, you should get permission from any parent or legal guardian present, but you should also persuade the child to let you help. Techniques for communicating with and treating children are described in the chapter on patient assessment.

When you provide emergency care, your legal status depends on whether you have a **duty to act**. Medical professionals who are on the job or at their place of employment where emergency care is normally provided always have a duty to act in an emergency, even if they are not on shift. In some countries, any bystander has a legal duty to provide assistance in an emergency (provided that it is safe to do so) but not in most states of the United States. The law does, however, recognize a duty to aid and protect anyone in a relationship of **dependence**, which would include participants of an organized wilderness trip, and imply that the leader has a duty to act.

Anyone with a duty to act is held to a **standard of care** depending on level of training; and failure to meet that standard on duty is **negligence**.

Negligence has four elements:

- Duty to act
- Breach of duty
- Cause
- Harm.

To prove negligence, an attorney has to prove all four elements:

- The care provider had a **duty to act**.
- There was a **breach** of duty, meaning that the provider failed to do something he or she should have done (in the **scope of practice** for the level of training and job responsibility), or did something NOT in the scope of practice.
- That act or omission was the **cause**
- of **harm** to the patient.

Every state in the United States has a **Good Samaritan Law** to encourage people who do not have a duty to act to help in an emergency. For example, the California law says: "No person who in good faith, and not for compensation, renders emergency medical or nonmedical care at the scene of an emergency shall be liable for any civil damages resulting from any act or omission." *California Health and Safety Code* 1799.102(a). The phrase "medical or nonmedical" was added in a 2009 amendment, in response to a 2008 court decision that the law did not cover pulling a victim out of a wrecked car because it was not medical care. Apparently the judge did not know that auto extrication is part of Emergency Medical Technician training.

The story of the Good Samaritan is told in Luke 10:30-37. A Jewish traveler was wounded by thieves, who stripped him and left him lying on the road, half dead. Two other Jewish travelers saw him, but "passed by on the other side." Then a Samaritan (a sect very hostile to the Jews in Biblical times) "had compassion on him, and bound up his wounds, pouring in oil and wine, and set him on his own beast, and brought him to an inn, and took care of him." *King James Version*

If you choose to act as a Good Samaritan, remember that the law has four elements, and that all four must be observed for the law to apply:

- You do NOT have a duty to act.
- You do emergency care.
- It is at the emergency scene.
- You do NOT expect or accept any compensation.

Once you choose to begin care as a Good Samaritan, you have a legal as well as moral obligation to continue care until relieved by someone of equal or greater training. Otherwise, you could be accused of **abandonment**. Moreover, in a serious wilderness accident, your situation could still be an emergency scene until the patient was evacuated to safety; and going out for help could be a necessary part of the emergency care.

In describing the standard of care expected from a Good Samaritan, the phrase "what any reasonable and prudent adult would do" is common. For wilderness emergencies, this translates into doing what you have been trained to do competently.

The **Volunteer Protection Act of 1997** (Public Law 105-19) is meant to protect volunteers for **non-profit organizations** against frivolous lawsuits, which were discouraging people from volunteering. It applies to volunteers who were acting "within the scope of the volunteer's responsibilities"; and who have any licenses or certifications that are required for that volunteer activity. However, the act does not apply to harm caused by operating any vehicle that requires an operator's license. And harm "caused by willful or criminal misconduct, gross negligence, reckless misconduct, or…indifference to the rights or safety of the individual harmed by the volunteer" is also excluded from the Volunteer Protection Act.

Learning to find the problems

You should learn and practice a basic patient assessment near the beginning of the class. Then you should develop each part of it to a more sophisticated level as you learn about what you are looking for. For example, before doing a splint, assume that you have done a complete assessment, but come back to the limb with the supposed injury and examine it in more detail. When you play victim, work out a plausible accident scenario including: mechanism of injury, damage, reactions of the vital systems, as well as signs and symptoms. Then get into the role, and act it out.

When you have learned about sudden illness, you can practice getting a more detailed medical history. You can also practice giving a sixty-second oral report or preparing a written report. Organizing, selecting, and putting information into categories, instead of giving a blow-by-blow narrative, is a valuable skill for emergency situations.

Injuries

Slides can be invaluable, especially if they show the accident scene (mechanism of injury) and close-ups of injuries (damage done). But the effect of gruesome injuries can be amplified if you are locked into a spectator role, which leaves you with nothing to do but react to the scene emotionally or try to escape. Avoid this problem by asking yourself and visualizing how to treat each injury.

In a real accident, taking positive action to help the victims redirects the mind, at least during the scene. That is why you must practice until basic skills become reflexive. These reflexes can carry you through the first emotional impact of the scene. Also, learning how injuries damage the body and affect the vital systems trains you in whole-accident response, rather than single-skill tunnel vision. You learn to treat the patient first and the injury second.

Sudden illness, trauma, and shock

Illness kills in two ways: by disrupting vital systems and by diminishing the victim's ability to avoid accidents. In working through accident scenarios, you should check for medical causes, especially if the accident does not otherwise make sense. By including false leads among the causes, instructors train students to consider all the evidence. For example, diabetes can mimic the effects of alcohol abuse.

Getting the history of the present illness is akin to reconstructing the mechanism of an injury. In both cases, you are finding causal connections that converge to a damaging event. Both lines of inquiry can uncover problems that you would otherwise have missed. Any problem that interferes with the delivery of oxygen to

the vital organs usually has first priority, and anticipating problems may give you the margin needed to save lives.

Begin by looking at the systems that deliver oxygen to the tissues: airways, lungs, pump, pipes, fluid, and signals that control them. Then you can work out what happens when different parts of the system are damaged or disrupted. For example, what effects can chest injuries have on breathing? How can the circulatory system compensate for loss of blood? What injuries can interrupt signals from the brain to the respiratory or circulatory system? A similar approach can be used to learn about sudden illness. Once you understand how an injury or illness affects different parts of the body, or disrupts vital systems, you can work out what signs and symptoms will be produced.

Environmental stress

When the body's internal environment is pushed to extremes, we need to re-examine our understanding of vital processes and emergency procedures. Until the 1960s, for instance, High Altitude Pulmonary Edema (HAPE) was routinely diagnosed as pneumonia and treated with antibiotics. Victims who were not promptly brought down to lower elevations often died. People have also died of undiagnosed heat stroke because, contrary to what the textbooks said, their skins were still pale and sweaty. We learn to begin CPR if we find no pulse, but what about a victim in deep hypothermia, who may have an impalpable pulse?

These examples teach us to focus on what is happening to the vital systems, just as with sudden illness. Shortage of oxygen during an ascent can have many unpleasant effects, including headache and nausea. However, if the respiratory or central nervous system is disrupted, then the victim needs to relieve the stress on the system by descending.

For instance, if one climber always remains fatigued and short of breath after resting, when others are ready to go on, then we should suspect HAPE. We needn't wait until we hear fluid gurgling in the lungs or the victim starts coughing up pink sputum. Similarly, if someone's mental functions and balance are seriously impaired after exposure to altitude, we should suspect High Altitude Cerebral Edema.

Heat exhaustion often looks like compensated, hypovolemic shock. In both conditions, blood volume is down because of fluid loss, and circulation is withdrawn from the skin and skeletal muscles. Hence the pulse (especially in the wrist) is usually weak, and the heart compensates for low stroke volume by speeding up. Skin is pale, cool and clammy.

The victim usually feels nauseated as well as weak, because circulation to the digestive system is a low priority for the body. Comparing heat exhaustion with shock, and working out the differences of mechanism and treatment, illuminate the circulatory system's two main functions – delivery, especially of oxygen, and heat transfer.

In heat stroke, there is a conflict between these functions since carrying excess heat to the skin takes circulation away from vital organs. If heat accumulates in the body, the temperature in the vital organs can get dangerously high even if the victim is still pale and sweating. In a conscious victim, irrational behavior is a more reliable danger signal than skin appearance, because the brain is very sensitive to temperature.

Behavioral changes may also be the first warning of hypothermia. Listing brain functions that become impaired as body temperature goes down (from reasoning to coordination to balance) yields a level of responsiveness table familiar from other contexts. Thinking about how to rewarm a hypothermia victim reminds us of how the body produces heat and controls temperature.

The controversy about doing CPR on a hypothermic victim with no perceptible vital signs illustrates an important principle of first aid instruction. Even established procedures like CPR, which instructors drill into students, are based on assumptions about the situation. When variables are introduced, as often happens in the wilderness, we may need to make judgments about procedures that we would do automatically elsewhere. If you start CPR, will it be physically possible to continue CPR during evacuation? Can you even maintain the victim's temperature while doing CPR, much less rewarm? How close are you to your own margin of survival? Working through hypothetical situations trains you to take nothing for granted in a wilderness emergency.

Biological hazards

Although snakes and bears are more dramatic classroom topics, arthropods and microorganisms cause far more problems. All wild water may be contaminated, and there is no perfect way to disinfect it. Boiling water requires fuel and time. Ceramic filters can crack if dropped or allowed to freeze when wet. Paper filters must be replaced when they clog up. Neither filter is certain to take out viruses. No chemical is completely reliable, and chemical disinfection is hindered by sediment or cold water.

There is much folklore and misinformation about bugs and snakes. Slash and suck snakebite kits, for instance, were sold for many years, and an article in 1991 advised shocking victims with DC current to "devitalize" snake venom. Also much folklore exists about insect repellents. Outdoor magazines have advertised everything from vitamin B pills to ultrasound generators. Yet the only repellents that have any effect in laboratory tests are chemicals like DEET, which appear to jam sense receptors of some insects.

Most wild animals, from wasps to bears, will not attack if we avoid provoking them. Staying out of their way requires that we understand something about their behavior and habitats. Blood-feeding arthropods like ticks and mosquitoes may seek us out, but humans are aberrant hosts for most of them. Abnormal behavior in wild mammals (e.g., friendliness) may be a sign of rabies. You need to educate yourself about the actual biological hazards where you will be going, and get up-to-date information on coping with possible damage.

Testing and putting it all together

It is easy to write and grade questions that test memory. Questions that require thinking and problem solving, however, bring you closer to emergency response behavior. Instructors should be asking themselves how the process of responding to each test question will help train you to cope with emergencies.

Skills tests should be learning tools as well as evaluation tools. Individual skills can be reviewed and checked, but you should go through several full-scale simulated accidents, realistically acted out and staged with full make-up, as well as many smaller scenarios. If no trained volunteers are available to stage an accident, you and other students can take turns playing the role of victims; but you need scripts based on plausible mechanisms of injury to make the accidents convincing and effective.

Navigating the body

In order to discuss and document injuries and medical problems, we need terms for directions on the human body and movements. Directional terms come in pairs. **Superior** means toward the head; **inferior** toward the feet. **Anterior** means toward the front of the body; **posterior** means toward the rear. **Medial** means toward the midline of the body; **lateral** away from the midline. So, for example, the nose is superior to the mouth, medial to the eyes, and anterior to the ears. For navigating the arms and legs, we need two more terms: proximal and distal. **Proximal** means closer to the heart; **distal** means further away from the heart. For example, the elbow is distal to the shoulder, but proximal to the wrist. When we check distal nerve functions and signs of circulation, we mean distal to an injury, because we want to know if the injury is affecting circulation or nerve functions. For purposes of anatomical description, we assume that the body is in the anatomical position: standing with arms at the sides, palms forward.

From that position, the arms and legs can **abduct** (move away from the midline of the body) or **adduct** (move toward the midline of the body). They can also **rotate**. Joints in the body and limbs also enable us to **flex** and **extend**, as the side view shows. Solid arrows point in the direction a part of a limb or the body moves when it flexes. Hollow arrows point in the direction a part of a limb or the body moves when it extends. Like abduct and adduct, flex and extend refer to opposite movements. Another way to think of it is that when we flex every part of the body, we are moving into the fetal position. When we extend every part of the body, we are moving away from the fetal position. The corresponding movements of the foot, however, are called dorsiflex and plantarflex, from the Latin *planta* "sole of the foot" and *dorsum* "back of the foot".

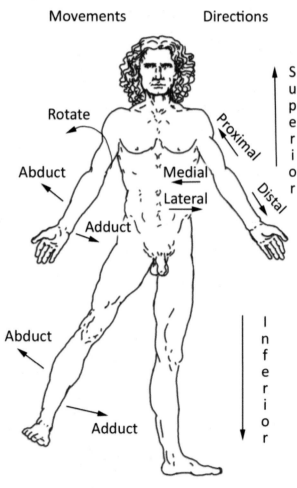

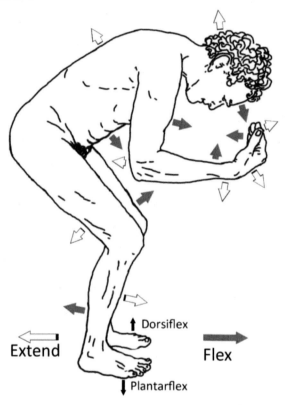

Using these terms for body directions and movements, we can describe the location of an injury or sign (such as swelling or deformity), a patient's position (e.g. arms flexed), and what an injured patient can and cannot do, e.g. can flex an injured forearm but not rotate it. These terms are also part of the vocabulary we need in order to learn about human anatomy.

Chapter 2. Patient assessment

To treat a patient effectively, you first need to find the problems and set priorities. This process of assessment begins as you approach the scene. In what position is the patient? How does he or she appear? Are there clues on the scene to the mechanism of injury? Are there hazards that would make it dangerous to approach? Urgent problems (such as severe bleeding) that you need to deal with immediately? Is the patient responding? Does the patient look at you spontaneously or only when you give a voice or touch stimulus? Is the patient oriented to identity, place, and time, and event (able to describe what happened?)

If the patient accepts your offer to help, you have two ways of finding the problems: physical examination and asking questions. With a responsive patient, however, both ways are forms of communication. You may see an open wound or deformed limb immediately, but the patient's response to your physical exam can alert you to other, less obvious injuries. A patient may be expressing pain or discomfort with body language. For example, someone having a heart attack may be clutching his or her chest and wincing; and someone with an injury may be guarding and protecting it.

Patients who are not responding vocally may still respond by flinching, grimacing, guarding or withdrawing from your touch. Lower levels of response may be involuntary, but they still tell you about the patient's condition. In a more responsive patient, even the pulse may change depending on whether you reassure or cause anxiety. Breathing may change if the patient becomes aware that you are observing it. Communication skills in assessment, therefore, include more than getting and giving information vocally. You also need to understand responses with the eyes or body, and the effects that your own words, body language, and manner may have on the patient.

Observation, especially visual, includes interpretation. We tend to see what we expect to see and often overlook what we do not expect. Practicing patient assessment in a standard way should link problem-finding techniques with understanding of the problems, so that you observe intelligently.

If the **mechanism of injury** (MOI) or **nature of illness** (NOI) is minor, and there is no sign of more serious problems, you will usually need to do only a focused assessment. For example, if someone twists an ankle (but does not fall), is the swelling interfering with circulation and nerve function in the foot? And in a wilderness situation, can the patient still walk? But if the mechanism of injury was a hard impact from a fall or collision, you should do a complete assessment, especially if the accident may have been caused by a medical problem. Similarly, any medical condition that is affecting vital signs can develop into an emergency in itself, or cause an accident by reducing mental and physical efficiency.

Patient assessment includes vital signs, medical history, and head to toe exam. **Vital signs** are observable measures of vital functions. For example, rate, depth, and apparent effort of breathing are measures of how well the respiratory system is working. Rate and strength of pulses in arteries that we can feel just under the skin are measures of how well the circulatory system is working. Skin color and temperature help you evaluate both respiratory and circulatory system function. If you have the equipment, you can also measure blood pressure and oxygen saturation, and listen to lung and heart sounds. How the patient responds to questions helps you evaluate brain function. **Medical history** should include any medical problems, previous injuries, or medications that could affect the patient's condition or your treatment. **Head to toe exam** should be thorough and systematic.

Playing the role of patient also helps you to learn assessment, because it trains you to connect mechanisms with injuries and symptoms with causes. Acting out the pain and anxiety of injury or illness gives insight into patient behavior and point of view, so that your patient communication and care will be more effective. Preparing patient scripts with plausible mechanisms of injury helps you to put it all together, so that in a real emergency you will be better able to find the problems and figure out what to do about them.

Age and vital signs

Age	Pulse rate/minute	Breaths/minute	Systolic BP
Infant (to 1 year)	100-160	30-60	70-95
Toddler (1 to 3 years)	90-150	24-40	80-100
Preschool (3 to 6 years)	80-140	22-34	80-100
School age (6 to 12 years)	70-120	18-30	80-110
Adolescent (12 to 18 years)	60-100	12-20	90-110
Early adult (18 to 40 years)	60-100	12-20	90-140
Middle adult (40 to 60 years)	60-100	12-20	90-140

Vital signs vary with age, though they are also affected by health and physical fitness. So the figures above are approximate. The tiny hearts of infants may beat very rapidly, and the resting pulse rates of toddlers and preschoolers can be much faster than those of adults; but their systolic blood pressure is typically lower than that of adults, partly because they have not had time to clog and stiffen their arteries with decades of poor living habits. The breathing rate of very young patients, with their small lungs and undeveloped intercostal muscles of the rib cage, is also more rapid than that of adults. By adolescence, vital signs usually stabilize at the adult level, and subsequent changes depend mostly on health and fitness, especially in older adults (over the age of 60).

Checking breathing and pulse

CPR training helps overall accident response by making the first part of patient assessment (responsiveness, breathing, and pulse) reflexive. Reflexes carry trained rescuers through the critical first few moments of an emergency, when untrained responders may freeze or act aimlessly. Although the sequence for assessing and treating an unresponsive patient with no signs of breathing changed with the 2010 Guidelines for CPR, the new mnemonic applies only to unresponsive patients who may have had a heart attack. **CAB** (**Circulation**, **Airway**, **Breathing**) means to start chest compressions if an unresponsive patient has no pulse or signs of breathing, then open the airway and ventilate. But for patients who are breathing, especially those with injuries, we still use the old mnemonic: ABCs for **Airway**, **Breathing**, and **Circulation** (including **severe** bleeding). Even a patient who is breathing may not be breathing adequately, and that is still a priority.

If the patient is breathing, you will want to learn more about it and other vital signs. Skin signs (color, temperature, turgor or skin tension, moist or dry) can be checked as part of the head-to-toe along with the appearance of the eyes. Checking the pulse and breathing, however, takes more time to do, so you should think of it as a separate module, which may also include breath sounds and blood pressure

When you push gently on an artery with your fingertips, you can feel and time the surges of blood pushed out by contractions of the left ventricle of the heart and moved on by contractions of the smooth muscle in the arterial walls. For an **unresponsive** adult or child, the carotid pulse is the easiest to find because the artery is big and close to the heart. Slide two or three fingertips into the groove between the trachea (Greek *traxus* "rough" because of its corrugated structure) and the slanting strap muscle of the neck, just below the jaw. You should always take the pulse on your side of the patient's neck. If you reach across the trachea (the mugger's grip) your action may be misunderstood, and you may unthinkingly squeeze the trachea between fingers and thumb.

On an infant, whose neck is short and small, find the pulse on the brachial artery where it passes over the bone on the inside of the upper arm. With a **responsive** adult or child, check the radial pulse at the wrist, because poking fingers into the neck might be both threatening and uncomfortable for the patient. The radial artery parallels the radius (the bone that enables you to rotate your forearm) and can be felt at the base of the thumb, in the groove between the bony edge of the wrist and the tendon that enables you to flex your index finger. If you cannot feel the pulse, press a bit harder with the downstream finger (closest to the thumb) to dam up the blood under the upstream fingers and create a stronger pulse. Count for 30 seconds and multiply by two or 15 seconds and multiply by four to get the rate per minute. The more fingertips you can lay on an artery, the easier it is to find a pulse.

What is a normal pulse? That depends on many factors including age. An infant's pulse may be as high as 160 per minute, twice as fast as an adult's. Pregnant women at term may have a resting pulse of up to 100. An adult marathon runner may have a resting pulse of 50. But in hypovolemic shock, one way that the circulatory system compensates for loss of blood is by increasing the heart rate. Even if you're not sure what is normal for a patient, therefore, an increase in resting pulse or a marked increase in pulse when the patient sits or stands is usually a sign of trouble.

In a responsive patient, you can take the radial pulse for 30 seconds with the wrist on the chest; then (without changing position) watch and feel chest movement for 30 seconds. A patient who thinks that you are still taking pulse is less likely to change the rate and depth of breathing. Pulse can be described in terms of its rate, strength, and rhythm. Breathing can be described in terms of its rate, depth, and rhythm. For an adult at rest, a breathing rate of 12 to 20 per minute is considered normal. Breathing may also be easy or labored, quiet or noisy. It may hurt to breathe deeply. Breathing may be unequal in the two sides of the chest, because of chest injury or problems with one lung. In an adult, breathing from the diaphragm alone, with no chest motion, may be a sign of cervical spine injury. Nerves controlling the diaphragm branch from the spinal cord high in the neck, so they are less likely to be cut off by a neck injury than the nerves controlling rib cage movement. In infants and toddlers, however, belly breathing (from the diaphragm alone) is normal because the intercostal muscles of the rib cage are undeveloped.

Capillary refill is a quick test of local circulation. Press on a nail bed (or skin if the patient has nail polish) and see how long it takes for the capillaries to pink it out with blood again. Two seconds is about normal. In cold weather, however, circulation to the extremities is usually reduced. Compensation for hypovolemic shock also includes withdrawing blood from the extremities, so you should do the capillary refill test on the forehead as well as the nail beds, and compare the results. With very dark-skinned people,

you will not be able to blanch the forehead, but gums and conjunctiva (inside the eyelids) on an unresponsive patient may be visibly pale and bloodless.

Pulse games

Practice counting the pulse in groups of three, with two people each taking one wrist of the third. After counting silently for 30 seconds, the two pulse-takers compare results. Rotate roles and continue this exercise until you and your partner consistently get the same numbers for the subject's pulse. This is also a good way to practice measuring blood pressure. Simultaneously measure blood pressure in each arm of the same person; then compare numbers.

Another exercise, which develops sensitivity, is to feel the difference in strength of two people's pulses, one with each hand. This exercise prepares you to compare distal pulses in the limbs of a patient when circulation in one limb may be impaired by a fracture or other injury. Developing sensitivity is also important because patients may have pulses that are weak and hard to find anywhere.

Brachial pulse

With the arm held palm up, the brachial artery (Latin *brachiolis* "arm") can be felt just medial to the big tendon that attaches the bicep muscle to the ulna, and just proximal to the crease of the elbow. That is where you put the bell of your stethoscope when you are measuring a patient's blood pressure. Distal to the inside crease of the elbow, the brachial artery branches into the radial and ulnar arteries, which pass under the tendon and an adjacent muscle.

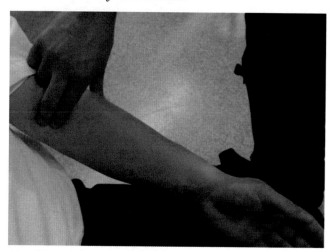

Checking the brachial pulse

Measuring blood pressure

Measure blood pressure with a sphygmomanometer (Greek *sphygmos* "pulse" + *manos* "sparse" + *metron* "measure"). First check the arm for injuries, then seat the patient with the arm at about heart level. Secure the cuff around a limb (usually the upper arm) and find the radial pulse with one hand.

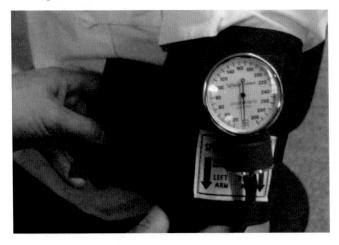

Inflate the cuff with the other hand past the point where the radial pulse stops. Watch the dial and slowly release pressure in the cuff until you feel the radial pulse return. That will give you the approximate **systolic blood pressure** by **palpation** ("feeling").

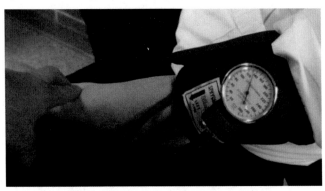

To measure systolic and **diastolic blood pressure**, you need a stethoscope (Greek *stethos* "chest" + *skopein* "to view"). "Systolic" comes from the Greek word for contract, and when more blood is pushed into the arteries by the contraction of the left ventricle against peripheral resistance, it increases blood pressure. Between contractions, blood pressure decreases, and "diastolic" is from the Greek word that came to mean a pause or relaxation. The difference between systolic and diastolic blood pressure, called **pulse pressure**, is a measure of arterial health.

Stiffening arteries increase peripheral resistance to blood flow, which increases systolic blood pressure. But elastic recoil of arterial walls (which increases diastolic blood pressure) is reduced by stiffening, so diastolic blood pressure usually does not increase as much as systolic pressure. Pulse pressure usually increases during exercise, but returns to normal in about 10 minutes. Resting pulse pressure of about 40 in an adult is normal. Pulse pressure of 60 or more is a risk factor for heart attack or stroke, independent of high systolic blood pressure.

Blood pressure can be increased by stress, transiently or chronically. For example, blood pressure may go up when it is taken by a doctor (white coat effect). A head injury with intracranial bleeding, or a brain tumor, can compress intracranial arteries enough to reduce circulation to the brain, so that oxygen demand drives up systolic blood pressure in response. It can also compress and disrupt the cardiac and respiratory control centers in the medulla. Then breathing becomes irregular and the heart (when sympathetic nervous system signals are cut off) slows down (bradycardia). These three signs (widening pulse pressure, irregular breathing, and bradycardia) are called **Cushing's triad**, after the doctor who first described them.

To measure blood pressure by auscultation ("listening"), place the bell of your stethoscope on the brachial artery, and inflate the cuff past the systolic blood pressure that you have measured by palpation.

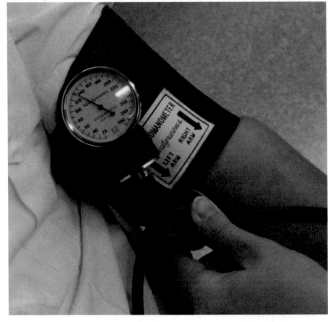

Blood forced through a partially constricted artery by each contraction of the left ventricle creates turbulence, which causes vibration, perceived as sound with the stethoscope. As you slowly release pressure, when you first hear a regular sound, the dial of the BP cuff will show the systolic blood pressure.

When pressure of the BP cuff drops enough so that the artery is no longer constricted, blood flows smoothly again with no turbulence, so the sound stops; and the dial will show the diastolic blood pressure. But if it is too noisy to hear the sound, you can still find systolic blood pressure by palpation.

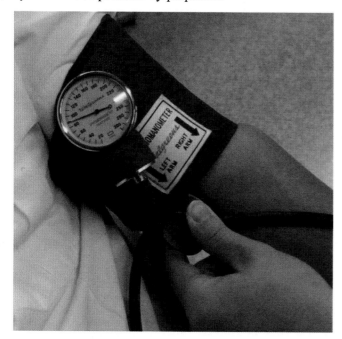

Hypertension and hypotension

Systolic blood pressure in most healthy adults ranges from 90 to 140, though a higher reading may be transient and caused by stress. So you should always reassess, and (for an elderly patient) check blood pressure in both arms. Also, ask about blood pressure medications, and whether the patient has been taking them on schedule. Regular aerobic exercise tends to lower blood pressure by clearing the arteries and reducing peripheral resistance. Even an unusually low reading may be normal for a fit athlete if there are signs of adequate perfusion: good skin color and temperature and capillary refill in two seconds or less. If blood pressure drops significantly when the patient stands up, however (**orthostatic hypotension**) then circulation is not adequate, and the patient may be hypovolemic from blood loss or dehydration.

Pulse oximeter

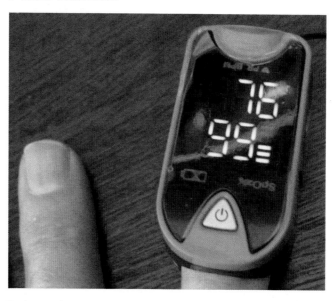

Pulse oximeters measure the oxygen concentration in the blood by the wavelength of light passing through bound hemoglobin in red blood cells (99% in the photo). They also measure the pulse rate (76 in the photo). However, pulse oximeters may give a falsely low reading in cold weather because circulation has withdrawn from the limbs (peripheral vasoconstriction); and they may be less accurate for oxygen saturation levels below 80%. Also, pulse oximeters cannot distinguish between hemoglobin-bound oxygen and carbon monoxide (CO), so they may give a false positive reading for anyone exposed to CO, e.g. from cooking in a tent. Pulse CO oximeters (which can distinguish O_2 from CO) are more expensive.

Level of responsiveness

Level of responsiveness (LOR) includes vocal, eye, and motor response. A simple mnemonic for LOR is **AVPU**: **Alert**; responds to **Vocal** stimuli; responds to **Pain** stimuli (a pinch); and **Unresponsive**. A more sophisticated measure of responsiveness is the **Glasgow Coma Scale** (GCS), which assigns numbers to how the patient responds with the eyes, the voice, and the body. An unresponsive patient gets a 1 in each test for being there, so the minimum GCS score is 3.

Eye Opening

Eyes do not open	1
Open only to pain stimuli	2
Open to vocal stimuli	3
Open already and tracking	4

Vocal Response

Silent	1
Sounds only (no words)	2
Inappropriate words	3
Confused or disoriented	4
Alert & oriented	5

Motor Response

Does not move	1
Extends both arms	2
Flexes both arms	3
Withdraws from pain	4
Localizes pain	5
Follows request	6

The **eyes** may already be open (4); open in response to speech (3); open only in response to pain (2); or not open at all (1). Similarly, a patient who **talks** alertly and is oriented to name, time, place, and event gets a 5 for vocal response. A patient who talks intelligibly but is less than fully alert or oriented gets a 4. For example, a patient may be oriented to identity, time, and place but not know what happened. Words that make no sense (word salad) get a 3. Sounds but no words get a 2. A silent patient gets a 1 for being there.

For **motor response**, a patient who moves a hand on request gets a 6; localizes (e.g. pushes your hand away when you pinch) gets a 5; withdraws from a pinch or poke gets a 4; flexes both arms (regardless of the stimulus) gets a 3; and extends both arms gets a 2. And a patient who does not move, gets a 1.

Edmison's Mnemonic

Mike Smith, in the *Journal of Emergency Medical Services*, described a simple way of quickly evaluating a patient, which he learned from James L. Edmison. The mnemonic is M.A.N.: Movement, Appearance, and Noise. Each one gets a score ranging from 0 to 2; then you add the numbers. Generally, a score of 4 to 6 means no immediate danger; scores of 2 or 3 mean serious problems needing immediate care; and scores of 0 or 1 mean poor chance of survival, especially in the wilderness. Here are the possibilities:

Movement

Still/not moving	0
Lethargic	1
Active	2

Appearance

Cyanotic (blue)	0
Pale	1
Pink	2

Noise

Silent	0
Moaning/groaning	1
Talking/crying	2

Getting the medical history

Assessment includes doing a head-to-toe exam and checking vital signs as well as asking questions. The SAMPLE mnemonic will guide you through the questions you should ask to get the patient's history.

• S stands for Signs and **Symptoms**. What signs of injury or medical problems do you observe (i.e., see, feel, hear, smell)? What symptoms does the patient describe (e.g., pain, discomfort, tingling, numbness)?

• A stands for **Allergies**. Ask whether the patient is allergic to anything, including medications, latex, foods, beestings, pollen, etc. Give examples to make sure you don't miss anything, especially latex allergy.

• M stands for **Medications**. Is the patient taking any? For what? When? Need to take a medication now? Can you assist? Any signs of substance abuse?

• P stands for **Pertinent** medical history, including Pregnancy. Give examples of medical problems to make sure that the patient understands the question.

• L stands for **Last** oral intake (food, water) and output (urination). When? What?

• E stands for **Events** leading up to the emergency. If it was a medical problem, what brought it on? If it was an accident, reconstruct the mechanism from clues at the scene and testimony from the patient and bystanders. Find out if an environmental or a medical problem helped cause the accident, e.g. heat, cold, altitude, hypoglycemia, seizure, etc.

Is a known disease causing the present problem? If so, what led up to it? For example, if the patient has heart problems, ask about (and look for) cardiac risk factors like high blood pressure, smoking and obesity. Also, has the patient had any other major diseases or injuries that might affect his or her present condition? Are you finding any signs and symptoms that suggest a medical problem? If possible, get the name, location and phone number of the patient's doctor.

Whether they come from the pharmacy or the street, drugs can cause life-threatening problems. Overdoses of depressants (including alcohol, barbiturates and narcotics) can cause respiratory arrest. Stimulants and hallucinogens can drive up blood pressure and bring on strokes or heart attacks. They can also cause repeated convulsions. Many other prescription medications can have serious side effects, and can even cause medical emergencies. So it is important to identify any drugs the patient has taken.

Patients' reaction to pain depends on their temperament, and may be affected by the impression you make. **Pain** can be described in terms of its quality, quantity, location, timing, setting and whether anything changes it. For example, a crushing pain in the chest is typical of a heart attack, whereas a sharp pain in the chest may be a blood clot in the lungs (pulmonary embolism).

Throbbing describes pain intensified by the pulse. The surge of blood through the arteries that increases blood pressure makes it worse. A pain may be localized or a diffuse ache. It may radiate (as pain from a heart attack often does) or even be referred (felt in another location). For example, pain from the liver may be felt in the right shoulder because the same nerves pass through both locations. You should also learn when the pain began, in what circumstances, whether it is constant or intermittent, whether anything makes it better or worse, and whether the patient has done anything to relieve the pain.

Checklist: Vital signs and history

HI: As you approach, check the scene for **Hazards,** patients, mechanism of injury/illness, position and appearance of patient(s) .
Introduce yourself and offer to help.

ABCs in the wilderness (EMS *NOT* available)
If the patient (with injuries) does not respond, check:
- **Airway**: No sign of breathing? Open the airway.
- **Breathing**? If not, start rescue breathing.
- **Circulation**: If no pulse, start CPR.
- **Serious** bleeding? Stop the leak.

For an apparent heart attack victim, however, the mnemonic is **CAB**, as described in chapter 29.

Spinal/head injury possible? Ask:
- Did you hit your head?
- Did you lose consciousness?
- Any pain in your head, neck or back?

SAMPLE history
Ask about:
- **Symptoms** (Pain? Discomfort? Nausea?).
- **Allergies**: To what? Medications? Latex? Bee stings? Foods?
- **Medications**: Taking any? For what? Need to take? Indications of substance abuse?
- **Pertinent** medical history, including pregnancy.
- **Last** oral intake (When? What?) and output.
- **Events** leading up to the accident: Mechanism of injury? Medical/environmental factors?

PAIN (OPQRST)
- **Onset**: What were you doing?
- **Provocation**: Anything make it better or worse?
- **Quality:** (Sharp or dull)?
- **Region:** Where is it? Does it **radiate**?
- **Severity:** (On a scale of 1 to 10)
- **Time:** When it started? Constant ? Throbbing?

LOR (Level Of Responsiveness)
Check the patient's level of responsiveness: The patient may respond with the eyes, speech, or body movement (Glasgow Coma Scale). **Oriented** to identity, place, time, event? Is the LOR changing?

PULSE and BREATHING
Check the **radial pulse** 30 seconds in a responsive patient and multiply by 2 to get the rate per minute. Then while pretending you are still checking the pulse, check **breathing** for 30 seconds: rate, depth, rhythm, easy/labored, noise, etc. Check blood pressure and breath sounds if you have the equipment.

SKIN SIGNS
Check the skin on the forehead with the back of your hand: hot or cool, sweaty or dry, elastic or loose when pinched? In a dark-skinned patient, check color in gums. If the patient is unresponsive, check inside the peeled-back eyelid.

Head-to-toe exam

When do you need to do a head-to-toe exam? A good guideline is: When in doubt, check it out. After any hard impact to the body (e.g., a fall or collision), it is important to do a complete exam, especially if level of responsiveness (LOR) is affected. As with other vital signs, changes in LOR may be more ominous than first findings. Was a blow to the head part of the mechanism of injury? Did the patient black out during or after the accident? A patient who is lucid when found, but whose LOR starts going down within about 30 minutes of the accident (**lucid interval**), may have bleeding in the skull that is gradually increasing pressure on the brain.

Novices are easily distracted from completing a head-to-toe exam. They often get no further than the obvious injury of which the patient is complaining. They may also miss injuries, because they hesitate to open clothing and look, using shears or a seam ripper if necessary. Experienced rescuers acknowledge the patient's discomfort but always complete their exam. They know that the most painful injury is not necessarily the most serious.

Experienced rescuers also keep talking to a patient even if there is no apparent response, and they never use scare words like "die," "bleeding," or "paralyzed" when a patient can hear. Instead of describing the patient's injuries, they discuss what needs to be done. You should never lie to a patient, but you can acknowledge a problem in general terms and redirect the conversation towards what you are doing to help.

Novices tend to be timid in their touch. You need to think about what you are trying to feel, and use enough pressure to feel it. This is another reason for not reading a checklist when you are practicing assessment. A head-to-toe exam is interactive – a conversation with the patient's body. While doing the exam, keep glancing at the patient's face, both to maintain rapport and to see non-vocal responses to pain such as wincing or guarding.

Head, face and neck

If the scalp has no open wound, spread the fingers of both hands over the skull and gently feel its contour for deformity. Blood coming from ears or nose may be from a skull fracture; clear fluid (cerebrospinal) is a more definite sign. To find out if cerebrospinal fluid is mixed in blood, capture some of the blood on a piece of absorbent cloth. If the stain is all red, it is just blood. However, if you see a yellowish ring around the red and perhaps some red fading to yellow towards the center, that is cerebrospinal fluid (halo or ring test). Blood from a fracture of the skull may seep into the tissues around the eyes (raccoon eyes) or behind the ears (bruised appearance known as Battle's sign).

Even if the skull is not damaged, the brain may still have been bruised by an impact that bounced it around inside the skull resulting in a concussion. Swelling in brain tissue or bleeding in the skull can impair sensory and motor functions. How does the face look? Is one side more mobile than the other? Is there weakness, paralysis, or rigidity of the limbs on one or both sides of the body? Is speech slurred or garbled?

Check the eyes. Some people have pupils naturally unequal; but grossly unequal pupils usually mean injury to one side of the brain. Pupils constricted even when not exposed to light may mean drugs or heat stroke. Dilated pupils may mean heat exhaustion or shock. If there is any suspicion of neck injury, you should hold the head still and tell the patient not to move before checking eye motion. Have the patient follow your fingers up, down, to each side.

Inability to move the eyes in one direction may mean fracture of a bone, inside the skull, to which eye muscles attach. Eyes that track with a jerky motion usually mean that the patient is under the influence of alcohol or some other drug that depresses the central nervous system. In a responsive patient, check vision by asking, "How many fingers?" Check pupil response with a penlight; or (in bright sunlight) by shielding and then exposing the eyes. Is the patient wearing contact lenses? Do they need to be removed?

Put the back of your hand to the forehead to feel for temperature and moisture. Pinch the skin--if it is loose and remains tented, the patient is severely dehydrated. Gently press the nose and facial bones to check for fractures. Can the patient open the jaw? Wiggle it from side to side? Stick out the tongue - is it straight or deviated? How does the mouth look? Are there foreign objects? Dentures? Missing teeth (where did they go)? If bleeding is in the mouth, can you position the patient on the left side to protect the airway? How does the breath sound? Is there an odor of ketones (fruity or acetone breath)? Is the patient a diabetic?

In the neck, tensed muscles suggest respiratory distress, from injury or disease. If one side of the chest is not moving or the trachea is deviated, then pressure in the lungs is unequal, and one lung is collapsing. Check immediately for a chest injury. Distended neck veins, however, suggest heart failure or (after blunt impact to the chest) cardiac tamponade [see chapter 12 on chest and abdominal injuries].

About 25,000 people in the U.S. have a hole in the front of the neck through which they breathe, because their larynxes have been surgically removed. Check for a medic alert necklace or bracelet. Finally, you should be able to feel at least the cervical spine (behind the neck) and part of the lumbar spine (the small of the back), no matter what position the patient is in. Is there deformity? Point tenderness? A fracture usually gives a sharp, localized pain response to the touch, whereas a bruise usually causes a dull, more diffuse pain.

Examining the shoulders and chest
Feel the collarbones (clavicles) for deformity and point tenderness. If the patient is sitting upright or standing, is there shoulder droop? Guarding? Inability to raise the arm? Press in and down on the shoulders, watching the patient's face for a reaction. Check the breastbone (sternum) with the edge of your hand for point tenderness. Now gently press both sides of the rib cage with your hands and ask the patient to take a deep breath. If that causes pain, ask the patient to point to where it hurts. A sharp pain response to pressure on the rib cage suggests a fractured rib.

In the chest, your main concern is for damage that may affect vital organ function, especially of the heart and lungs. A puncture in the chest wall (sucking chest wound) needs to be sealed. Pressure (from an air leak or bleeding) between the lung and the chest wall can also collapse the lung. Coughing up blood or pink-tinged sputum is a dangerous sign, whether it is caused by injury or by High Altitude Pulmonary Edema.

An impact to the chest can also bruise the heart. If the heart bleeds inside the pericardium ("around the heart") the accumulating blood will crowd the heart and gradually muffle the sound of the heartbeat (cardiac tamponade). This pressure can only be relieved by draining the excess blood with a hypodermic (a medical technique).

If there was an impact to the chest, it is important to question the patient about the mechanism of injury. Young children may develop breathing or heart problems up to 24 hours later. Since their rib cages are more flexible than an adult's, they transmit more of the impact to the organs underneath.

Examining the abdomen
The liver is mostly in the upper right quadrant of the abdomen but extends beyond the notch at the base of the rib cage. Damage to the liver or other solid organs like the spleen, which are full of blood, can cause serious internal bleeding and shock.

On the left side of the upper abdomen is the spleen, which recycles worn-out red blood cells. In the rear of the upper abdomen are the pancreas (which produces insulin) and the kidneys (which remove waste products from the blood). Blood in the urine suggests kidney damage.

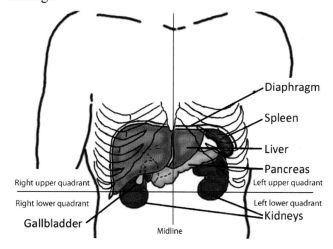

If the patient is spitting or vomiting up blood, the stomach may be injured. Bright red blood may be from the esophagus. Alcohol abuse often thins the lining of the esophagus, exposing blood vessels there to damage. Blood mixed with digestive juices, however, suggests damage to the stomach, which is in the upper left quadrant of the abdomen. Like the liver, the stomach is partially protected by the rib cage.

Whole blood irritates the body's tissues. Internal bleeding, therefore, whether or not it includes organ damage, can cause pain, guarding, and rigidity of the abdomen. If the hollow organs of the digestive system are ruptured, they may release toxins and infectious microorganisms, which can cause distension or bloating as well as abdominal pain.

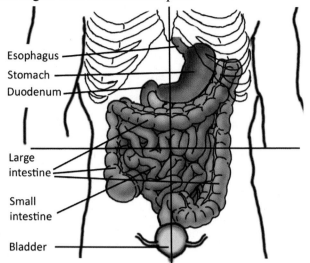

Esophagus
Stomach
Duodenum

Large intestine

Small intestine

Bladder

Sharp pain in the lower right quadrant, with a board-like abdomen, suggests appendicitis. Intestines fill much of the lower abdomen, and in the center is the urinary bladder. Above the bladder in women is the uterus. Internal bleeding in women, especially bleeding from the vagina, may be related to pregnancy, so rescuers should always ask if the patient is pregnant. Bright blood in feces is probably from hemorrhoids, but dark, partially digested blood suggests bleeding higher in the intestines.

To check the abdomen, feel with the flats of the fingers on your dominant hand and use the other hand to press your fingers in. Divide the abdomen into four quadrants by visualizing horizontal and vertical lines running through the navel. Then press slowly but firmly on each quadrant – one prod per quad – while watching the patient's face for a pain reaction. If the patient is complaining of pain in one quadrant, check that quadrant last and look for signs of injury.

Rescuers are usually reluctant to examine the genital organs, but if signs of injury are there and the patient will be in your care for some time, you should tactfully look. Priapism (uncontrolled erection) after an accident may be caused by spinal injury, which you should corroborate by checking other spinal functions in hands and feet (sensation, movement, strength). You should also feel as much of the spine as you can without moving the patient. Head or spinal injury may cause incontinence of bowels or bladder.

Examining the pelvis and limbs

If the patient is complaining of pain in the pelvis, probe carefully to locate the injury, or pull gently on one leg – if that elicits pain in the pelvis, suspect a pelvic fracture. If not, press in and down on both pelvic bones, watching for a reaction. With both hands, work down one leg at a time. If you get no pain reaction, press firmly because the femur is buried in masses of muscle. With an older patient, however, watch for varicose veins, especially in the calf muscle. Pressure could release blood clots. If one part of the leg seems injured, check the rest of the leg first, and then cautiously check the suspected area. Pain and guarding from an incautious probe could mask any lesser injuries in that leg.

If there are indications of a leg injury, expose that leg and both feet. The mnemonic for checking distal functions in the limbs is CSM: Circulation, Sensation, Movement. Signs of distal circulation include pulse strength, capillary refill time, and skin color and temperature. Simultaneously compare these signs in both limbs. One pulse is found in the hollow behind the medial ankle bone (posterior tibial). Another pulse is found on the top of the foot, just lateral to the tendon that enables you to raise the big toe (dorsalis pedis) [Photos in Chapter 7: Bone injuries and splinting].

To check sensation, ask, "Which toe am I touching?". If the patient cannot feel a soft touch with the finger, try a sharp touch with your fingernail or a pinprick. Then ask the patient to wiggle the toes in both feet. If you find no bone or joint injury in the leg, ask the patient to press up then down with both feet against your hands.

A fracture or dislocation may interfere with circulation and nerve functions distal to the injury. Hypothermia and some kinds of shock reduce circulation in the extremities. Frozen tissues have neither circulation nor nerve functions. A head injury may cause weakness, loss of sensation, or paralysis, usually on one side of the body.

Check and compare distal functions in the hands. Compare strength by having the patient squeeze with both hands. To avoid injury to your hands, offer only your first two fingers, crossed over each other. Finally, if you have ruled out spinal injury, roll the patient over if necessary so that you can check the back for injuries.

Head-to-toe exam
Photos courtesy of Ruth McConnell

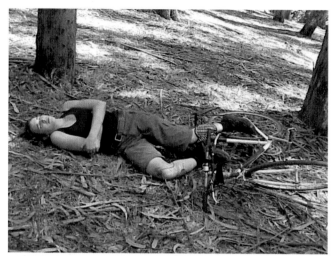

1. A mountain biker has had an accident.

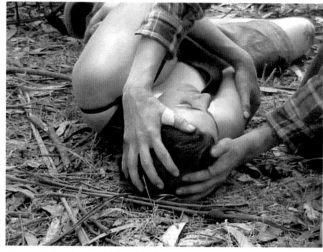

4. Feel the top of the skull.

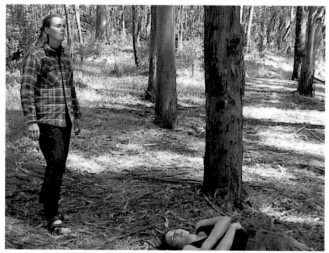

2. Check the scene.

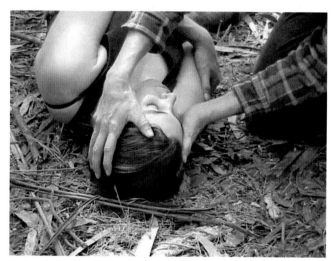

5. Feel the back and sides of the skull

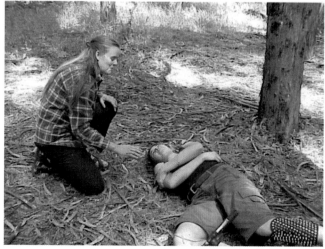

3. Check responsiveness. Ask what happened, introduce yourself and offer to help.

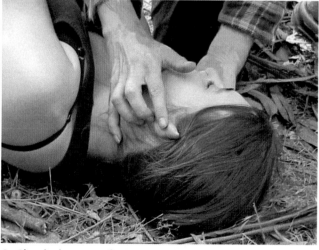

6. Check the ears, face, nose, jaw, and mouth: Fluids? Bruising?

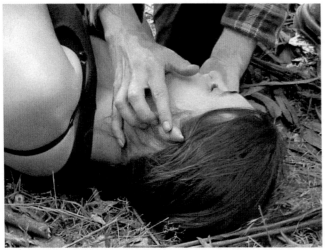

7. Check for raccoon eyes. Also compare pupil size and shape, check light response and eye movement.

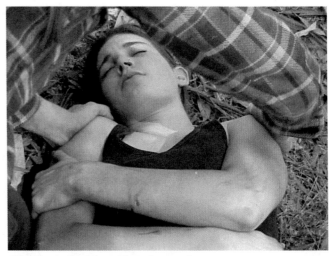

10. Press the shoulders inward.

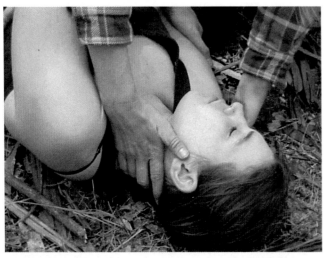

8. Check the facial bones, jaw, and neck. Feel the cervical vertebrae for deformity and "ouches."

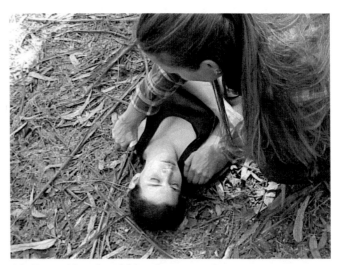

11. Press the shoulders downward.

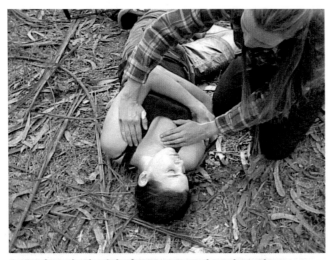

9. Feel each clavicle from one end to the other.

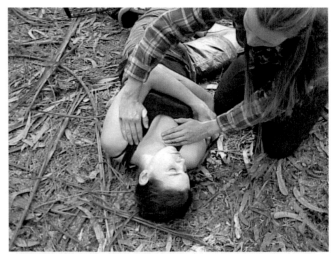

12. Feel the sternum (breast bone) inch by inch. Watch for signs of pain.

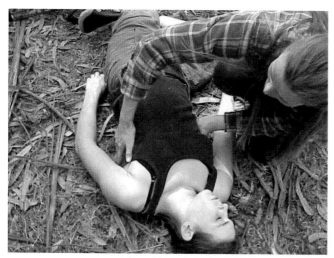

13. Press in on the rib cage. Ask the patient to take a deep breath and point to where it hurts.

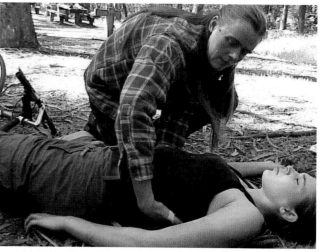

16. Reach under the small of the back and feel the lumbar spine for deformities and "ouches".

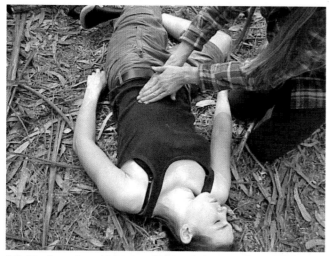

14. Feel each quadrant of the abdomen for rigidity, distension or signs of tenderness.

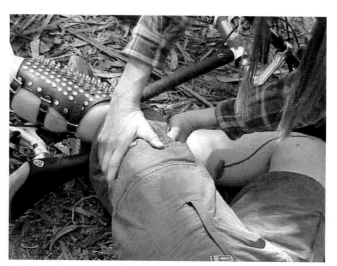

17. Check each leg for deformity and tenderness, working around where the patient says it hurts.

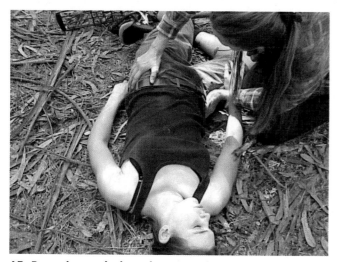

15. Press inward, then downward on the pelvis.

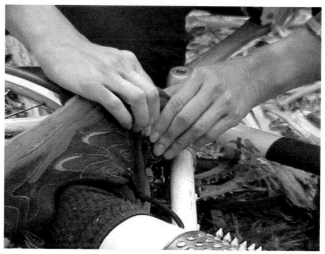

18. Ask, "which toe am I pressing?" "Can you wiggle your toes?" Check and compare signs of circulation.

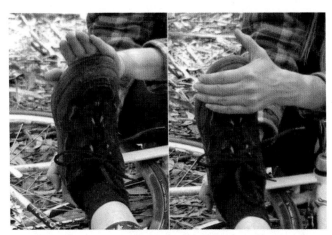

19. Ask the patient to press down and up on your hands with both her feet. Compare strength.

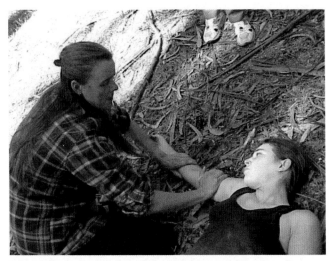

20. Feel each arm for deformities and "ouches."

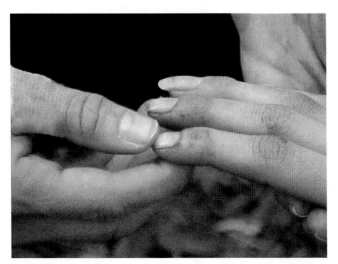

21. Check capillary refill and other signs of circulation (distal pulses, skin color, temperature) in the fingers.

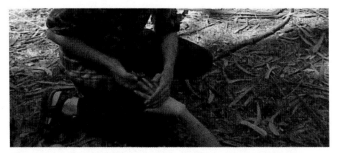

22. Ask "Which finger am I touching? Wiggle your fingers?"

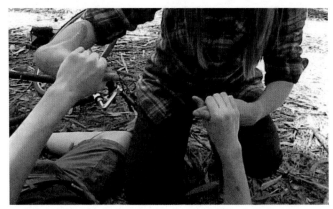

23. Ask, "Can you squeeze my fingers?" Compare strength in the patient's two hands.

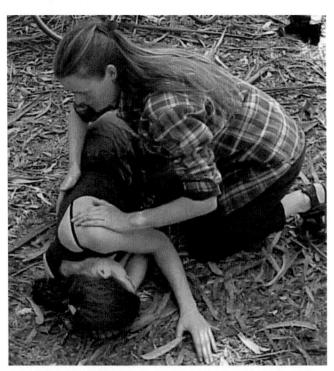

25. If the patient shows no sign of spinal injury, roll her towards you and check the back for injuries.

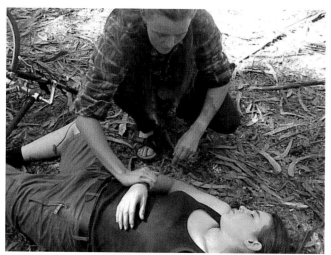

26. Check the radial pulse for 30 seconds. Then (without telling the patient), count breaths for 30 seconds. Multiply by 2 to get the rate per minute. Check blood pressure and breath sounds if you have the equipment.

Checklist: Head-to-toe exam

Always go to skin if necessary to find out what the injury is. If clothing cannot be unbuttoned or unzipped, use a seam ripper or shears.

HEAD

Scalp: Look for bleeding or open wounds.
Skull: If no obvious wound, feel for depressions.
Forehead: Hot? Cold? Moist? Feel with backs of fingers. Turgor? Pinch the skin.
Pupils: Dilated? Constricted? Unequal? Glazed? Light response? Contact lenses?
Eyes: Hold the head: "How many fingers? Follow the fingers." Raccoon eyes?
Nose: Broken? Clear or blood-tinged fluid draining?
Facial bones: Deformity? Bruising? Point tenderness?
Ears: Bruises behind (Battle's sign)? Clear or blood-tinged fluid draining? Capture patch of bloody fluid on white cloth (halo or ring test).
Jaw: "Can you open it? Wiggle it from side to side?"
Tongue: "Can you stick it out?" Straight or twisted?
Mouth Bleeding? Foreign objects? Check alignment of teeth. Missing or false teeth?
Breath: Odor?

NECK

Trachea Deviated? Check for chest/lung injury.
Muscles: Tensed? Check for other signs of respiratory distress/disease.

Veins: Distended? Suspect right heart failure.
Stoma? Look for small hole or tube near base of neck.
Cervical spine: Feel for point tenderness & deformity.
Medic alert tag: On chain around neck?

CHEST & SHOULDERS

Clavicles: Feel for point tenderness & deformity.
Shoulders: Press in, then back. Any pain?
Sternum: Feel for point tenderness & deformity.
Rib cage: Gently press in with both hands as victim takes a deep breath. Pain? Where?
Motion of chest: Asymmetrical? Paradoxical? Guarding? Diaphragm or chest movement only?

ABDOMEN

Look: Bleeding? Wounds? Bruising? Guarding? Distended?
Feel (one prod per quad): Rigidity? Distension? Pain?

SPINE

Feel as much as you can without moving the patient. Deformity?
Watch the patient's face and **listen** for an "Ouch!"- point tenderness?

PELVIS

Look and **smell** for incontinence (loss of bowel &/or bladder control).
Pelvic bones: Press in, then down. Any pain?

LEGS

Look: Bleeding? Bruising? Angulation? Deformity?
Feel down each leg with both hands, firmly. Pain? Point tenderness?

FEET

Look & feel. Signs of injuries in legs or feet? Check
Circulation: Check color, warmth, capillary refill (press nail beds).
Pulse: Posterior tibial (behind inside ankle knob) & dorsalis pedis (top of foot). Equal in both feet?
Sensation: "Which toe am I touching?" Make sure patient can't see it.
Movement: "Can you wiggle your toes?"
Strength: "Can you press up, down against my hand?"

ARMS

Look: Bleeding? Swelling? Deformity? Medic alert bracelet?
Feel down each arm with both hands, firmly. Pain? Point tenderness?
Pulse : Radial (wrist, near base of thumb). Equal in both wrists?

HANDS
Signs of injury in legs or feet? If so, check
Functions: Sensation, finger movement, strength.
Circulation: Check color, warmth, capillary refill.
BACK
Look: Bleeding? Bruising? Deformity?
Feel: Deformity? Point tenderness in spine?

Format for an accident report

Name, age, gender, and appearance of the patient
Chief Complaint: What bothers the patient most?
Vital Signs should include LOR, pulse, breathing, skin
signs as well as blood pressure and breath sounds if
you have a BP cuff and stethoscope. **Record the
results and times,** and note any changes.
SAMPLE history
- **Symptoms**: Pain? Discomfort? Vertigo? Nausea?
- **Allergies**: To medications, latex, foods, beestings, pollen, etc.?
- **Medications**: Prescribed? For what? Over the counter? Herbal/alternative? Last taken?
- **Pertinent** medical history: Medical problems? Past injuries? Pregnant?
- **Last** oral intake: Food or drink, including alcohol.
- **Events** leading up to the emergency: Medical? Environmental? Physical (e.g., fall, collision)? Reconstruct **mechanism of injury** (MOI).

Physical exam & treatment
- General Appearance, body position, apparent level of distress.
- Head-To-Toe Exam: What observable signs of injuries or medical problems did you find? What pain or discomfort did the patient express with body language?
- Treatment: Briefly report what you did.

Putting it all together

With practice, you should be able to do a complete
patient assessment in two or three minutes. If the
problems seem to be injuries, you may start the head-
to-toe exam immediately after checking ABCs and
taking care of any immediately life-threatening
problems. If level of responsiveness is going down,
however, you should get as much medical history as
you can while the patient is still answering questions.
With experience, you will be able to ask questions as
you do the physical exam. Check pulse and other vital

signs regularly and write down the results, along with
the time. Be sure that you find all of the problems and
set your priorities before starting treatment.

Oral report

When you turn over care of the patient, tell the new
care giver what he or she needs to know immediately
about the patient. Organize what you observed and
were told into categories: patient's name, age, and
general appearance; chief complaint; SAMPLE history;
vital signs; injuries; treatment. It should take you no
more than one minute to present the facts, with no
unnecessary words. Details belong in the written
report, which should go with the new care giver.
Example:
"This is John Doe. He's 28 years old. John was found
sitting at the base of a boulder and complained of pain
in his right ankle. He is alert with a GCS of 15, pulse
70, and respirations 12. He denies any allergies; carries
an inhaler for asthma, but denies any other medical
problems; had an energy bar for lunch; fell when he
was bouldering and injured his ankle. We splinted it
and carried him out."

Written report

Record what you observed and what you were told by
the patient or witnesses. Organize information into the
same categories that you use to perform the
assessment: Patient; general appearance when found;
chief complaint; vital signs (including any changes you
recorded in the time the patient was under your care);
SAMPLE history; results of head to toe exam;
treatment. A factual report will help those who take
over the patient to provide good care, and document the
patient's condition when found and what you did, in
case there is any legal question later. Even if you use
an accident report form, organize the information in
your mind before recording it. Then your focus will be
on the patient, not just on filling in the blanks.

Remember that any information you obtain from
the patient in your role as an emergency care provider
is **confidential**, and should be shared only with the
EMS or medical professionals to whom you transfer
the patient. When patient information is used for
medical research or teaching, all details that might
identify the patient must be removed.

Age, development and behavior

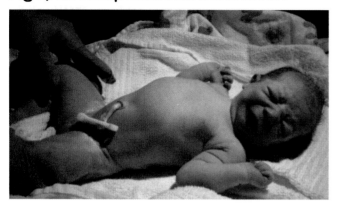

In their first two months, **infants** tend to sleep when they are not eating. By the third month, they are usually becoming more active. Their eyes track, and they begin to recognize faces. They are very sensitive to temperature change because of their small size, which means relatively little heat-producing volume compared to heat-radiating surface area. So you need to keep them warm and dry. Though they are usually not afraid of strangers, by the sixth month they may show separation anxiety. So it is best to examine an infant in the mother's arms or with the mother nearby. At about six months, infants also begin to babble, though most infants don't use words until about a year of age. But persistent and inconsolable crying or irritability may be a sign of serious illness.

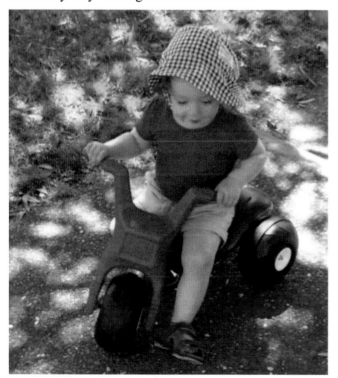

Toddlers (1-3 years) usually show separation anxiety, so a parent should be present when you assess them. They also usually show stranger anxiety, so you should limit touching and start your physical examination at the feet, while talking to the toddler in a soothing voice. Toddlers are very self-centered, so talk to them about themselves to gain their cooperation, and let them choose what you examine next. They may not like having clothing removed, so get the parent or care giver to help, and replace clothes as soon as possible. But they are curious, so you may distract them by giving them something to play with. Language use varies with age and development of the child, and their thinking is magical rather than logical, so they may not be able to describe their pain clearly. But they can understand (or misunderstand) more than they can express, so watch what you say in their hearing.

Preschoolers (3-6 years) have active imaginations and are rapidly learning language, but understand it literally. They may think that injury or illness is their own fault, or punishment for their behavior. So explain things to them clearly and simply. Let them see and (if possible) play with equipment before using it to examine them. Start the physical exam at the feet, as with toddlers. Preschoolers are afraid of pain, injuries, and blood, so cover any open wounds quickly.

School age children (6-12 years) are usually talkative and can think logically – they understand cause and effect. They can also understand that you are there to help them. So explain to them in simple terms what the problem is, and what you are going to do to make it better. Also make sure that you have privacy for the assessment, but ask if the child wants a parent or caregiver present. Remember, however, that injury or illness can make a child regress emotionally, and behave like someone much younger.

Adolescents (12-18 years) can be rational and able to express themselves logically (though injury or illness can make them regress). So explain honestly (but in neutral terms) to the patient what injuries or medical problems you find in your assessment. Also encourage the patient to ask questions, and help in his or her own care. Give choices when possible, so that the patient will feel more in control. Usually, adolescents are starting to behave more independently, which often includes risk taking. Peer approval is becoming more important, and fear of being embarrassed before their peers, so ensure privacy. If possible, have someone (or ideally two people) of the same gender do the assessment.

Changes in older patients

Vital signs in older patients (over 60) vary, depending on health and exercise habits. As vital systems age, they tend to become less efficient. But anyone doing activities that require strength and endurance is likely to be more physically fit than average, and may have vital signs typical of someone younger. So it is useful to distinguish **chronologic age**, **pathologic age** (based on changes caused by disease and degenerative processes), and **functional age** (based on changes of function from impairment caused by disease or degenerative processes). For example, a patient with coronary artery disease will have circulation problems, which will give him a higher pathologic age. That will reduce his work and exercise capacity, which will increase his functional age. But a patient with no medical problems who has maintained fitness with regular exercise is likely to have a pathologic and functional age less than his chronologic age.

The aging heart tends to become less responsive to the nerve impulses that control contraction of the ventricles and heart rate. So with advancing age, the **pulse** may become weaker and slower. You should check the radial pulse in both arms, however, to rule out a blockage of blood flow in one arm. If you cannot find a radial pulse, you can measure heart rate by listening to the heart with a stethoscope. Elderly patients are more likely to have **arrhythmias** – irregular pulses.

Heart rate is also affected by some medications, especially **beta blockers**, which block sympathetic nervous system signals that would normally increase heart rate and blood pressure. Aging arteries tend to stiffen, which limits the ability of the circulatory system to control blood pressure and can cause **orthostatic hypotension** – a drop in systolic blood pressure as the patient stands up. Poorer circulation in older adults slows **wound healing**. It also limits their ability to dissipate heat in warm weather, along with reduced activity of the sweat glands; which makes them more vulnerable to **heat illness**.

Vital capacity in the elderly may be reduced by weakening respiratory muscles and stiffening of the rib cage, as well as chronic respiratory diseases such as emphysema. This may make chest rise and breathing rate harder to assess. Less vital capacity means more **residual volume** of stagnant air left in the lungs with each breath, which reduces the percentage of oxygen in the alveoli, and therefore makes gas exchange less effective. With age, chemoreceptors for carbon dioxide and oxygen in the blood become less sensitive, which can lower **oxygen concentration** in the blood, so that a pulse oximetry reading of 93% to 95% may be normal for a patient over 65. These changes reduce endurance and maximal performance, and make it harder to compensate for the effects of injury or illness.

Muscle mass and **bone density** tend to decrease with advancing age, as well as viscosity of the synovial fluid lubricating the joints. So the elderly tend to lose strength as well as flexibility, and become more

vulnerable to fractures. In the eyes, lens translucency and pupil size decrease, increasing the need for illumination, and decreasing visual acuity and night vision. The number of auditory neurons decreases, resulting in **hearing loss** and reduced ability to tell the direction of a sound. The number of cochlear hair cells also decreases, which affects **balance**.

Assessing older patients

Any assessment includes checking the environment for hazards and clues about the mechanism of injury or nature of illness. For urban situations the **GEMS** mnemonic reminds us of possible differences in older patients' living conditions and situations as well as their vital functions and vital signs. G stands for **Geriatric**: older patients may have experienced significant physical, psychological, and physiological changes; but they must be treated with respect, which means addressing them formally and listening patiently to what they have to say, especially if you are a generation younger than the patient. E stands for **Environment**: check an older patient's home for hazardous conditions, livability, access to a telephone, and any special equipment such as walkers, wheelchairs, or oxygen. M stands for **Medical history**, which may be complex. Older patients may have several chronic medical problems, and be taking many medications. Are the medications all current and from the same doctor? S stands for **Social**: Are the patient's needs being provided for adequately? Does the patient have a social network?

Patients with disabilities

Many people with sensory, physical, or developmental disabilities engage in outdoor activities. On the ski slopes, for example, you may see blind skiers with guides ahead of them calling the turns, one-legged skiers on monoskis, and paraplegics in ski sleds. People with physical disabilities also do other outdoor activities, such as hiking and mountain climbing.

Over six million people in the United States have visual disabilities, meaning that they have trouble seeing even with glasses; and over one million are **legally blind**, with vision of 20/200 or worse. About one million people in the United States are functionally **deaf**, and nearly ten million are hard of hearing. **American Sign Language** (ASL) is the third most used native language in the United States, after English and Spanish.

Developmental disabilities can affect mental, sensory or motor functions. The most common causes of developmental disability are abnormalities in or damage to the developing brain, usually before birth, which can be from infection, bleeding, hypoxia (too little oxygen), maternal drug or alcohol use, maternal malnutrition, or a hereditary condition. Depending on which parts of the brain are damaged, it can affect mental, motor, or sensory functions, and make the patient liable to seizures. This type of disability is called **cerebral palsy** ("brain paralysis"), and affects up to one million people in the United States. Traumatic brain injury can cause similar loss of function.

Patients with impaired motor functions may be using canes or walkers, or be in wheelchairs. They may have impaired speech, but that does not necessarily mean their intelligence is affected. Moreover, most people with disabilities value their independence, and must be treated with respect. So it is important to communicate clearly and make sure you have their permission.

Assessing the deaf and blind

Members of the deaf community usually do not consider themselves disabled. But very few of them can read lips (contrary to popular folklore), especially the lips of strangers. So unless you know their language (ASL), you need to communicate with them in writing, and keep it simple. Those who were born deaf, or went deaf at an early age, tend to have a low reading level because it is hard to learn how to read without phonetics. You also need to be careful to stay within deaf patients' range of vision, so that you can maintain communication and they know what you are doing. Two web sites can help you learn some useful ASL signs for communicating with the deaf: www.signingsavvy.com and www.lifeprint.com. Both web sites have video dictionaries of ASL.

If you need to help a blind person walk to safety, offer your arm or shoulder and let the patient hold it. Describe what is happening and the terrain ahead. When assessing blind patients, it is especially important to tell them exactly what you are going to do before you touch them, what you are doing as you proceed with the assessment, and why. Although blind people often learn to compensate with their other senses, any serious injury or medical problem disrupts the feeling of control over one's own life. Good communication, and giving the patient choices whenever it is possible, can help restore that feeling of control.

Conclusion

Patient assessment includes observation, physical examination, measuring and recording vital signs, and the art of asking questions that elicit information about the patient's condition and problems.

Recovery position

A patient who is unresponsive but breathing, and has no indications of spinal injury, should usually be left in the recovery (left lateral) position. A supine patient who feels nauseated should also be rolled into this position to protect the airway. Since the stomach is on the left side of the body, the recovery position keeps stomach contents below the esophagus; and vomit is less likely to be aspirated into the lungs.

Moving a patient into recovery position

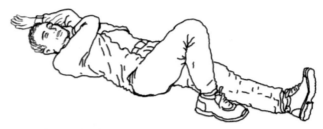

Raise the right knee, lay the left arm alongside the head, and place the right hand on the left shoulder.

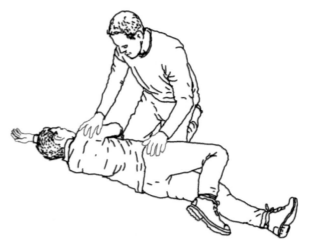

Grip shoulder and hip, and roll the patient towards you onto his side.

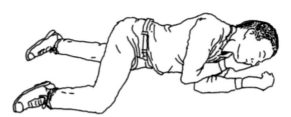

The patient's right knee and right elbow keep him in a stable position that helps to protect the airway.

Chapter 3. Wilderness first aid kits

Many people who do wilderness activities give little thought to first aid kits, until they learn the hard way that they are not prepared to deal with wilderness accidents. Emergency care training should give you some skill at improvising. But without the proper equipment, you will be handicapped at best, and at worst, you'll find yourself unable to treat injuries effectively or prevent complications.

For practical purposes, injuries are of three types: those that will kill the victim unless something is done immediately; those that cause serious damage and that may kill or disable the victim in time; and minor injuries, which would normally cause only temporary discomfort. In the wilderness, however, even minor injuries like foot blisters can be disabling. And infections are much more of a hazard when you are far from help, since they have more time to develop and become dangerous.

Wounds, dressings and bandages

Anything that stops breathing or circulation will kill within minutes at normal body temperature. In these situations, a first aid kit may not be of much help – what you need is training in CPR (cardiopulmonary resuscitation). To control serious arterial bleeding, which can also kill within a few minutes, you need a bulky dressing and something to hold it in place or (if that fails) a tourniquet.

For most bleeding wounds, 4" x 4" sterile gauze pads work well. For severe bleeding, surgical dressings (trauma pads) are very absorbent, with a non-stick layer to cover the wound.

Triangular (cravat) bandages are very versatile. They can apply strong pressure on a bleeding wound, as well as holding a dressing in place. Triangular bandages can be bought, or made, by cutting a piece of fabric (perhaps an old bed sheet) at least 40" square, on the diagonal. This will give you two triangular bandages. Hem the cut edges to prevent fraying. Cotton muslin and cotton-polyester blends work well, but slippery synthetic fabrics do not.

Rolls of stretchy gauze are good for general wrapping – the 4" width is most versatile, and 2" rolls

are good for finger bandages. You should also have two rolls of tape: a narrow (1/2" - 3/4") roll of porous athletic tape, which can hold dressings in place without cutting off air flow; and a roll of 2" wide duct tape.

For activities that carry a high risk of serious open wounds, your kit might also include two battle dressings – antiseptic pads with long bandages attached, which can quickly be secured to almost any part of the body. An expedition kit might also include very large gauze pads (8" x 10").

Bandage dressings with adhesive strips will cover most small wounds. For wounds in which bleeding is not a problem, non-stick pads on the dressings are best.

Butterfly closures are often used even by doctors to close gaping cuts, as an alternative to the traumatic technique of suturing. These sterile adhesive strips with narrow bridges in the center hold wounds shut without pressing on them. Tincture of benzoin (made from the sap of a tree) will make the skin adjacent to a wound tacky, and help the adhesive to stick. Superglue has long been used by trainers to close cuts on boxers, and there are formulations made for wound closure. But wounds should not be sealed in wilderness settings unless necessary for function, because of the danger of sealing in infection.

Disinfecting and cleaning agents

In the old days, we anointed open wounds with tincture of iodine or mercurochrome. This killed many of the intruding bacteria (and did much to build character); but it also damaged the surrounding flesh. Mild antiseptics like povidone-iodine and benzalkonium chloride are sold in foil packets as well as bottles. Use the liquid form, which will spread through the wound area, not the ointment. However, these antiseptics are not as effective as **honey** (see chapter 5).

Irrigating a wound effectively requires a forceful jet of water (7-8 psi) to flush out debris. A wound irrigation syringe with a blunt needle will do the job best. A 30 ml syringe is a good size, though a 10 ml syringe will fit better into a small kit. An 18-gauge plastic catheter tip will also work. A plastic squeeze bottle with a screw-on cap and a very narrow nozzle (in which liquid condiments are sold) will also produce a forceful stream. Squeezing a ziplock bag with a pinhole in a bottom corner will produce about 2 psi of pressure.

Use biodegradable liquid soap to wash your hands before treating a wound. In the absence of water, benzalkonium chloride antiseptic pads can do a reasonable job of cleaning your hands as well as the skin around a wound – but remember to wipe away from the wound.

Gloves help to protect you and your patient from sharing infections. Synthetic gloves, such as nitrile, avoid the danger of latex allergy in you or your patient.

Fractures and splints

Splints can be improvised from poles, ice axes, the staves of internal-frame backpacks, rolled-up foam pads – anything that will support and immobilize the fractured limb. Splinting is easier, however, with a splint designed for the job.

- SAM splints (www.sammedical.com) designed by an orthopedist, are thin strips of flexible aluminum (4.25" by 36") with foam on both sides. Forming the splint into a half-cylinder gives it structural rigidity, as well as fitting it snugly to the limb. It weighs 4 oz. and rolls or folds up compactly.
- You can make a wire splint by cutting a 6" piece off a 30" roll of hardware cloth (1/4" wire mesh, available at a hardware store). Trim the projecting wires from the cut edges and cover them with duct tape. This kind of splint functions like a SAM, but needs padding and is less durable.
- Another option is the air splint, a double-walled plastic sleeve that fits over the limb. It is inflated until it supports the limb without cutting off circulation. Advantages are that it can be applied quickly, it is transparent, and its uniform pressure helps to control the internal bleeding caused by a fracture. Disadvantages are that it is comparatively expensive and heavy; air pressure must be adjusted if you go to higher or lower altitudes, and a leak or defective valve will make it useless. Also, it cannot be used for a bent limb splint.
- Traction splints are expensive, and too bulky for a small first aid kit. They can be improvised, however, from ski poles, a hiking staff, or a long paddle. (See chapter 8.)

To hold splints in place, you can use cravat, gauze roller, or elastic bandages. You can also secure them with duct tape, though that would make it difficult to adjust the tension when the fractured limb swells. For an arm fracture, a triangular bandage will make a sling, though you can improvise with the bottom of the patient's shirt or jacket – fold it up to cradle the arm and safety pin it together. Even without a splint, this will help stabilize a fractured arm.

In freezing weather, the hand or foot of a fractured limb is very vulnerable to frostbite. Damage to blood vessels by the broken bone ends, constriction by splint fasteners, and the victim's inability to move the splinted limb all tend to interfere with circulation. In this case, one or two hand warmers, well wrapped and secured, may be the only way to keep the extremity from freezing. Cheap, disposable warmers weigh less than 3 ounces and give up to 20 hours of heat.

Medications

You can avoid most discomforts that might tempt you to use medications in the back country by taking care of yourself: putting enough water and fuel into your system; disinfecting drinking water; acclimatizing to heat or altitude; and dressing properly. Used with caution, however, medications can prevent a trip from becoming an ordeal, and free you from distracting discomfort.

Aspirin is anti-inflammatory as well as analgesic (pain-killing). It may be needed for burns and wear-and-tear injuries, which involve swelling or inflammation, especially in heavily used joints like the knees. Enteric-coated aspirin are more durable, and less likely to cause stomach irritation. Acetaminophen (500 milligram tablets)is a stronger medication for relieving moderate pain. Tylenol with codeine is an oral narcotic for relieving severe pain. One painful injury, sunburn, can usually be prevented by carrying extra lip balm and sunscreen.

Antihistamines or decongestants may help if narrowing or clogging of the air passages makes breathing and sleeping difficult. Epinephrine, in an inhaler or epipen, might save the life of a victim with a severe allergic reaction to insect venom or other foreign protein by opening constricted breathing passages.

Gastrointestinal miseries, although they are usually preventable, are debilitating and common. A laxative can relieve constipation, and Lomotil might be used to relieve diarrhea if it is dangerously dehydrating the victim. An oral rehydration mix with electrolytes is better, if it can keep the victim hydrated while the disease runs its course.

For infections on a long trip, an oral antibiotic may be a lifesaver. For altitude illness, acetazolamide or dexamethasone may help. Hydrocortisone cream relieves itching, and oil of cloves can ease toothache. For a long trip, a dental first aid kit is a good idea. Anti-fungal powder or ointment will help to control athlete's foot and other fungal infections.

Prescription medications (Rx) must be obtained from a physician, for one's personal use. For a long trip, the leader can give participants a list of types of medications to get from their own physicians, e.g., oral antibiotics, to avoid the medical risk of giving people drugs to which they may be allergic, and the legal risk of practicing medicine without a license.

Pills have expiration dates on them because it is required by law. If the exact dose is critical, as with a prescription medication for a chronic illness, then these expiration dates may matter. Other pills, however, can generally be used until they crumble, although they may lose some of their potency with time.

Tools

In emergency care, as in any other craft, you can do a better job and do it more easily with the right tools. One basic operation is cutting – dressings, bandages and (if there is no other way to get at an injury) clothing. For a pocket kit, you can make do with the tiny scissors on your Swiss Army knife. A larger kit, however, should include a set of universal shears (also called paramedic or EMT shears), available from medical supply stores and some hardware suppliers. They are offset, self-sharpening bandage scissors made of stainless steel, with plastic-covered grips large enough for your whole hand. The tip of the bottom blade is blunted to slide harmlessly on skin.

If you do need to take apart clothing, it will be easier to stitch it together again if you open the seams with a seam-ripper (which you can find with other sewing supplies) rather than shredding the fabric.

Safety pins can hold the clothing together until it is repaired. Diaper pins are the strongest safety pins.

Sterilized in a flame, a needle from your sewing kit can be used to remove splinters, but Uncle Bill's Sliver Grippers are designed for the job. Short and broad, they are easy to manipulate and come to a sharp point, so that you can grip and pull out even tiny hairs of metal or fiberglass. They can also be used to remove ticks that are attached to the skin. Tick Spoon and Tick Pliers are more specialized tools that can be used to grip a tick and pull it out.

Needle nose vise grips can be used to remove large cactus spines, as well as for equipment repair. To remove tiny, hair-like spines and nettles from the skin, spread rubber cement over them, let it set, and peel it off. If you lack rubber cement, you can use duct tape.

Body temperature may be elevated by fever or heat exposure, or depressed by cold exposure. But it is questionable how useful thermometers are on a wilderness trip. First, only a rectal thermometer will give a good reading of the temperature in the body core, and that is awkward to use, especially if the patient is not cooperative. Secondly, the signs and symptoms of conditions that change the body's temperature should tell you more than a thermometer would. An ordinary oral thermometer can measure moderately elevated or lowered body temperatures. Alternatively, a high-reading hyperthermia thermometer and a low-reading hypothermia thermometer will cover the whole range of body temperatures between them. Glass thermometers are fragile, but fairly accurate. Cheap digital thermometers are less fragile, but not very accurate.

Snakebite kits seldom help, and can cause serious damage if they require people to make incisions. Plastic suction pumps, such as Sawyer's Extractor, do not require incisions, but there is no published evidence that they actually extract venom.

A CPR mask will protect against infection when doing mouth-to-mouth respiration. For a small first aid kit, a disposable mask is the most compact. It will fit in a shirt pocket or on a key chain.

For taking notes, include a notepad with water-resistant plastic paper, and a number 2 pencil or space pen (developed for NASA).

Containers

Before selecting a container for your first aid kit, ask what it needs to do. Must it be rigid to resist crushing, or would a flexible container be easier to pack? Must it be completely waterproof? Must it float (e.g., for rafting or boating)? A small, personal kit can go in a transparent plastic envelope with a zipper or a small freezette container secured with a nylon strap.

Another option is a nylon zipper bag with compartments, preferably the kind that folds out when opened so that all your equipment is easily accessible. For a large expedition, a military surplus ammunition box (available in three sizes) makes an almost indestructible container. Any large kit should be organized into smaller modules in labeled containers, so you can select the modules needed for a trip, and quickly find things in an emergency.

Small ziplock bags can organize and protect dressings, bandages, and other small items. Small transparent plastic containers hold pills. For liquids, such as disinfecting solution, use plastic squeeze bottles with flip-up squirt caps (1 or 2 oz. size for small kits). Wrap the threads of the bottles with PTFE thread seal tape (available in plumbing supply sections of hardware stores) before screwing on the caps, so that they will not leak.

Survival

Equipment for personal survival may also help your patient survive. If you have to bivouac or do a long evacuation, protection against the elements may be more important than emergency care. For survival, you may need spare clothing, shelter-building supplies, fire-starters, and spare sunglasses. To find your way out or attract help, you may need a compass, watch, maps, signal mirror, whistle, and coins for a phone. A GPS can pinpoint your location, but you always need backup navigation tools in case the GPS fails, or your lines of sight to the satellites are blocked by the terrain. To transport a patient, you may need materials for building a litter or sled.

Putting it all together

Drug stores and online stores will have many of the supplies you need. Outdoor stores often stock the more wilderness-oriented items. For some items, you may have to go to a medical supply store or online catalog.

Putting your own kit together is worth the trouble, for several reasons. First, it makes you think about what you need and whether you have the training to use it. Second, if you buy a commercial first aid kit, you will still have to spend time and money adding and subtracting things to make it functional. Third, you will need to restock your kit periodically anyway, so you might as well find your supply sources now.

However, no matter how well trained and equipped you are, remember that you cannot be a walking hospital. Even physicians may not be able to give adequate medical care in the backcountry. Your priorities are to try to save lives, to minimize damage from serious injuries and to minimize discomfort and complications from minor injuries. In other words, an artistic bandage won't do much good if, while you're applying it, the victim is dying of shock or hypothermia. On the other hand, having adequate first aid equipment and training will help you to handle emergencies quickly and efficiently so that you can then turn your attention to surviving (and even enjoying) the rest of the trip.

List of supplies

Some of the items in this list may be kept in your repair kit or elsewhere. The quantity of supplies you include depends on the kinds of problems that are most likely encountered on a trip, as well as the length of the trip, number of people, and possibility of replacing what is used up.

If you repackage medications, copy both the expiration date and dosage information onto the new label and cover it with transparent tape for protection. Note, however, that pills can generally be used until they disintegrate, unless the   exact dosage is critical (e.g., a medication for a serious ongoing illness). Basic items are in boldface. More specialized items are in lightface. The uses of an item are in italics.

Tools

Swiss Army knife or multi-tool – *Cutting, equipment repair*
EMT shears: *Cutting bandages, clothing, boots, etc.*
Seam ripper: *Opening clothing to expose injuries*
Uncle Bill's Sliver Grippers: *Removing slivers and wound debris, can also be used to remove ticks*
Tick Spoon or Tick Pliers: *Removing ticks*

Needle nose vise grips: *Equipment repair, gripping needles, removing large cactus needles*
Diaper pins: *Fastening bandages, closing ripped seams in clothing*
Sewing kit with button and carpet thread: *Repair of clothing, sleeping bags, tents, packs, etc.*
Small flashlight: *Checking light response in patient's pupils, doing assessment in the dark*
Small magnifier: *Removing slivers, ticks, specks from eye*
Pencil or pen
Notepad
Hand/body warmers
CPR mask (small disposable one)
Cotton-tipped applicators
Mini marshmallows: *Removing contact lenses*
Rubber cement: *Removing small cactus needles and nettles*

Containers
Vinyl zipper envelope: *Personal kit*
Nylon zipper bags with compartments: *Group kit*
Ammo boxes: *Expedition kit*
Ziplock bags: *Organize items*
Small plastic containers: *Organize pills*
Squeeze bottles: *Liquids, e.g. disinfectant*

Cleaning and disinfecting
Nitrile gloves (non-allergenic))
Liquid soap
Honey: *Disinfecting wounds*
Povidone iodine (liquid): *Disinfecting*
Benzalkonium chloride prep pads: *Cleaning and disinfecting hands, skin around wound*
Syringe with catheter tip: *Wound irrigation*

Dressings and bandages
Sterile gauze pads: *Wound dressings*
Trauma pads/battle dressings: *Bleeding control*
Band Aids (non-stick): *Wound protection*
Adhesive pads (non-stick): *Wound protection*
Triangular bandages: *Securing dressings and splints*
Gauze rollers (4"): *Securing dressings or splints*
Gauze rollers (2"): *Finger bandages*
Bias cut stockinette: *Securing dressings*
Butterfly bandages: *Wound closure*
Knuckle bandages
Fingertip bandages
Eye patch

Moleskin: *Blister prevention and treatment*
Mole foam: *Blister prevention and treatment*
2nd Skin: *Blister and burn treatment*
Athletic tape (3/4")
Duct tape: *Quick securing of splints, equipment repair*

Splints
Wire splints
SAM splints
Air splints
Traction splint: *For fractured femur*

Medications
Aspirin: *Mild pain & inflammation*
Acetaminophen (500 milligram tablets): *Moderate pain*
Rx Tylenol with codeine: *Severe pain*
Antihistamine: *Allergy/asthma*
Rx Epinephrine inhaler: *Severe asthma or anaphylactic reaction*
Rx pseudoephedrine: *Decongestant*
Laxative: *For constipation*
Rx Lomotil: *For diarrhea*
Electrolyte mix: *Rehydration*
Rx erythromycin: *Moderate infection*
Rx ampicillin or cephalexin: *Severe infection*
Hydrocortisone cream (1%): *Relieve itching*
Oil of cloves: *Ease toothache*
Antifungal powder/ointment
Lip balm

Dental first aid kit
See Chapter 10

Survival
Steel mirror and whistle: *Signaling*
Shelter or materials to make it
Extra clothing
Fire starters
Emergency food and water disinfecting system
Sun, insect protection

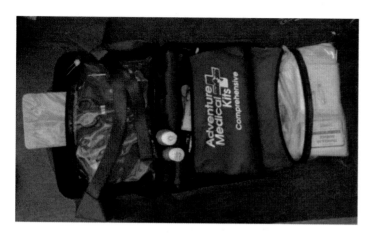

First aid kit opened

- On left: SAM splint, tools, and waist strap.
- Plastic squeeze bottles with disinfectant are in elastic loops.
- The center compartment holds medications, emergency dextrose tablets, and other supplies.
- The compartment at right holds bandages and dressings.

First aid kit tools
From the top

- Universal shears
- Seam ripper
- Sliver grippers with case
- Multi-tool
- Diaper pin
- Pen light
- Plastic pill container with O-ring seal in top
- Plastic squeeze bottle with flip-up squirt cap, threads wrapped with PTFE tape
- Space pen and pencil
- Notebook with water-resistant plastic paper

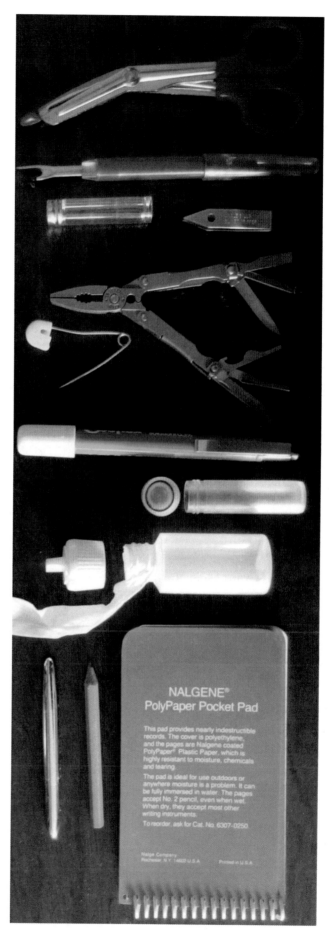

Chapter 4. Shock

Photos courtesy of Ben Schifrin, M.D.

Injuries can kill people in two ways: by damaging or destroying vital organs outright; or by interfering with the delivery of oxygen and other substances to the vital organs by the circulating blood. If the vital organs are not getting enough oxygen to maintain themselves, they start to die. This condition is called shock. It can happen in many ways, and depending on how it happens, medical textbooks give shock different names. For example, "neurogenic" shock means that the problem originates in the nervous system. But even though the initial signs and symptoms may differ, the final effect is the same. A rescuer's first priority, after taking care of the ABCs and scene safety, is usually to prevent or minimize shock.

Mechanisms of shock

How can injuries interfere with oxygen delivery?

- Loss of blood volume can cause **hypovolemic shock** ("too little volume"). Blood volume can be depleted by severe external or internal bleeding (**hemorrhagic shock**), or by severe dehydration.
- Circulation will become sluggish if a cervical spine injury or a neurotoxin cuts off signals from the brain that increase heart rate and constrict blood vessels (**neurogenic shock**). The arteries will dilate, causing blood to pool.
- Damage to the heart from a heart attack that blocks blood supply to part of the heart muscle (**cardiogenic shock**) will also reduce circulation by making the pump less efficient.
- Allergic reaction to intrusion of a foreign protein (**anaphylactic shock**) will reduce the supply of air to the lungs by constricting airways and make circulation sluggish by dilating the arteries.
- An infection that spreads through the whole body can do so much damage to blood vessels that they leak fluid into surrounding tissues (**septic shock**).

Treating for shock

In many cases, you can prevent or at least minimize shock by identifying and treating the cause:

- Stop serious bleeding from an open wound.

- Reduce pain and prevent further damage by splinting a fracture.
- Prevent further damage if you find signs and symptoms of a spinal injury. See the chapter on spinal injury management.
- Help a heart attack victim to take prescribed medications and avoid exertion while waiting for evacuation.
- Help someone with an allergic reaction take prescribed medications.
- Prevent, or at least identify and treat infection, before it spreads through the body. If infection has spread enough to cause septic shock, the patient has little chance of survival.

If shock is likely, you should begin treating for it as soon as possible. Do not wait for signs and symptoms to appear. In a wilderness situation, there are four important things that you can do:

- Guard the patient's airway, since shock victims may be nauseated and level of responsiveness may be going down. Vomiting and aspirating the vomit into the lungs is always a danger.
- Give oxygen if you have it, since the main problem with shock is shortage of oxygen in the vital organs.
- Maintain body temperature with ground insulation and covers, since any problem with oxygen delivery slows down metabolism and heat production.
- Give psychological support and reassurance, since the patient's emotional state (as discussed in the first chapter) affects functions controlled by the autonomic nervous system, which can make shock more or less severe.

Friedrich Trendelenburg, in an 1873 surgical textbook, recommended tilting patients head down for abdominal or pelvic surgery, so that abdominal viscera slide towards the diaphragm. During WWI, Walter Cannon suggested that the **Trendelenburg position** might also shift blood from the legs to vital organs for patients in hypovolemic shock. By the time he changed his mind, this practice (and the modified Trendelenburg position of just raising the legs) had become standard for treating shock. But clinical studies [see the bibliography] have shown the amount of blood shifted by this position is negligible (1.8%), because blood has already been shifted by the circulatory system's response to hypovolemia. Also, the position could aggravate some injuries and medical problems; so it is no longer recommended.

Hypovolemic shock

If bleeding or severe dehydration reduces the blood volume, the circulatory system will usually compensate in several ways. These compensations are often listed, confusingly, as the signs and symptoms of shock. But so long as compensation works, the circulatory system may continue to deliver enough blood and oxygen to the vital organs to keep them alive. If the circulation cannot fully compensate, however, or compensation begins to fail, vital organs will also begin to fail. Then you will see much more ominous signs and symptoms. So it is important to recognize when vital systems are stressed and to support them promptly.

Another consideration is that compensation for hypovolemic shock varies depending on age and physical fitness. A healthy child may compensate so well that you will not realize the problem until compensation fails. Then the child's condition can get worse very fast. Elderly people however, especially those with poor circulation or limited lung capacity, have much less margin to compensate for loss of blood volume. Therefore, you may see the effects of poor circulation and oxygen shortage in the elderly much more quickly.

An adult has about a quart of blood (a little less than a liter) for every 25 pounds of body weight, so a 150-pound adult has about six quarts of blood, of which about half is liquid. How do you tell if somebody has lost a significant amount of blood? On a hard, non-absorbing surface, like concrete or a bare floor, a fairly small amount of blood may look like a lot. But outdoors the ground may soak up blood even from a severe wound, so that a lot will look like a little. Similarly, it is hard to estimate the amount of dehydration, especially if it is caused gradually by failing to replace water lost through sweating and respiration. But you can get a good idea of lost blood volume from the effects on the patient.

- Circulation withdraws from the skin to concentrate on vital organs, so the skin gets cool and pale. In dark-skinned persons, check the gums. Skin may also get sweaty, because that is part of the body's automatic fight or flight reaction triggered by the release of adrenaline.
- Respiration speeds up to blow off accumulating carbon dioxide in the blood and becomes shallow when the chest does not have time to expand or contract fully.
- The patient may feel anxious and agitated because of the adrenaline coursing through the system.

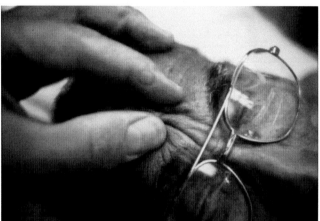
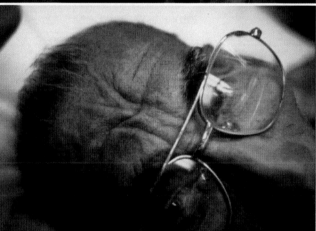

In severe dehydration, the skin loses elasticity, so that it remains tented when pinched.

As shock progresses and the body continues compensating:
- Pulse becomes weak because of reduced blood volume and rapid because the heart speeds up to compensate.
- Blood pressure may drop, because blood volume is down and circulation is withdrawn from the limbs.

33

- Pulse may speed up significantly, and blood pressure drop further, after the patient sits or stands up, especially in the elderly (postural hypotension).
- Capillary refill (when you press on the nail bed or forehead) may slow down - it takes longer for the pink to come back.
- Pupils dilate (the relaxed position of the iris muscles) because of reduced blood flow and respond more slowly to light.
- Nausea and thirst signal the withdrawal of circulation from the digestive system.
- Urine production decreases or stops.
- Weakness and possibly trembling in the arms and legs signals withdrawal of circulation from the muscles.
- Level of responsiveness drops because of poor circulation to the brain, and the patient usually becomes disoriented.

If compensation and your efforts to support the vital systems fail:
- Skin will become mottled (from patchy, pooled blood) and cold, and sweating may stop.
- Pulse will be fast, and you may not feel it.
- Blood pressure may not register.
- Breathing will be agonal (gasping and irregular).
- The patient will soon become unresponsive.

A patient who has lost 25% or less of the total blood volume will usually be given crystalloid by paramedics to replace the liquid part of the blood. This patient will continue to need oxygen, because it will take time for the body to replace lost red blood cells. A patient who has lost 30% or more of the blood volume will have a very weak pulse and need a transfusion.

Other mechanisms of shock

If a cervical spine injury or a neurotoxin cuts off sympathetic nervous system signals from the brain, then the circulatory system cannot compensate (**neurogenic shock**). The heart will slow down (**bradycardia**) because the adrenal glands, with no signal from the brain, are not releasing epinephrine; but parasympathetic nerves are releasing acetylcholine (which slows the heart rate). Blood vessels will dilate, so the skin will remain warm and flushed for a while, but level of responsiveness will drop as circulation gets more and more sluggish.

In **anaphylactic shock** (described in Chapter 23), the immune system over-reacts to the intrusion of a foreign protein. Air passages constrict, swell, and congest, which can dramatically reduce the amount of air inhaled.

In **cardiogenic shock** (heart attack), one or more of the arteries supplying the heart muscle with blood is blocked. Even if the patient is still breathing and has a pulse, the heart muscle will be damaged, and may be pumping less blood with each contraction. Usually the circulatory system will compensate (as in hypovolemic shock) by withdrawing circulation from the skin (making it cool, pale and clammy) and from the skeletal muscles (which will make the patient feel weak). If the digestive system is deprived of circulation, the patient may become nauseated and vomit, so you need to protect the airway.

The pulse may be weak or irregular. Damage to the heart muscle can cause back pressure in the pulmonary veins returning oxygenated blood from the lungs to the heart (**congestive heart failure**). Then fluid will accumulate in the lungs (pulmonary edema). Breathing rate may increase to compensate for less oxygen getting through soggy lung tissue to the blood, and you may be able to hear breath sounds with a stethoscope as air is forced through frothy fluid in the bronchioles. Give the patient oxygen if you have it.

The patient may feel a dull pain or discomfort that does not subside. It is usually in the chest, but may radiate down the left arm, or be referred – felt in the jaw or back. Some patients, however, feel no pain from a heart attack, especially if they are elderly.

Usually a conscious patient suffering a heart attack will be most comfortable in a sitting or semi-sitting position, especially in congestive heart failure, because that position drains the fluid to the bottom of the lungs; whereas lying down would spread the fluid over more lung surface and reduce oxygen delivery to the blood. An unresponsive patient who is breathing can be propped in a semi-sitting position.

Patients surviving their first heart attack may be in denial. But any exertion could cause a second, probably fatal heart attack. So the most important thing you can do for them (especially in a wilderness situation) is to persuade them not to exert themselves, and wait for evacuation.

Chapter 5. Wilderness wound care

Photos courtesy of Ben Schifrin, MD

In both wilderness and urban situations, you need to stop serious bleeding immediately and protect yourself from possible blood-borne diseases. In the wilderness, even minor wounds can easily become infected and turn into major emergencies if you do not treat them properly. So wilderness rescuers also need to know how to clean wounds and keep them clean with effective dressings and bandages.

Stopping the leak

The best way to stop serious bleeding is to squeeze the leaking blood vessels by pressing firmly on the wound, using thick dressings, a clean bandana, or a gloved hand to apply direct pressure; then replace manual pressure with a pressure bandage. If that doesn't stop the bleeding, then for an injury in a limb you can supplement the direct pressure with a tourniquet, depending on your training and the equipment at hand.

When is bleeding serious?

Blood from a cut artery spurts with every contraction of the left ventricle, until blood volume and blood pressure drop. So until arterial bleeding is controlled, it can prevent the formation of a clot. Bleeding from a cut vein does not spurt, and is therefore usually easier to control; but if it is more than a trickle, the patient can still lose enough blood to go into shock. Clotting, the body's mechanism for sealing an open wound, can take 10 minutes or more even for minor wounds.

Pressure points

A pressure point is a place on a limb where you can press an artery against the underlying bone. Manual pressure on a pressure point is no longer recommended for controlling bleeding, because it is difficult to maintain, and bleeding from peripheral circulation will usually start within 30 to 60 seconds. But a pressure point might be useful as a temporary supplement to direct pressure while someone else prepares a pressure bandage or an improvised tourniquet. For an arm wound, the best pressure point is on the brachial artery inside the upper arm, between the biceps and the triceps muscle. If your hand is big enough, you can

grab the arm from below and behind, midway between the shoulder and the elbow, and clamp the artery against the bone with the flats of your fingers. You will feel it pulsing against the upstream fingers but not against the downstream fingers. You can also monitor the radial pulse in the wrist with your other hand. When it stops pulsing under your fingers, you have clamped the brachial artery effectively. On a big arm, you may have to use two hands to squeeze or clamp the arm in the crook of your elbow.

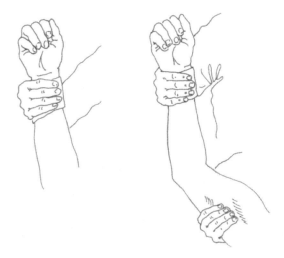

The main pressure point for the leg is on the femoral artery, which runs down the inside of the thigh and is as thick as the thumb. Your landmark is the line from the groin to the hip that creases when you flex the leg. Kneel alongside the supine patient's thigh, facing the head. Put the heel of your hand on that line, lock your elbow, and use body weight to apply pressure.

Tourniquets

Tourniquets (constricting bands around an arm or leg that shut off circulation to the limb) were used in the Roman legions, and continue to be used by the military because in combat situations, there may be no practical alternative for quickly controlling severe bleeding. Some military uniforms even incorporate tourniquets, which can be tightened with one hand by the patient.

Contrary to the traditional belief that applying a tourniquet always means sacrificing the affected limb, their use in the military has caused little damage to limbs, even when they stayed on longer than the recommended limit of two hours. So tourniquets are becoming a standard tool in urban emergency medical services, where patients are rapidly transported to a hospital. Since commercial tourniquets can be applied very quickly, they free EMTs to deal with other aspects of patient care.

Most commercial tourniquets are made of webbing, between one and two inches wide. Wider is better, because it controls bleeding with less pressure. To apply the tourniquet, put it around the limb two inches proximal to the wound (but not on a joint), and pull the webbing through the buckle until it is tight. Twist the attached rod to increase the pressure until the bleeding stops (and there is no distal pulse), then secure it. One tourniquet design applies pressure by squeezing a bulb to inflate the band (like a blood pressure cuff) instead of twisting a rod. Arterial bleeding will stop when the compression equals systolic blood pressure, and there is no distal pulse. Even for severe venous bleeding, however, you should tighten the tourniquet until there is no distal pulse. Otherwise, arterial blood can continue to flow into the limb and be trapped, causing compartment syndrome.

Once successfully applied, a tourniquet should not be loosened until the patient is in the hospital, because loosening it could not only cause bleeding to resume, but also release blood clots into the circulation.

You can improvise a tourniquet with a folded triangular bandage or other strong piece of cloth. After tying it snugly around the limb, pass a stick through the knot, twist the stick until bleeding stops, and secure the stick with the tails of the bandage. After applying a tourniquet, you should write a large T on the patient's forehead with a sharpie pen, as well as the location (e.g. RA for right arm) and the time applied.

There are also **junctional tourniquets** to control bleeding from wounds too close to the proximal joint for a regular tourniquet to fit. They have inflatable bladders that fit over a pressure point and apply pressure to an artery.

Hemostatic agents

Hemostatic agents (substances that help control bleeding) have a long history. Some herbs, such as yarrow, were used for that purpose by the ancient Greeks, and are still used by herbalists. Surgeons use substances such as bone wax (a mixture of beeswax,

paraffin, and other ingredients) and oxidized cellulose to control bleeding in their patients while operating. And there have been efforts, starting in WWII, to isolate and package the body's clotting substances. The American Red Cross developed a sealant that contains purified thrombin and fibrinogen.

Most hemostatic agents now used in the field are made from either **zeolite** (inert mineral granules that speed clotting by absorbing the liquid part of the blood) or **chitosan** (made from shrimp shells) whose positively charged particles attract and bind to negatively charged red blood cells, forming a glue-like seal over the wound. Chitosan is also antibacterial. Because of its origin, however, chitosan should not be used on a patient with a shellfish allergy. Since loose hemostatic granules could simply be flushed out of a bleeding wound, most hemostatic agents are now sold as coatings on trauma dressings.

While these products can help to control bleeding, they do not replace the traditional methods; and they are not cheap. To use a hemostatic dressing, first control the bleeding with direct pressure, or have our partner or the patient do it while you unpack the dressing. Start pressing the hemostatic dressing into one side of the wound, and keep packing it into the wound to replace the direct pressure. Then keep direct pressure on the hemostatic dressing for 3 to 5 minutes, cover it with more dressing (hemostatic or regular), and secure the dressing with a bandage.

Protecting yourself

Blood may carry disease organisms such as hepatitis B or C, so you should protect your hands with gloves and your eyes with goggles, if necessary.

For many years, latex, made from the sap of a tropical tree, was the standard for impermeable gloves that are also light and flexible. Unfortunately latex contains proteins that can cause allergic reactions. Even a minor allergic reaction can cause the skin to crack, scale, or blister. Although rare, a severe reaction can cause anaphylactic shock, which is often fatal. Powdered latex gloves are especially dangerous, because pulling them out of the package and putting them on releases a latex tainted aerosol, which an allergic patent or bystander could inhale. Because of the growing allergy problem, latex is being phased out of the health care industry.

As with any allergy, before you can suffer a reaction to latex, you must be sensitized by repeated exposure. In 1988, when AIDS was first publicized, the number of latex gloves imported into the United States each year jumped from one billion to eight billion. Health care workers, people trained to do first aid and emergency care, and even people in the food industry began wearing them regularly, which greatly increased exposure. Synthetic gloves, however, give the same protection without risk of allergy. The standard synthetic alternative to latex is nitrile.

Preventing infection

A healthy immune system can usually protect living tissue in minor wounds if they are not too dirty. But it does not protect dead tissue or foreign matter. These become colonization sites for bacteria, which can then multiply until they overwhelm the body's defenses. So the only way to prevent infection in the wilderness is to clean the wound and keep it clean. And the only safe way to clean an open wound in the field is to irrigate it with a forceful jet of water. This may not be pleasant for the patient, but it is essential for preventing infection.

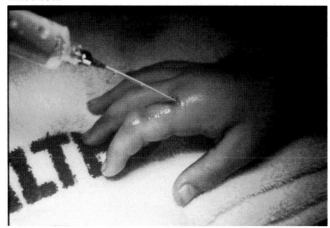

Wound irrigation syringes with blunt needles or plastic tips are sold by medical supply companies, and through the internet. They produce 7-10 psi (pounds per square inch) of pressure. To avoid splash-back, you can run the syringe or the needle through the bottom of a plastic cup or something else that will act as a shield.

A plastic squeeze bottle with a screw-on cap that has a narrow opening for squirting out a thin stream of liquid can also be used for wound irrigation. Another alternative is a large heavy-duty ziplock bag with a pinhole in the bottom corner. Just fill it up, seal the top, and squeeze. However, it will not produce nearly as much pressure as a syringe. Whatever device you use, keep irrigating until the wound is as clean as you can get it. Disinfected water from your water bottle is ideal, but use the cleanest water available.

If you see dirt or debris embedded in the wound that does not flush out, then you need to pick it out with clean tweezers. After removing the debris, irrigate again. Lacerations from a clean knife or other sharp object are least likely to become infected, because they leave relatively little crushed dead tissue in the wound.

Puncture wounds are at high risk of infection, because they may carry contaminants deep into the tissues and are hard to clean. If possible, apply hot compresses to a puncture wound (20 minutes every 2 hours) for a day or two, to draw out contaminants.

Disinfectants and "antibiotic" ointments

Antiseptics will not completely disinfect a wound, but they may slow down bacterial growth. Povidone-iodine (a buffered 10% iodine solution) and benzalkonium chloride are the two standard antiseptics (Greek *anti* "against" + *sepsis* "putrefaction") for hospital and emergency care use. They also come in sealed antiseptic towelettes, which are good for scrubbing the skin around a wound and for cleaning your hands if water is short. Povidone-iodine is dark red and stains. Benzalkonium chloride does not. To carry either solution in your kit, use a 2 oz. plastic squeeze bottle with a hinged squirt nozzle in the cap. Wrap the threads with Teflon tape (found in the plumbing section of hardware stores) to prevent leaking. Tincture of iodine, mercurochrome, and hydrogen peroxide are no longer recommended, because they may cause some tissue damage; and alcohol doesn't work.

Honey has been used in wound dressings for thousands of years. Many studies have shown that it is effective, even on organisms that are resistant to antibiotics. Dark manucca honey from New Zealand (Medihoney) has been approved for medical use because it has an especially high level of anti-microbial activity. The ingredient that makes it superior has not been identified. But all unprocessed honey reduces wound infection and promotes healing by several mechanisms. The sugar dehydrates bacteria by drawing out the fluid osmotically across cell membranes. Since honey is acidic, it disrupts the membranes of gram negative bacteria. And an enzyme in dark, unprocessed honey (glucose oxidase) releases a low level of hydrogen peroxide (not enough to cause tissue damage). Honey also helps keeps the wound moist, which promotes healing.

While some unprocessed honey may contain spores of the bacteria that cause botulism, there have been no reported cases of infection from it. Heating breaks down some ingredients that make honey effective as wound dressing, so Medihoney is sterilized by gamma radiation. Much of what is sold as honey in stores, however, is mixed with high fructose corn syrup. Moreover, some imported honey from Asia is contaminated by lead (from soldered seams of metal containers) and animal antibiotics. So it is best to buy locally produced unprocessed honey for both nutritional and medicinal purposes.

Antibiotic ointments are widely used and included in many first aid kits, but they do not actually kill bacteria. They may help to protect against infection by forming a barrier, but so will any ointment. A study of surgical wounds in the hospital by Smack and his colleagues [see the bibliography] divided the patients into two groups. One group had their wounds treated with a common antibiotic ointment, bacitracin. The other group was treated with white petrolatum, a neutral ointment that looks the same.

No significant difference was found in the healing or infection rate. Another problem with antibiotic ointments is that they may cause allergic reactions. So while antibiotic ointments will probably not do any harm, you should not depend on them to prevent infection. There is no substitute for irrigating a wound thoroughly, and then keeping it clean, especially in the wilderness.

Just a scrape

On a two-week backpacking trip in Hawaii, a woman scraped her knee on the first day of the trip. She just washed it with a little water and continued. Over the next few days, the knee became somewhat stiff and swollen, but she insisted it was fine. The assistant leader thought that the wound was infected, but the trip leader said it was healing. Even when the whole area above and below the knee became red and hot to the touch, the trip leader attributed it to the stress from hiking up and downhill. Only when the woman became feverish with a rapidly increasing temperature, and the knee had swollen into a throbbing ball of pain, did the leader recognize the problem and call for evacuation. Then it took five days on intravenous antibiotics in the hospital to knock down the infection. But if the patient had thoroughly cleaned the wound when it happened, and kept it clean, it probably would have remained just a minor scrape.

Signs of infection

If bacteria in a wound are increasing and multiplying, the body responds in several ways. It sends chemicals to the area that increase circulation (so that the skin around the wound becomes red) and that loosen the bonds between cells in blood vessel walls. White blood cells slip out of the blood vessels to attack and devour the bacteria. Fluid accumulates, causing swelling, which in turn causes pain by putting pressure on nerves. The swollen wound site will also be pressure-sensitive. All the chemical activity produces heat, so the area around the wound will feel warm. Fluid with dead white blood cells (pus) may leak out of the wound. Hot soaks can help draw out the pus from puncture wounds that are hard to clean by irrigation.

If the infection spreads, you may see red streaks going towards the heart, as dead red blood cells and other debris drain through the lymph vessels, causing inflammation. Lymph vessels have filters or nodes that remove solids from the fluid, so these nodes may swell. Large lymph nodes are in the armpits and groin, for example. Another reaction of the body to spreading infection is fever - raising the temperature may make the body less hospitable to some bacteria and viruses.

For an infection that is spreading in spite of wound cleaning and disinfection, an oral antibiotic may help. These are prescription drugs, however. So for a trip where you will be more than a day or two from medical care, you could have every trip member bring his or her own prescribed oral antibiotic just in case of uncontrolled wound infection.

Closing the wound

Any wound large enough to require evacuation, or showing signs of infection, should be left open unless it must be closed to control bleeding.

If you decide to close a clean minor wound, the simplest way is with butterfly bandages. You can make your own butterflies out of athletic or adhesive tape, or duct tape for a large wound. Just make a center section non-sticky by cutting part way in from the edges and folding them over. Before applying tape, dry the skin around the wound with sterile gauze and paint it with tincture of benzoin – a sticky red fluid derived from tree sap – to make the skin tacky. Do not put ointment on the wound if you want to close it with tape, because then the tape will not stick. Stick one or more pieces of tape to one side of the wound, use the other ends to pull the wound shut, and stick them down.

Another option for closing minor wounds is superglue, which has been used for many years to close facial cuts in boxers between rounds. Now a special formulation for wound closure is available. But the trick in using it is to hold the wound closed and spread the glue over the skin, not to squirt it into the wound, where it would just act as a foreign body and retard healing. Large or gaping wounds may have to be sutured, but this requires training and is best done in a hospital.

Wound healing

As the first step in wound healing, the blood delivers thrombin and fibrinogen, proteins that forms a matrix of fibers in the wound. This matrix does two things: forms a clot that stops bleeding, and provides a framework into which living cells can migrate, from the bottom of the wound up, pushing the fibrous material toward the surface to form a scab.

Some types of wounds heal more easily than others. A clean, straight cut made with a sharp edge is easy to align, and will usually close without complications if you keep it clean. A jagged cut with crushed tissue is less likely to heal by itself. Also, wound healing slows down at high altitude, because even when you are acclimatized, the blood delivers less oxygen to the tissues than at sea level. Above about 18,000 feet, without supplemental oxygen, wound healing stops.

Another problem with wounds outdoors is that the very parts of your body most likely to be injured, because you use them so much, are for the same reason hard to keep clean - the hands and feet especially. A trecker in Nepal found this out the hard way. His story was reported in the journal, *Wilderness & Environmental Medicine*. A spider bit him on his finger. The bite did not seem venomous, so he paid

little attention to the small puncture wound. But it became infected, and when he finally staggered into Kathmandu, his hand was swollen to twice its normal size. The local doctors were going to amputate when an American hand surgeon, who was vacationing in the area, saved the hand with a marathon operation by lantern light.

Types of wounds

Different mechanisms of injury can cause different kinds of damage. A sliding fall or skid can scrape off layers of skin. Granite rash from sliding down a rock slope, or road rash from a bicycling accident, are typical. Abrasions (from Latin *abradere*, "to scrape off, to shave") tend to be painful because of the number of nerve endings affected, and laborious to clean if grit or dirt is ground into the damaged skin. Also, a small first aid kit is unlikely to have enough sterile dressings to cover and protect a large abrasion.

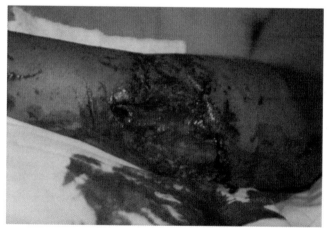

Wound caused by abrasion, deep enough to damage underlying tissues.

Lacerations (from Latin *laceratio*, "a tearing or mangling") can damage underlying structures as well as skin, such as large blood vessels, nerves, tendons, muscles, or bones. Once you have treated the wound, you should check distal functions for the effects of any damage: circulation, sensation, and movement (CSM).

The word "incision", for a clean cut made by something very sharp, usually refers to a deliberate cut made by a surgeon, as the Latin *insidere* ("to cut or carve into") suggests. Such a wound is less likely to need debridement (removal of dead tissue) by a doctor to prevent infection, than a more ragged wound; but a sharp object is more likely to cut deeply and cause damage to underlying tissues, such as blood vessels, nerves, muscles, or tendons. So it is important to check and document sensory and motor functions that may be affected by the wound after controlling bleeding.

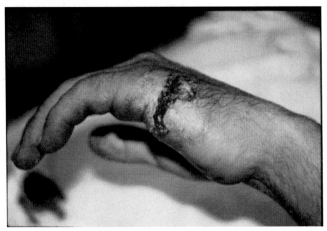

Laceration

Avulsions (from Latin *avulsus*, past participle of *avulsere*, "to pull away, tear off") are wounds in which living tissue is partially or completely torn away. If there is no serious bleeding, avulsed tissue that is not completely separated can be bandaged in its normal position after cleaning.

Amputations (from Latin *amputatio*, "a pruning") are probably the most dramatic of wounds, and you might have to use a tourniquet to control bleeding, although when blood vessels are completely severed their muscular walls tend to constrict them. After controlling the bleeding, wrap the amputated part in sterile gauze, and seal it in a water-tight plastic bag. Keep the bag cool during evacuation by putting it in ice, if available. Otherwise, wrap the bag in thick cloths and keep the cloths wet.

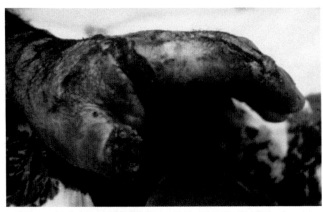

Amputation of a thumb

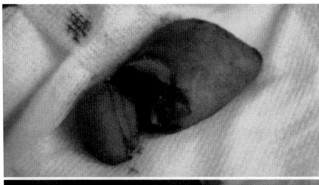

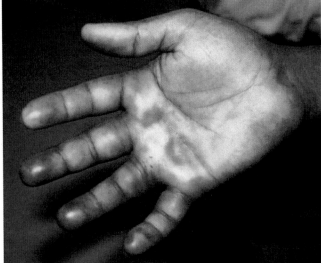

Amputated thumb, reattached by a surgeon

Bandages and dressings

Bandages (from Anglo-Saxon *banda* "to bind") hold dressings in place. Dressings "dress" a wound, protecting it from contamination. A scab (formed by the clotting proteins in the blood) is no barrier to bacteria, so the wound still needs to be protected. In fact, a scab can be a colonization site, since it is not living tissue. If possible, dressings should be sterile. But in a wilderness emergency, any clean cloth is better than nothing, and you can boil dirty cloths.

For serious bleeding, bulky dressings soak up blood and help form a clot. For other wounds, especially burns, non-stick dressings are best. Some non-stick dressings have a porous non-absorbent film over the absorbent layers. Others are coated with ointment. A wound that exposes internal organs (e.g., in the abdomen) needs moist sterile dressings to keep the organs from drying out.

You can secure a small dressing with tape. Many specialized dressings have attached adhesive strips or bandage tails, ranging from the small band aid to the thick battle dressing developed by the military, which can quickly be tied to any part of the body.

A trick for removing tape and stuck dressings painlessly (and avoid ripping out body hair) is to lift up a corner and start dabbing the adhesive with an alcohol wipe. If body hair is under the tape, pull in the direction that the hair is oriented (e.g., toward the hand or foot on a limb). The alcohol will dissolve the adhesive or clot as you peel the tape or stuck dressing. This is perhaps the only real use for alcohol wipes, which are worthless as antiseptic.

There are two types of bandages: stretchy and non-stretchy. Stretchy bandages conform to the body, so they are good for holding dressings on wounds that just need to be protected from contamination. Non-stretchy bandages are good for applying quick pressure to stop bleeding and are also more rugged. They resist being pulled loose while scrambling or bushwhacking.

The most common and versatile stretchy bandage is the gauze roller, which comes in several widths. For finger bandages, the 2" width is convenient, and the 4" width works for bandaging other parts of the body. Surgical roller bandages are also stretchy and cling to themselves. Elastic bandages are stronger, used mostly to wrap swollen joints.

The classic non-stretchy bandage is the cravat, so called because it was the predecessor of the necktie. Cravats are still part of the Boy Scout uniform. They are triangular pieces of cloth, which can be folded into strong strips for bandaging, splinting or securing a patient to a litter, or spread out to cover a large area of the body. You can improvise cravat bandages with any large piece of cloth.

Bandaging with gauze rollers

Urban-oriented courses seldom spend much time on bandaging, even at the professional level, because if the wound is serious enough that the patient needs to go to the hospital, the bandage only needs to stay on for a 10-minute ambulance ride. But in the wilderness, your bandages may need to stay on and keep the dressing in place during vigorous physical activity or a long evacuation.

To bandage an arm or leg, start on the narrow end of the limb, distal to the wound, and wrap up-limb. The following drawing shows a figure 8 spiral, which puts more uniform pressure on a bleeding wound. Angle the

roller alternately up-limb and down-limb about 20° with every other wrap. The interlocking pattern makes a secure bandage that will stay in place as the patient uses the limb.

- Leave one corner of the gauze sticking out on the first wrap, then fold it over and lock it down with the second wrap. This anchors the bandage.
- Hold the roller so that it unrolls onto the limb and maintain even tension as you wrap.
- When you have almost covered the dressing, fold the last exposed corner of it over the gauze roller and lock the dressing down with the next wrap.
- Continue wrapping well past the dressing.
- To tie off, fold the roller back over your finger so that you have a single end and a double end to tie together. If you don't have enough roller left, tear it down the center line to create two ends, or tape it to itself.

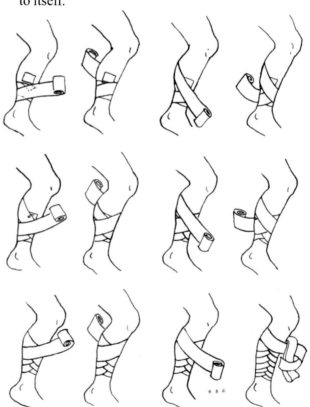

If you are improvising a roller bandage from a strip of non-stretchy cloth, use a reverse spiral to cinch the down-limb edge of the bandage. For a reverse spiral, do a half-turn toward the narrower end of the limb with every wrap.

To bandage a wound on the point of the elbow or knee, anchor the gauze roller distal to the joint. Then, holding the dressing in place with your other hand, angle the bandage diagonally across the dressing and wrap the bandage around the limb proximal to the joint. Diagonal back across the dressing, locking down its corner and making an X, then do another wrap around the limb distal to the joint

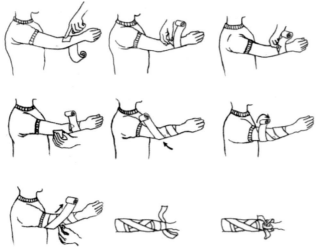

To bandage a wound on the hand with a gauze roller, anchor it at the wrist, and wrap diagonally to the hand to secure the dressing.

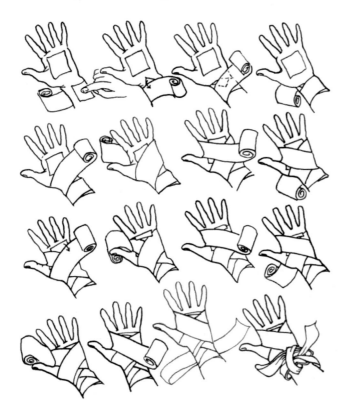

If the wound is in the hollow of the palm, add some extra layers of dressing or clean cloth to fill the hollow so that the bandage will exert pressure on the dressing. After covering and securing the dressing, wrap

diagonally back to the wrist in the other direction to make an X. and tie off the bandage at the wrist.

For a severely bleeding hand wound, fill the hand with several rollers or other padding (after applying sterile dressing) so that the patient's fingers wrap around the padding in the relaxed position of function, with the tip of the thumb even with the tip of the index finger, then anchor a gauze roller at the wrist, and wrap it diagonally around the loose fist to hold the fingers in place. This is also a good soft splint for a smashed hand or multiple fractured fingers.

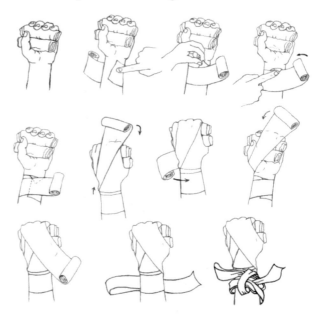

To do a good finger bandage:
- Cover the wound with sterile dressing, separating the fingers with dressings if several are injured.
- Anchor a gauze roller at the wrist, wrapping in the direction that will take the roller diagonally across the back of the hand to the injured finger, so that closing the hand will tighten rather than loosen the bandage. If the little finger or ring finger is injured, for example, the wrap starts from the thumb side of the wrist.
- Spiral up and back down the finger(s) to secure the dressing. If the fingertip is injured, secure the dressing over the tip with some up and down wraps, then anchor them with more spiral wraps.
- To add more layers, you can also take a couple of wraps up and down the length of the finger, then lock them down with more spiral wraps.
- From the base of the finger, inside, bring the roller back to the wrist and anchor it.

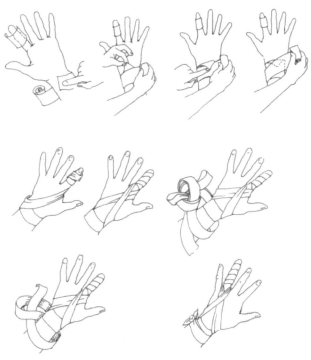

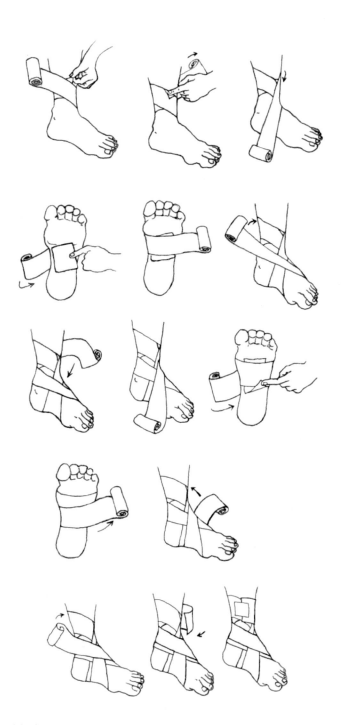

If the tip of the finger is injured, do some up and down wraps to hold part of the dressing over the tip and secure them with more spiral wraps before anchoring the bandage at the wrist.

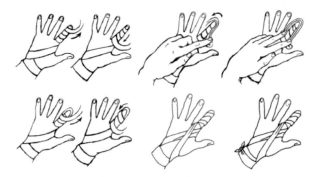

To bandage any part of the head or face, a gauze roller also works, but you may have to alternate vertical and horizontal wraps to make it secure. When going around the back of the head, be sure to pass below the bump at the base of the skull so that the bandage won't slip off.

A figure 8 roller bandage can also secure a dressing to a wound on any part of the foot, including the sole. Anchor the bandage at the ankle, then wrap it over the top of the foot and around the sole, capturing the dressing. Wrap diagonally back over the top of the foot and around the ankle. With the next wrap around the sole of the foot, lock a corner of the dressing, and continue to wrap until the wound is securely covered. If there is not enough bandage left to tie it off, tape the end of the bandage to itself.

Making a triangular bandage

Use cotton muslin or any other fabric that is not slippery or bulky. Scavenge old bed sheets, or go to a fabric store. Start with a square 40" on a side (or 42" for a large bandage). Cut on the diagonal. For durable bandages, hem the edges.

Folding the triangle into a cravat

For most bandages, you need to fold the cravat. If you have a clean surface on which to lay it out, fold the point to the long side and continue folding it in half until it is the width that you want. If you are outdoors, you can drape the cravat over your thigh to fold it. Or you can use a technique that requires a little practice

- Drape the long side over the fingers of your left hand and the point over the fingers of your right hand, keeping your thumbs out.
- Flip the center of the cravat outward, bringing your hands together.
- With your left thumb, clamp the cloth hanging inside your right fingers.
- Reach out to the end of the fold with your right hand and pinch grip the cloth.
- Now flip the cloth outward with your left thumb as you pull your right hand toward you.

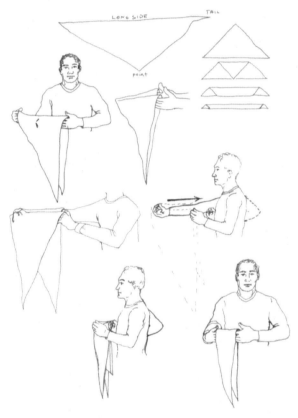

Square knot & quick release

To tie a square knot, the mnemonic is: Right over left, left over right. In the following picture, the right tail has gone over the left (and around and through). Then the tail on the left goes over the tail on the right (and around and through). If you look at the resulting knot (top right), you'll see that it is square and symmetrical – two U-shaped bends of the cravat intersecting each other. To do a quick release, pull one tail away from the standing end until it straightens out, converting the square knot into a slip knot. Then slip the knot off.

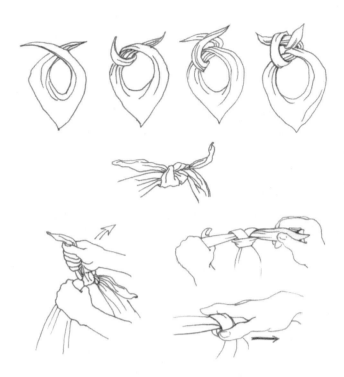

Bandaging with cravats

To do a good bandage with a cravat or other non-stretchy cloth, you need to maintain the tension as you wrap, which often requires you to pass the tails from hand to hand without ever letting go. You can't wrap a bandage loose and sloppy and expect to tighten it up at the end. To control bleeding with a pressure bandage, capture the dressing with the center of the bandage, wrap the tails around the limb a few times, then tie them together right over the dressing so that the knot puts extra pressure on the wound. Always use a square knot. You can use the same pressure bandage to hold a dressing on the forehead, making sure that the tails pass below the bump at the base of the skull so that the bandage doesn't slip off.

To secure a cravat pressure bandage over the point of the elbow or knee, you need to anchor it up-limb and down-limb. After capturing the dressing with the center of the bandage, wrap one tail around the limb proximal to the joint and the other tail around the limb distal to the joint. Then the dressing will stay in place even when the patient flexes the joint. Next, bring the tails back toward each other and cross them before doing the final wrap, then tie them on the outside of the joint - a knot right on the point of the elbow or knee would slip off as you flexed the joint.

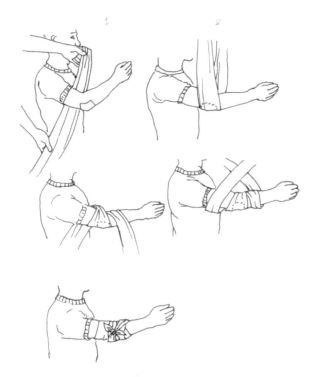

the back or side of the wrist to avoid pressing on the radial artery or nerves.

For a scalp wound, you can hold dressings in place with a turban bandage. Lay the triangle over the head with the point hanging down behind. Position the long side just above the eyebrows, and wrap the two tails around the head, crossing just below the bump at the base of the skull. Then bring the tails around and tie them in front. Now grip the point of the cravat that is hanging down the back and tug it till the bandage is snug over the scalp. Finally, tuck in the excess.

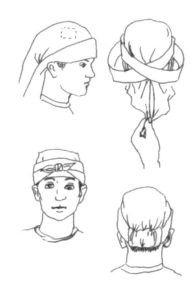

Preventing foot Blisters

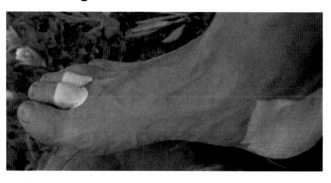

As your feet move inside your boots, friction on the outer layer of skin can shear it from the underlying layer, and as fluid accumulates between the separated layers, you grow blisters. Prevent blisters by:

- Proper boot fitting.
- Padding boots to fill gaps and cover rough edges.
- The 2-sock system (plus a cushioned insole).
- Covering hot spots (or potential hot spots) with Moleskin or tape before they grow into blisters.
- Tightening boots before walking downhill so your toes don't slide forward.

To apply pressure to a bleeding palm with a cravat, put a bulky sterile dressing and padding over the cut, for the patient to grip. Clenched fist palm side up, lay the bandage over the wrist, wrap one tail diagonally across the back of the hand, capture the two fingers on the far side of the fist, then bring the tail back diagonally across the front of the fist. This will pull the fingers closed. Maintain tension as you wrap the other tail diagonally across the back of the fist, making an X, capture the other two fingers, and bring it diagonally across the front of the fist (making another X).

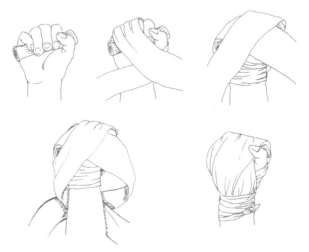

Wrap both tails around the wrist, making sure that the second tail passes up-limb from the first so that it can't slip off, and tie them in a square knot. Put the knot on

Leather boots mold themselves to your feet slightly during the break-in period. But they should be comfortable from the start – otherwise don't buy them. Plastic boots must fit very well from the outset, because they are rigid. Cases of frostbite have been reported from rented plastic mountaineering boots that didn't fit properly and impaired circulation to the feet.

If one of your legs is a bit shorter than the other, or your feet roll excessively when you come down on them, you may need to consult a podiatrist (foot specialist) or a podarthist (specialist in analyzing and correcting gait problems) and get customized boots.

When fitting boots, wear the socks that you would normally wear: thin synthetic inner socks that cling to your feet like an extra layer of skin (and reduce friction on your skin); and one or more thick socks of wool or synthetic. With the boots unlaced, you should be able to slide your foot forward enough to fit two or three fingers in the space behind your heel. After lacing up the boots, test them:

- Walk. Do leg stretches. Any pressure? Excessive heel lift or movement of toes?
- Stand on the inclined surface of one or two fitting stools, toes angled down. Do your toes slide forward and touch the fronts of the boots? If so, the boots are too loose.
- Plant one foot on the incline with the toes up and step up (balancing with the other foot in the air). Does your heel lift more than a fraction of an inch? If so, you have too much heel slop.

If the boots you own have heel slop or rough edges inside where two pieces of leather are joined, you can pad them with Mole Foam, a sheet of adhesive cloth with foam padding. When your boots are clean and dry, cut pieces of Mole Foam to fit, and press the adhesive firmly onto the leather. Going uphill, heel lift may cause blisters, so cover your heels and Achilles tendons with large pieces of Moleskin or tape to protect them from friction. Before going downhill, tighten your laces so that your toes don't slide forward, and wrap vulnerable toes with tape or moleskin.

Several types of tape are made specifically to help prevent blisters. KT Tape, for example, is thin and stretchy, so it can adhere better to curved or flexing parts of the foot. And foot lubricants that can be rubbed or sprayed on reduce friction. For expert advice on blister prevention, see: www.fixingyourfeet.com.

Treating blisters

Once blisters have formed, they can be treated in two ways. You can try to prevent them from popping or puncture them. If a blister on the heel or side of the foot is still small, you may be able to protect it:

- Cut a donut of mole foam to fit around the blister and take the pressure off it.
- Lay a piece of Spenco 2nd Skin® on the blister, fitting inside the hole.
- Cover the donut with Moleskin or tape, sealing in the 2nd Skin.

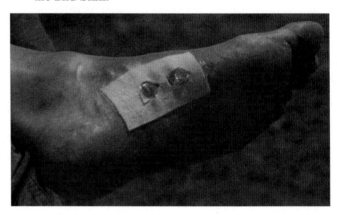

If a blister has started to form on the bottom of the foot, any thick covering would make walking uncomfortable. So the best way to protect the incipient blister from friction is with a large piece of duct tape - put a small piece of duct tape in the center of the sticky side, so that the tape will not stick to the blister.

To puncture a blister, sterilize a needle and pierce the blister at the base. You may need to enlarge the hole to prevent it from re-sealing and the blister from filling up again. Let the blister drain, irrigate, and disinfect it as you would any open wound. Afterwards, use the same technique described above to protect it against further abrasion.

Conclusion

Bleeding control is the same in wilderness and urban situations: apply direct pressure. If that is inadequate or impractical because of an underlying fracture, apply a tourniquet. Prevent infection by cleaning the wound with forceful irrigation and keeping it clean. Mild disinfectants or honey can also help. Bandaging supplies and skills are essential for protecting wounds during evacuation.

Chapter 6. Burns & wilderness fire hazards

Photos courtesy of Ben Schifrin, MD

In the wilderness, the most common cause of burns is cooking accidents. This includes minor burns to the hands from grabbing hot metal; potentially major burns from stove flare-ups; and scalds from tipping over pots of boiling liquid. If you cook in a tent, flare-ups can start a fire, even though tent fabrics are supposed to be flame retardant. Wildfires are the other way to get burned in the wilderness.

Avoiding and preventing wildfires

If you build campfires in the wilderness, do it on mineral soil, not soil that is blended with decaying forest vegetation and threaded with roots from surrounding trees. Fire can work its way down through vegetation debris to tree roots and travel along the roots. Careless campers have awakened to find that the surrounding trees had turned into giant torches.

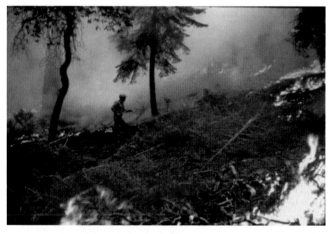

To escape a wildfire, you need to get behind it. You can't outrun a wind-driven fire, especially if it is going uphill. Wind flowing upslope compresses the layer of moving air, which increases its velocity. Also, smoke and superheated gases are pushed up ahead of the fire, especially through gullies (natural ascent routes), which act like the flume of a fireplace. In hilly terrain with narrow valleys between ridges, fire can even jump from crest to crest.

But fire needs fuel. In a shallow fuel area, such as grassland, fire will burn through fast, and you may be able to get behind it through a gap. But forest fires, especially in areas that have accumulated a lot of deadwood because of fire control, burn long and deep.

If you can't get around or through them, or find a large bare area, your only hope may be to jump in a stream or lake. Heat moves upward, so the water will keep you cool, though you need to get as far as possible from a fire to breathe relatively clean, oxygenated air.

If you are trapped, get rid of synthetic clothes because they can melt into napalm. Soak remaining clothes with water if you have any, get low and breathe through a wet bandana. Some smoke jumpers have survived fires by digging in and covering themselves with reflective space blankets, but this is a desperate tactic to use only when there is no alternative.

Thermal burn factors and damage

Thermal burns can be caused by exposure to flames, contact with a hot object, scalding by hot liquid, or steam. Burn damage depends on the temperature and conductivity of the heat source, contact time, and contact area. Hot liquid or metal can cause a much more serious burn than an open flame of the same temperature, because they transmit heat much faster than air. However, chefs can plunge their hands into boiling water for a second without harm. But an elderly person trapped in a bathtub can suffer serious burns in water at a temperature as low as 113° F, because of greater contact time and contact area. Firewalkers can walk barefoot over a bed of porous red-hot charcoal if they don't stumble, but they would not last long if they tried the same stunt on a red-hot griddle of iron, which conducts heat much more efficiently.

Burns can damage or destroy one or more layers of skin directly by heat. The inflammatory response of the body then causes accumulation of fluid to the burn, which raises blisters in a partial thickness burn. When a large part of the skin is damaged or destroyed, fluid can ooze out and dehydrate the patient. The human body is about two-thirds water, and one function of skin is to hold it in.

To take an extreme example, serious burns over half the body area of an average sized man would leak and evaporate 4-5 liters of water per day; and serious burns over 10% of the body would evaporate about a liter per day. Each liter of water that evaporates from a burn takes away about 570 Kilocalories of heat, which is as much heat as the body produces in an hour of vigorous activity. So a burn patient can easily become hypothermic as well as dehydrated.

The smoke and heated gases from fires can damage the air passages and lungs if inhaled, and cause the most deaths in burn victims. Inhalation injuries are most common in enclosed spaces, but can happen in forest fires or accidents inside a tent. Carbon monoxide (produced by all fires) can be deadly even in low concentrations, and burning synthetic fabric gives off hydrogen cyanide. Steam can burn not only the air passages but also the lungs, because water vapor has more heat capacity than air and is more conductive.

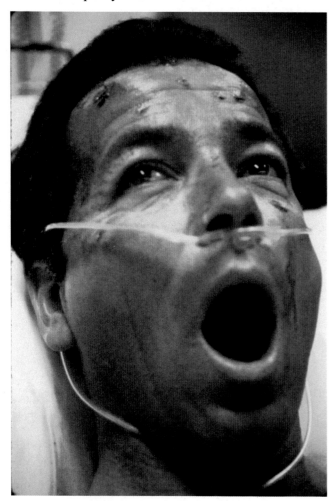

Facial burns with inhalation injuries

Serious burns also put stress on vital organs. Shortage of blood and oxygen can cause ulcers in the stomach. Kidneys can be overloaded with proteins dumped in the blood from damaged tissues. And fluid can leak into the lungs because of damage from inhalation injuries. Also, since the skin is a barrier against microorganisms, serious burns leave the patient open to infection, which may develop within days.

Assessing thermal burns

Most textbooks give the rule of nines for estimating the percentage of skin area covered by burns. Each major part of the body (e.g., an arm or the front of the torso) has either 9% or 18% of the total skin area. There are two problems with this rule: it is hard to remember, and burns seldom neatly cover one part of the body completely. So the rule of ones is much more useful. The patient's hand, from wrist fold to fingertips but excluding the thumb, is about 1% of the patient's total skin area. So estimate how many hands of skin the burn covers.

If a burn is superficial, skin will redden because of increased circulation to the injury, but it will turn white when you press on it (forcing the blood away), then turn red again as the circulation comes back. Superficial burns may not require dressings because the living layers of skin are intact. Only the transparent, non-living outer layer may peel off.

In a partial thickness burn, several layers of skin are seriously damaged, and the rush of circulation to the damaged layers pushes them apart to form blisters. These burns are extremely painful, because the damage triggers so many nerve endings. Full thickness burns do not hurt because all tissues in the skin, including nerves, have been killed. The skin may be charred, deep red, or white; or it may be burned away, exposing deeper tissues. Full thickness burns may be surrounded by partial thickness burns, however, which will hurt.

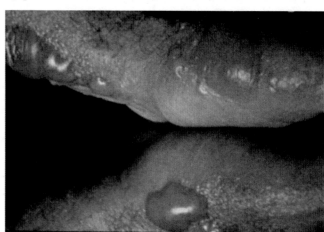

Partial thickness burn with blistering

How do you decide whether a burn requires evacuation? Any full thickness burn is serious; and any partial thickness burn that covers more than 5% of the total skin area, or any significant part of the face, hands or genitals, requires evacuation. Even a superficial burn may be serious enough to require evacuation if it covers more than 20% of the skin area. When in doubt, the patient's condition should make your decision clear. A burned patient who is shivering, vomiting, or feverish urgently needs to be evacuated.

Burns that impair function are also more serious. Facial burns can affect the eyes, and inhalation of smoke or superheated gasses can affect the airway and lungs. A circumferential burn to a limb can impair distal circulation. And any serious burn to the hand or foot can cause permanent loss of function.

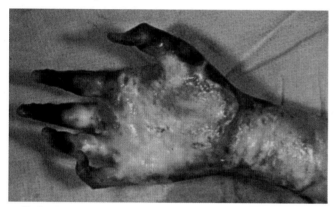

Full thickness burns to fingers

Treating thermal burns

Immediate care for a thermal burn is to stop the burning by removing the patient from the source of heat; then cool the burned area with water. If clothes are burning, smother the flame. If scalding liquid is saturating clothing, get the clothing off immediately, because it will still be broiling the victim's skin. Then cool the skin with water, because (like a roast just out of the oven) it will still be cooking.

In the wilderness, your first concern after cooling the burn will be pain control. An expedition doctor would probably give morphine to someone with a severe burn. Over the counter painkillers are not as effective, but you should use the strongest that you have if a burn patient is in severe pain.

A non-stick dressing is best for a burn. Spenco 2nd Skin is soothing, though it is not sterile. It is a sheet of gel (96% water) that you take out of a sealed package and expose by peeling away a plastic film. Other non-

stick dressings are also good. If you do not have any, you can use a moist dressing on any burn less than about 10% of total body area. It will be more soothing than a dry dressing. For a larger burn, however, a wet dressing could chill the patient into hypothermia. Change the dressing regularly.

After pain control, your next problem with a serious, extensive burn is fluid loss. If the patient is alert enough and not too nauseated to swallow safely, you should provide fluids with electrolytes (runner's drink or Oral Rehydration Salts, diluted to half-strength) and make sure that the patient drinks regularly. An occlusive dressing, made by taping a piece of plastic over a regular dressing, may reduce fluid loss as well as preventing further contamination of the injury through the dressing.

Electrical burns

Electricity, like other forms of energy, follows the path of least resistance. Nerves, blood, and muscle are more than half water, so they are good conductors of electricity. Bone, fat, and dry skin (especially calloused skin) have less water, so they are more resistant. If your body becomes part of an electrical circuit, the current flowing through it can cause serious damage by heating the tissues. Damage depends on the voltage and current, as well as the duration of contact and which part of the body it goes through.

Voltage is the potential difference in electrical energy between two points in a circuit. According to **Ohm's Law**: Voltage = Current times Resistance. So the greater the resistance, the more voltage it will take to force a given current through. Current is measured in amperes (amps).

Household circuits in the United States are usually 110 volts and 15 to 20 amps, though some appliances require 220 volts. This voltage usually causes only contact burns. Industrial voltage (over 500 volts) can cause severe damage to muscles and organs as the current flows through the body, which will not be apparent from the entrance and exit wounds. It can also cause **cardiac arrest** if the current crosses the chest or **respiratory arrest** if the current affects the respiratory center of the brain. Power cords in household and industrial circuits are insulated with material that has high resistance, so they can be safely handled. High tension power lines, however (20,000-100,000 volts) are insulated only by air. Current from power lines can arc through the air, creating its own conductive pathway of ions, to make you part of the circuit. So it is not safe even to approach a downed power line.

Direct current (DC), which was championed by Thomas Edison, flows in one direction. Contact with it usually causes a single muscle contraction that can blow the patient away from the source. But most power is transmitted by alternating current (AC), which changes direction 60 times per second, because AC (based on inventions by Nicola Tesla) can be stepped up to very high voltages and transmitted over long distances with little power loss. Contact with AC can cause sustained muscle contraction that can lock the patient on to the electrical source.

Never touch a patient who may still be in contact with an electrical source until the current is turned off. Remember that electrical burns, especially from industrial current, will have both entrance and exit wounds, which should both be covered with dry sterile dressings. Give oxygen if you have it, and check for any breathing problems or irregular pulse.

Chemical burns

Some chemicals can damage skin and underlying tissues on contact. Strong acids break down proteins in cells and solidify the tissues into a scab, which can limit penetration. Since the damage resembles the damage of thermal burns, injuries from contact with strong chemicals are also called burns. Strong bases liquefy skin and underlying tissues, so they can penetrate more easily into underlying tissues. Strength of acids and bases is measured by the pH (power of hydrogen) scale, since their reactions involve the exchange of hydrogen ions (protons). Acids give up protons, and bases bind protons. The strongest acids have a pH of 1; the strongest bases a pH of 14. Pure water has a pH of 7, which is neutral. Skin has a pH between 5 and 6, which is just slightly acidic.

Sulphuric acid is found in some toilet bowl and drain cleaners, as well as car batteries. Hydrofluoric acid is found in rust removers and tile cleaners. Hydrochloric acid is found in swimming pool cleaners and some toilet bowl cleaners, as well as the stomach's digestive juices. Common bases include sodium and potassium hydroxide, found in some drain and oven cleaners; sodium and calcium hypochlorite in household bleach; ammonia, in some cleaners and detergents; and phosphates in many household cleaners and detergents. Most of the household products are too dilute to cause serious contact burns to the skin. But they can cause severe damage to the eyes, and are very toxic if swallowed. Some of them can also give off dangerous fumes, especially if you mix ammonia and bleach, which produces chlorine gas.

Immediate treatment for a chemical burn is to remove the patient from the source and remove any contaminated clothing if you can do so without exposing yourself. Then continue flushing it with cool water for at least 15-20 minutes after the patient is no longer feeling a burning sensation, though if the chemical is in powder form, you should first brush it off before flushing. Flush each eye from the inner corner to the outside, so as to protect the tear duct and the other eye. If both eyes are affected, you can position a nasal cannula over the bridge of the nose and connect it to a container of water or sterile saline so that it flushes from the inside corners outward.

Chemical fumes can irritate or damage the airways so that they swell, and inhaled chemical fumes can damage the lungs. So after any exposure to hazardous chemicals, you should monitor the airway and breathing, and administer oxygen if necessary.

Conclusion

Serious thermal burns can cause dehydration as well as damage to skin and underlying tissues, and partial thickness burns are among the most painful of injuries. Anyone who has been burned in a fire should also be assessed for inhalation injuries. In a wilderness or remote situation, after cooling the burn, you need to keep the patient warm and hydrated and (for an extensive burn) reduce fluid loss with occlusive dressings. Industrial electrical current passing through the body can cause much more damage than is apparent from the entrance and exit wounds, and affect breathing or heart function. So after making sure that the patient is no longer in contact with the source of electrical current, you may need to do basic life support. Many chemicals can cause burn-like injuries as well. Treatment is to brush away dry chemicals and flush wet chemicals with cool water.

Backpacking stoves: Function and safety
With the technical assistance of Stephen M. Hibbs

"We first felled a...butternut tree 10 inches in diameter...For 'night-wood,' we cut a dozen birch and ash poles from 4 to 6 inches across...then we denuded a dry hemlock of its bark...We had a bright, cheery fire from the early evening until morning..."

In the century since "Nessmuk" described his campfire technique, wilderness has shrunk, and campers have proliferated. So most campers now carry stoves. Otherwise little wilderness would be left to enjoy. To select the right stove and use it safely, you need to understand how stoves and their fuels work.

Fuels

Most popular backpacking stoves use either liquid fuels, or LP (liquified petroleum) fuels that are sold in pressurized containers. They all produce about 20,000 BTUs (British Thermal Units) of heat per pound of fuel. The common liquid fuels are naphtha (white gas) and kerosene. These are available in gallon cans, and you must transfer them to smaller bottles. Naphtha is very volatile, which makes it explosive. Kerosene is less volatile, which makes it safer, but also harder to light when cold, and messy if spilled. Don't use any kind of automobile gasoline. Besides clogging your stove, byproducts from its additives will be as toxic at close range as your car's exhaust.

The available LP fuels are normal butane, isobutane, and a butane-propane mixture. Below 32° F, normal butane generates no vapor inside the canister and will not light. Butane lighters have the same problem, though keeping them in your pocket may warm them enough to light. Altitude lowers this threshold temperature somewhat, but butane stoves are still sluggish in cold weather. Isobutane, however, will still vaporize at a temperature of 12° F, 20° colder than normal butane.

All these fuels produce carbon monoxide when they burn, so it is important for the cooking area to be well ventilated. Since carbon monoxide bonds very strongly to the hemoglobin in the blood, it reduces oxygen-carrying capacity for hours after exposure, so even if the dose is less than lethal, it reduces the body's ability to do work and generate heat, which increases the risk of both hypothermia and altitude illness.

Burners

There are two burner types: the strike plate and the ported burner. In the strike plate, vaporized fuel jets upward from a metering orifice, drawing up air with it, and strikes the bottom of the plate. The resulting turbulence mixes fuel and air for burning. In the ported burner, the jet of fuel vapor draws air into the stem through a vent hole, and mixing takes place inside a hollow disk. The mixture burns from many tiny holes around the rim of the disk.

With a strike plate stove, simmering is difficult because a weak vapor jet doesn't create enough turbulence for efficient mixing. A ported burner allows simmering because its enclosed mixing chamber is efficient at all settings. Efficient mixing makes a steady blue flame. The unsteady yellow flame from poor mixing produces soot and extra carbon monoxide.

Stove designs

Liquid-fuel stoves can have burners of either type. The Svea 123, which was the first portable backpacking stove (introduced in 1955), has a strike plate, while some MSR and Coleman stoves use ported burners and vaporizing tubes that pass through the edge of the flame. These can only burn naphtha (white gas). The Svea and Coleman stoves have integral tanks that you must fill from a separate fuel container. The Coleman is pressurized by a pump, while the Svea's tank must be heated by pouring a small amount of fuel into the primer pan and lighting it to draw and vaporize fuel from the tank.

Several MSR models and some other stoves draw fuel directly from a fuel bottle, which is pressurized by a pump you screw in to replace the cap. The fuel valve is in the pump. Because the fuel bottle is separate from the burner, it can be shielded from the heat.

All LP-fueled stoves use ported burners. Some models punch a hole in the butane fuel canister when they are connected and then seal it with a rubber ring. The MSR Rapidfire and several others connect to a threaded fitting on an isobutane canister. Fuel canisters are reusable, and empties must be packed out of the back country.

Lighting

An LP-fueled stove is convenient to start. Just hold a match near the burner and open the fuel valve. But liquid-fueled stoves must be primed by burning a small amount of fuel in a cup at the base of the burner. This heats the burner base so that fuel will be vaporized before passing through the orifice. Just before the flame dies, open the fuel valve, and the stove should start. Over-priming, however, can cause a flare-up and opening the fuel valve too far can spill burning fuel around the stove.

When cooking on snow, you need insulation under the fuel tank, or it will remain too cold to vaporize fuel efficiently. For a stove with a pump that screws into a separate fuel bottle, the bottle can be wrapped in insulating foam, but an unsupported burner will melt the snow. Several lightweight metal platforms are available for MSR and other stoves, which support either the stove alone or the stove and fuel tank above the snow.

Stove safety

Most backpacking stoves are only used occasionally. Tiny orifices can become clogged in storage, so test the stove before each trip. If your stove won't work, you will eat cold food, and in winter, be unable to melt snow for drinking water.

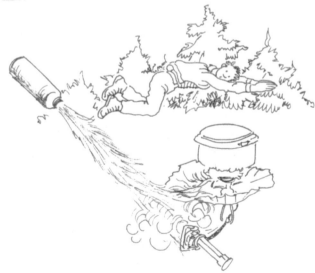

On stoves that connect to a separate fuel bottle, if the connection is weakened by worn or crossed threading on the pump, the bottle can be blown off the pump when you pressurize it. If the stove is running, the bottle can become a flaming rocket. Check the threads before a trip or anytime the pump does not

screw in easily. Also, the bottoms of cheap fuel bottles may bulge and burst under pressure, and their threads may be defective.

LP stoves with threaded canisters can be safely disconnected anytime; but those without threaded canisters cannot be disconnected until the canister is empty; and the connection can be dangerously stressed during packing and transportation. Stoves with integral tanks can be transported either filled or empty, but be sure their fuel valves are securely closed. Stoves that connect to separate fuel bottles can travel with the pump screwed in the bottle but not under pressure. They can be primed by momentarily opening the fuel valve, letting a little liquid fuel squirt out. Some stoves with strike plates, like the classic Svea 123, must be primed with an eye dropper, from either the stove's tank or a fuel bottle - a method that invites spills and burns. Keep your gear and your face away and upwind of the flame. Priming paste is safer to handle and burns more gently.

The low, wide profiles of stoves that connect with pumps to separate fuel bottles make them fairly stable. But stoves mounted on fuel tanks are tall with narrow bases, making them easy to upset along with a pot of hot food or water. Pot-and-windscreen kits widen a narrow stove's footprint, making it much safer.

A stove with a built-in tank can explode if wind shielding and the pot reflect too much heat into the tank.

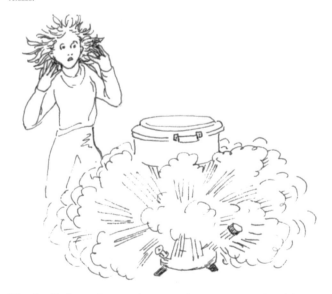

The built-in safety valve on the gas cap should vent enough pressure to avoid an explosion from an overheated gas tank, but the venting can send out a jet of flame, which will destroy the seal and make the stove inoperable unless you have a spare cap. You should turn the gas cap away from you when operating the stove.

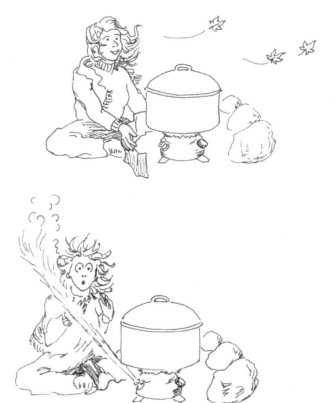

Cooking In tents

Many accidents can occur in tents, from trying to fill a tank before the stove has cooled or pouring fuel too near a flame. Stoves primed with liquid fuel frequently flare up when lit. The flare can burn a tent. Liquids boiling over or upset pots of boiling liquid can cause second or even third degree burns where people have no room to dodge.

Carbon monoxide poisoning is always a danger when cooking in a small enclosure (either a tent or a snow shelter). It has probably played a role in many deaths attributed to hypothermia.

Instant frostbite

Frostbite is an injury not usually associated with stoves and cooking. Yet LP fuel escaping from pressurized canisters can cause frostbite in any weather if it strikes your skin, because it is chilled by expansion. Also, evaporation of liquid fuel on bare hands can quickly chill them below the freezing point of water in wind or cold weather. Spills are more likely if your hands are already numb from the cold. If you pour fuel in cold

weather, protect your hands by pulling thin rubber gloves over your glove liners. These are the types of gloves used by health care professionals.

With an MSR or LP canister stove, you won't have to pour fuel. But metal fuel bottles and canisters can cause contact frostbite, especially if they've been out in the snow all night, and the fuel inside is chilled below the freezing point of water. So wrap them with duct tape, which also helps prevent dents and scratches that can weaken the fuel bottles.

Minimalist stoves

Alcohol burning stoves (such as the Trangia) are very light, quiet, and clean burning. Disadvantages are that alcohol generates only half as much heat per ounce as petroleum-based fuels, and may not burn well in sub-freezing weather. Another cheap and lightweight option is a stove that burns twigs. That also will generate much less heat than petroleum-based fuels, and is dependent on a supply of dry twigs. There are several commercial models of twig-burning stoves. But both alcohol-burning and twig-burning stoves can be made at home from sturdy cans (zenstoves.net).

Conclusion

Cooking with campfires requires dry firewood, which may not be available; and there are many restrictions on campfires in national parks and forests because of fire danger. So most campers carry stoves for cooking. No stove is absolutely safe or unsafe, under all conditions. To use stoves safely, know their hazards before you buy, and learn how to minimize the hazards when you are cooking. To pick the best stove for your activities, consider temperatures in the seasons when you will be camping, the size of your group, weight of stove and fuel, and whether your goal is to boil water rapidly or simmer gourmet meals.

Chapter 7. Bone Injuries and Splinting

While the human body is about 60% water overall, bone is only 20% water. In an adult, the structural material of bone is about two-thirds mineral and one-third tough protein fiber, a composite that combines density and rigidity with resistance to bending stress. Children's bones have less mineral and more protein fiber, which makes their bones more flexible and less likely to break. They also have growth plates at the ends of their long bones, however, and injury to these plates can stunt growth of the bone.

Under a magnifying glass, a cross-section of bone shows a honeycomb structure, with material following lines of stress. Red blood cells are made in the spaces of this honeycomb at the ends of long bones, and in the ribs and vertebrae. Each bone is enclosed by a membrane called the **periosteum** ("around the bone") containing nerves and blood vessels that penetrate the bone through a network of canals. So cracked or broken bones bleed, and broken bone ends can cause more bleeding by cutting blood vessels. Fractures also hurt and continue to hurt, though the pain may be masked for a while by the epinephrine rush of an athletic activity. Finger pressure on the fracture causes a sharp, local pain (**point tenderness**), which helps distinguish the injury from the diffuse pain of a bruise.

Keeping bone Strong

Many elderly people are very vulnerable to fractures because they have **osteoporosis** ("porous bone"). They have lost so much bone mass and mineral content that the honeycomb structure you see under a magnifying glass is mostly air. These fragile bones can break even before the victim hits the ground. Women past menopause are especially vulnerable to osteoporosis.

To prevent osteoporosis, you need enough calcium in your diet to maintain the mineral content of your bones. But you also need to do regular weight and stress-bearing exercise to stimulate the replacement of calcium. Bone responds (within limits) to the demands that you put on it. Thus as you get older, your choice is to use it or lose it. Running and other sports that weight and impact the leg bones will help maintain their bone mass and density, but do little for the upper body.

Weight lifters generally have the strongest, densest bones, and even elderly people have regained some lost bone mass by regular resistance exercise, providing that they increased the weight as they grew stronger. So if you don't get enough resistance exercise for your whole body in your work or recreational activities, weight lifting is a good way to keep your bones strong and reduce the risk of fractures.

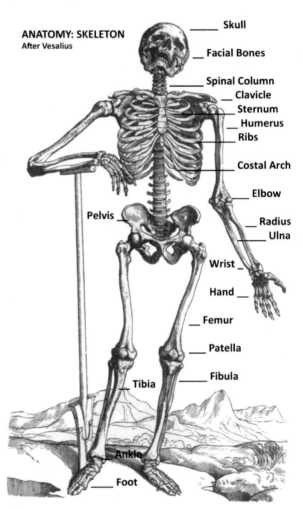

ANATOMY: SKELETON
After Vesalius

Skull
Facial Bones
Spinal Column
Clavicle
Sternum
Humerus
Ribs
Costal Arch
Elbow
Pelvis
Radius
Ulna
Wrist
Hand
Femur
Patella
Fibula
Tibia
Ankle
Foot

Mechanisms of bone injury

Bone can be damaged by many mechanisms of injury, and visualizing the mechanism will give clues to the damage. A direct blow from a fall or collision or the impact of a fast-moving object can crack a bone or break it completely. A crushing blow can shatter bone into fragments. An indirect blow radiating up an extended arm or stiffened legs can injure any bone or joint in the limb and beyond.

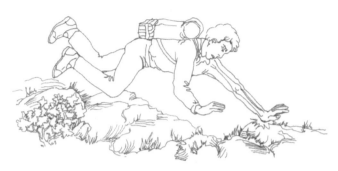

A bending force, caused for example by a ski wedged in heavy snow or a foot jammed between rocks as the body continues to move, can snap a bone. A slow twisting fall on skis, when the bindings do not release, can break the bone in a spiral pattern. Repetitive impact stress from backpacking or running can cause a hairline or displaced fracture in the foot.

The victim of a fracture may have heard something crack, and if spasming muscles are moving broken bone ends against each other, you may hear a faint grating sound (**crepitis**). The patient will probably be **guarding** the injured bone – cradling it or at least unwilling to move it. But remember to check for other injuries that could have been caused by the accident, or by underlying medical problems, before focusing on the most obvious injury.

Assessing bone injuries

The pain of a fracture may mask other injuries, so you should do a quick assessment of the whole body after acknowledging and looking at the bone injury that is probably the patient's chief complaint. As you do the assessment, visualize the mechanism of injury and ask yourself what other injuries are likely from the same mechanism. Specifically:

- Radiating injuries can be caused by an impact transmitted along a bone (e.g., falling on an outstretched arm or on the feet from a height).
- Associated injuries can be caused by the same mechanism (e.g., the twisting force that causes a spiral fracture can also tear ligaments in an adjacent joint).
- Check for injuries common to the type of accident (e.g., snow boarders often injure their wrists and arms by reflexively sticking out their hands to break a fall).

When checking the injured limb, first ask where it hurts and work around that area to check the rest of the limb. Open clothing if necessary to see any injuries underneath. Also remember to check circulation and nerve functions on the distal side of the injury, as described in the chapter on patient assessment: circulation, sensation, motor (**CSM**). Motor functions include movement and strength. To check movement, ask the patient to wiggle fingers or toes on both limbs, and compare. Then ask the patient to push down and up on your hands with both feet or squeeze crossed fingers with both hands, and compare.

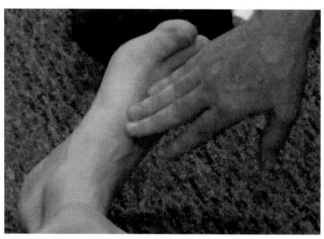

Dorsalis pedis ("top of the foot") pulse: just lateral to the tendon that enables you to raise the big toe.

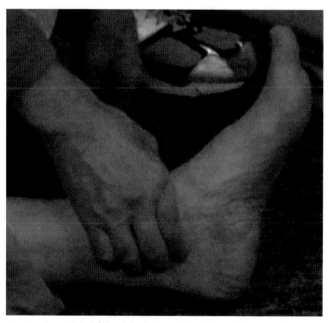

Posterior tibial ("behind the tibial knob") pulse.
Photos courtesy of Lynn Garcia.

A fracture can crimp or damage arteries and nerves. If any distal functions are impaired (weaker than on the uninjured limb) or absent, you should apply gentle inline tension to the fractured bone then check again. Grip the limb near the joints and gently stretch it out. After splinting, re-check distal functions to ensure that the splint is not impairing circulation or nerve function.

Signs of a fracture

- **Angulation**: A fractured limb may be bent at the break, making an angle.
- If the broken bone ends are shifted sideways, you may see a **step deformity**.
- If the muscles spasm, they may move the broken bone ends like an extra joint (**false motion**).

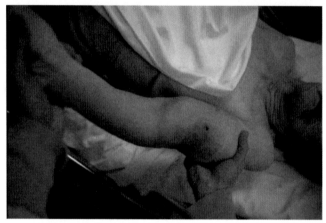

Angulated open humerus fracture.
Photo courtesy of Ben Schifrin, MD

Rotation

- In a hip fracture, the leg and foot are usually rotated outward. A spiral fracture of the lower leg from a twisting fall could also rotate the foot.

Shortened limb

- The bone may be impacted, which means driven into itself or its socket by an impact on the extended limb.
- In a femur fracture, spasming muscles can also shorten the limb by driving broken bone ends past each other into the soft tissues.

Other signs

- You may see tenting – a broken bone end pushing up under the skin – or blood under the skin.

As you feel a limb, you are checking for point tenderness as well as deformity, so you need to grip with both hands and feel every inch.

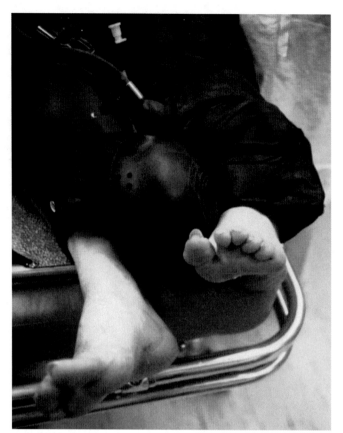

Femur fracture shortened leg. *Photo: Ben Schifrin, MD*

Keep one eye on the patient's face and back off if you get an "Ouch!" Otherwise, you should grip firmly enough to feel the bone. Some bones, such as the femur, are sheathed in thick layers of muscle, but other bones are more accessible. For example, you can feel most of the humerus on the outside of the upper arm and the tibia (shinbone) on the front of the lower leg.

When checking a fracture in the upper arm (humerus), have the patient make a fist and then extend the fingers of the injured arm. If the patient can do this, then the **radial nerve**, which wraps around the humerus, is intact. Touching the tip of the thumb to the base of the little finger tests the **median nerve**. And spreading the fingers into a fan tests the **ulnar nerve**. Given this information, an orthopedist may not need to operate to repair a nerve, even if the patient develops wrist drop later because swelling is compressing the radial nerve.

Open and closed fractures

Any fracture that has a deep open wound near it has an open pathway for infection all the way to the bone marrow, even if the bone is not sticking out. So the first problem is to treat the wound. If the bleeding is serious, you may not be able to put much direct pressure on it, so you might need to use a tourniquet. If bleeding is not a problem, then you need to irrigate and protect the wound first, then position the splint so it does not put pressure on the wound. A **closed fracture** is still enclosed by the skin and underlying tissues.

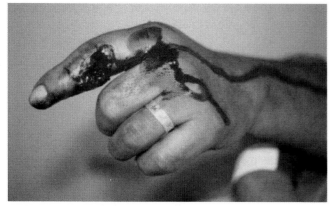

Open finger fracture. *Photo: Ben Schifrin, MD*

Principles of splinting

Not only does a fracture bleed and hurt; the broken bone ends can cause further damage to the soft tissues around them as the limb moves or the muscles spasm. To prevent this damage, you need to immobilize the broken bone ends. Since muscle attachments go across joints, you also need to immobilize the joints adjacent to a fracture. Otherwise the muscles contracting to move those joints would put leverage on the broken bone ends. After splinting a fractured limb, you should elevate it if possible to reduce swelling.

A splint is anything that immobilizes the injured bone and adjacent joints. Narrow boards or stiff cardboard are the traditional splints for urban first aid, though a magazine wrapped around the limb or anything else that gives support can do the job. In the wilderness, if you are not carrying a ready-made splint, you can improvise with a stick, tent pole, ice ax, metal stave from an internal frame pack, foam pad, or any other materials at hand.

If you use something hard as a splint, it is important to pad it, for several reasons:

- To fill any empty space between the splint and the limb, e.g. at the wrist, providing firm and even support along the whole length of the limb;

- To prevent pressure damage to the skin and to nerves that pass over bone close to the skin;
- To insulate a metal splint, especially in cold weather.

Think about which bones you are trying to immobilize and where they lie when you are positioning the splint. For example, to splint the forearm a flat splint should usually be on the palm side, so that it will be closest to both bones and can support the hand in a relaxed position. To secure a splint to the limb, you can use cravat bandages, cloth ties, gauze roller bandages, surgical wrap, tape, or anything else that is wide enough to distribute the pressure over the limb, and not cut off circulation.

You can wrap a stretchy bandage the whole length of the splint, adjusting the tension for the patient's comfort; but if the ties are non-stretchy, you should avoid putting them over the break. Think about where you put the ties. To immobilize a broken bone end, a non-stretchy tie should ideally be a few inches from the break – far enough away so that it does not press on the break, but close enough to apply maximum leverage and immobilize the bone end. Put the knots on the outside of the splint, where you can reach them – with a board or other rigid splint, they should be just between the edge of the splint and the limb, so they do not dig into the flesh.

For a forearm splint, the hand should be in the **position of function** - the relaxed position that equalizes muscle tension on both sides. If you hold your forearm up vertically and relax the hand, you will see that the wrist is slightly extended (bent back) and the fingers half curled. To keep the hand in this position when the arm is splinted, you can place a roller or a wad of padding under the palm, or let the fingers curl around the end of the splint. In a leg splint, the knee should be slightly flexed, not hyperextended.

Handling a fractured limb

Before you start to splint, organize and lay out your equipment, so that once you begin you can continue without interruption until the limb is secured. If you are using cravats or cloth ties, you can drape them around your neck to keep them clean and in reach. An assistant or the patient can stabilize the injured limb or hold the splint in place as you are securing it to avoid jiggling. If you are splinting a leg, however, and the patient is on the ground, you can usually get ties into place without moving the limb - just slide them under the spaces behind the knee or ankle and into place.

If you do need to move a fractured limb to get the ties or splint in place, you should support it so that you will not put a bending stress on the fracture. If the patient has long pants or sleeves, have your partner gather up the slack of the cloth in both hands, on either side of the fracture, so that the clothing is snugly wrapping the limb, and then lift. If you are working alone, slide a stick or pole inside the pant leg and then grip the cloth around the stick to lift the leg.

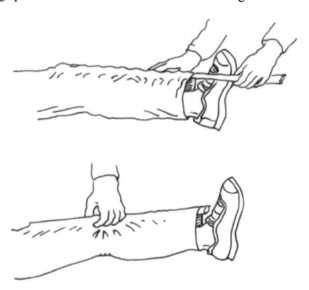

Another way is to grip the limb near the joints and apply gentle inline tension (pulling apart) to prevent the break from sagging as you lift.

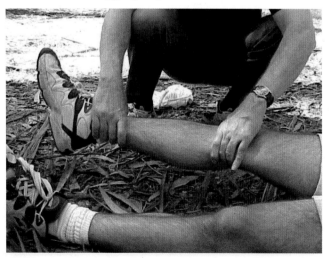

Using gentle inline tension to lift a fractured leg
Photo courtesy of Ruth McConnell

But you should never just pick up an unsplinted, fractured limb by one or even both ends, because the fracture could sag, causing pain and possible further damage. While you lift the limb, your partner can put the splint in position.

If the fracture is angulated, you should align it for splinting by applying gentle inline tension, especially if the angulation is interfering with circulation or nerve function to the limb.

Types of ready-made splints

Large groups that do not have to carry everything on their backs may carry **air splints**: double-walled sleeves of transparent plastic that fit over the injured limb and inflate until they apply enough pressure to immobilize the limb without stopping circulation.

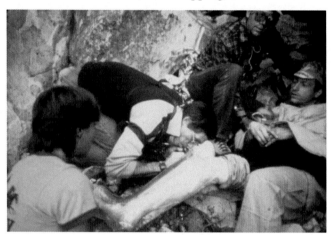

Air splint. *Photo courtesy of Ben Schifrin, MD*

Their advantages are that they can be applied quickly, need no fastening, reduce swelling by putting pressure on the entire limb, and are transparent, so that you can check the appearance of the limb. Their disadvantages are that they are relatively heavy and expensive, they can leak, they trap perspiration and stick to the skin, and if you are gaining or losing altitude, you need to adjust the pressure.

SAM splints (www.sammedical.com), developed by Dr. Sam Scheinberg, are much lighter and more versatile alternatives and are carried by many ski patrollers and wilderness rescuers. They are made from a thin sheet of aluminum padded with foam on both sides, 4" by 36," can be folded up or rolled for carrying and weigh just 4 oz. They are also radio-lucent, so they don't have to be removed for x-rays. You bend the splint into a half-cylinder to give it strength, then mold it to the uninjured limb to get an exact fit before applying it to the injured arm or leg. You can fold it into a sugar tong so that it wraps both sides of a limb, as shown in the two photos below.

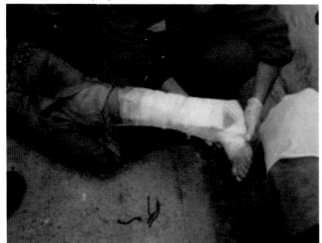

SAM splint applied to a lower leg fracture

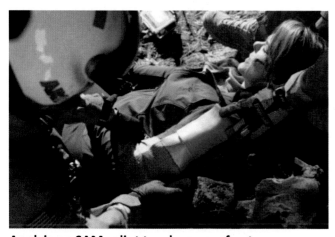

Applying a SAM splint to a humerus fracture.

Another option for a forearm or wrist fracture is to fold the SAM splint double and fit it under the palm side of the forearm, with padding under the palm to keep the hand in the relaxed position of function. You can combine two SAM splints to make an extra-long sugar tong splint for the leg. You can also shape the SAM splint into a rigid triangle to support a locked knee or a dislocated shoulder that is locked in an awkward position. SAM splints have illustrated directions printed on them, and instructional videos can be downloaded from their web site.

Soft splints for leg and ankle

For a fractured lower leg or ankle, a foam sleeping pad makes an excellent splint. Lift the leg, using one of the techniques already described, and slide the foam pad underneath so about half of the length is on either side of the leg. Then roll up the pad on either side until the two rolls are snug against the leg. If you are working alone, kneel below the patient's feet and clamp the two rolls against the leg with your knees. Slide two or three cravats or other ties into position under the pad and fasten them with the knots in accessible positions.

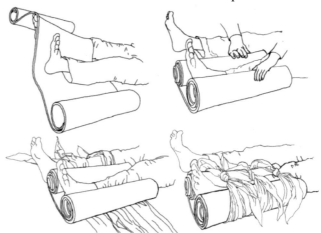

A blanket or bulky garment can make a good splint for an injured ankle. In cold weather, you could leave the boot or shoe on for warmth and additional support, but loosen the laces and check regularly to make sure that swelling is not impairing circulation or nerve function.

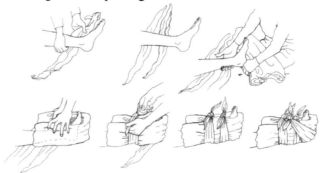

Fold the blanket or jacket into a rectangle about 1' x 3'. If the patient is sitting or lying on the ground, slide two cravat bandages under the ankle, slipping them through the space behind the Achilles tendon. Then fold the blanket around the bottom of the foot so that it wraps the ankle and lower leg on both sides. Now slide one cravat up almost to the upper edges of the blanket and tie it, pulling it as tight as is comfortable for the patient. Tie the second cravat around the ankle.

Spread out the third cravat so that it cups the bottom corner of the blanket, bring it diagonally to the instep and tighten it as much as the patient will tolerate. This tie really snugs up the splint. If you are using a rolled up jacket instead of a blanket, and it does not give enough support, add a figure 8 bandage: loop the center of a cravat around the ball of the foot, cross the tails, pass them around the splint and under the ankle, bring them back up and tie them.

The swivel hitch

If you are improvising a splint with sticks or poles, the swivel hitch is a helpful technique. If you just wrap ties around both the stick and the much thicker limb, the stick can slide around within the wrap. If a fractured leg is already on the ground in a good position, you can usually apply a splint without moving the leg.

Start by sliding the ties in place under the leg. For a supine patient, use the spaces behind the knee and Achilles tendon, then slide the ties into position. Leave about 2/3 of each tie on the outside. You can use a single stick or pole (on the outside), or one on each side. Then slide the stick(s) or pole(s) under the ties, next to the leg, and wrap each tie around the stick(s). Put padding in place, e.g., a spare jacket draped over the leg so that it will hang down between the leg and the stick(s). Then bring both ties across the leg, bring the outer tie under and around splint and leg again, tighten as snugly as is comfortable for the patient, and tie the ends together on the outside just above the stick.

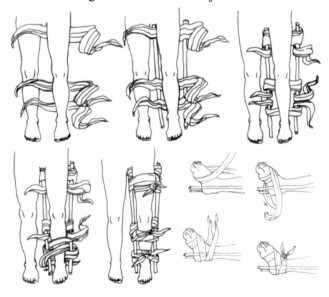

The stick(s) can rolled up or down to align with the central axis of the bone. A figure 8 bandage around the foot (lower right) stabilizes the ankle

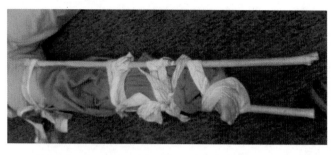

Sticks secured with the swivel hitch can also be swiveled to any angle with the limb - essential if you are splinting a joint injury that locks the limb in a bent position. By securing one or two sticks to the proximal and distal ends of the limb with a swivel hitch, you will complete the third side of the triangle and immobilize the injured joint. Secure the ends of the sticks to the leg near the ankle and the hip with the same technique shown in the previous splint. Lay a wide cravat across the sticks, secure it as shown in the following drawing, and fill the space between the cravat and the back of the knee with padding.

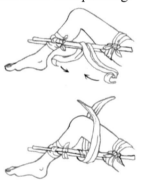
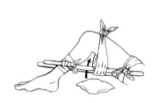

If the patient is on a stretcher or litter, another way to stabilize a locked knee is to lay a rolled blanket or bulky jacket over the good knee, pick up the injured leg (maintaining the angle of the knee) and cross the ankle over the ankle of the uninjured leg, so that the injured knee is supported by the rolled blanket. Then lash the ankles together with a cravat. This splint will stabilize an injured knee while the patient is being evacuated on the stretcher or improvised litter.

An ice ax also makes a good lower leg splint. Put padding (if available) between the shaft and the leg. Immobilize the ankle with a figure 8 bandage - One loop of the figure 8 secures the toe of the boot to the pick of the ax; the other loop wraps the splinted ankle.

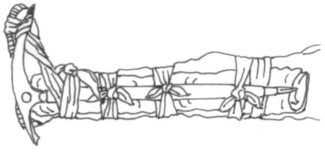

Ice ax splint for lower leg

Fractured clavicle

If a clavicle (collarbone) is fractured, a figure 8 bandage that holds the shoulders back in the military at attention position will help stabilize it. Wrap a cravat or piece of webbing around the injured shoulder, cross it in an X on the back, then wrap it around the other shoulder and tie it. A pack with the shoulder straps cinched tight can also serve as a figure 8 bandage. Use padding under the bandage if it presses uncomfortably on the injured side. While a sling is more comfortable, and is preferred by most orthopedists for stabilizing the clavicle as it gradually heals, in a wilderness accident the figure 8 bandage has the advantage that it enables the patient to use both hands while hiking, bicycling, or skiing out of the wilderness.

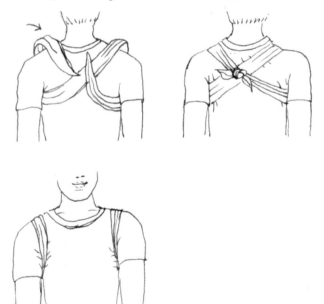

Arm splints

To splint a fractured forearm, you can use a padded stick or pole on the palm side, so that the relaxed fingers either curl around the end or are supported by padding between the palm and the stick. With either technique, you need to immobilize the wrist by wrapping the hand up to the first knuckles. A padded stick or pole can also be used to splint a fractured humerus, by placing it on the outside of the upper arm, where it will be close to the bone.

A SAM splint can immobilize an arm fracture more comfortably and securely. First bend it into a half cylinder, then use the uninjured arm to mold it into shape, so that it fits when you apply it to the injured forearm or upper arm.

For a forearm or wrist fracture, measure the splint on the uninjured arm (flexed at least 90° with the palm parallel to the chest) by wrapping it around the elbow so the splint encloses the forearm on two sides. If there is enough extra splint on the palm side, roll it up under the palm to hold the hand in the relaxed position of function. If the other side of the splint is long enough, it can go past the wrist to immobilize that joint; if not, immobilize the wrist by wrapping the hand.

If a sugar tong splint presses uncomfortably on the fracture, you can fold the SAM splint double, and place it on the palm side only of the forearm. Secure the splint with cravats, bandanas, coban (a self-adhering bandage), or a gauze roller bandage. A gauze roller bandage is usually the most comfortable way to secure a SAM splint, and the gauze can stretch to accommodate swelling. Do NOT, however, use tape to secure a SAM splint, because when you remove it, the tape will shred the foam padding of the splint.

To splint a fractured humerus with a SAM splint, one technique is to fold about a foot of the splint double, and bend the doubled part into a horse shoe to go around the elbow, so that it will extend about half-way up the inside of the upper arm. Leave a little space under the elbow, however, so the splint doesn't press broken bone ends together.

Check distal circulation, sensation, movement and strength before and after splinting and compare them to the uninjured arm. Also do three additional tests that check the function of three nerves: ulnar, median, and radial. **Ulnar**: make a fan with the fingers; **median**: touch the tip of the thumb to the base of the little finger; **radial**: extend the fingers and hand. If the patient already is showing wrist drop (cannot extend the wrist at all) then radial nerve function is impaired.

Since the radial nerve wraps around the humerus before continuing down the arm, it is most likely to be injured in a humerus fracture. By the time the patient gets to the hospital, distal nerve functions may be impaired by swelling. But if you documented that these functions were unimpaired before and after splinting, then the patient will probably not need surgery to repair the nerves.

Slings

An injured arm, even after being splinted, needs to be supported by a sling, which you can improvise by pulling the bottom of patient's shirt or jacket up around the arm and safety pinning it to itself. A triangular bandage, however, makes a much more versatile sling. Twist the point of the bandage into a rat's tail and tie an overhand knot in it (or use a safety pin) to create a cup for the elbow. Then ease the triangular bandage between the splinted arm and the patient's chest so that the upper tail goes over the good shoulder, with the knot toward the elbow of the injured arm, and the lower tail hangs down the chest inside the injured arm. Bring up the lower tail to wrap and support the forearm. You have three choices of where to go with that tail before tying it to the other tail:

- Bring it around the other side of the neck (American style).
- Bring it around the outside of the injured arm (French style) so it cradles the arm.
- Bring it under and through the armpit of the injured arm (British style).

Both the French and British style slings take pressure off the neck and make it easier to get good wrist elevation, which is important for reducing swelling before the arm is put in a cast. Generally, the French style is best for a lower arm fracture. The British style is useful for an upper arm fracture, because it does not put any pressure on the injury.

After tying the sling, secure the arm to the body with a swathe – another triangular bandage (with the cup fitted over the shoulder) or a wide strip of cloth wrapped around the arm and the chest, to prevent the injured arm from flapping as the patient walks or is transported. Spread out the cloth over the arm to distribute the pressure and tie the tails together behind the patient's body.

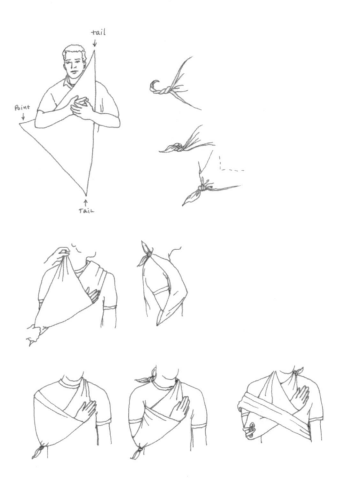

Finger splints

A broken finger can be splinted to one or two adjacent fingers, using athletic tape or a narrow gauze roller to secure it. If possible, keep the finger in the relaxed and slightly flexed position of function. Straight splints such as tongue depressors are less comfortable but can be used for up to 48 hours.

Soft splint of the hand

If several fingers or hand bones are broken, you can stabilize the whole hand in the position of function, with the tip of the thumb near the tip of the forefinger, by filling the hollow of the palm with padding or rolled up bandages, then wrapping the whole hand with a stretchy gauze roller or surgical wrap. Anchor the bandage at the wrist, then wrap diagonally over the back and palm sides of the hand to the wrist, gently holding the fingers curled around the padding in the palm. Then wrap diagonally around the palm side and back of the hand to the wrist to secure the remaining fingers, and tie or tape the bandage at the wrist. A sling will support the stabilized hand in comfort.

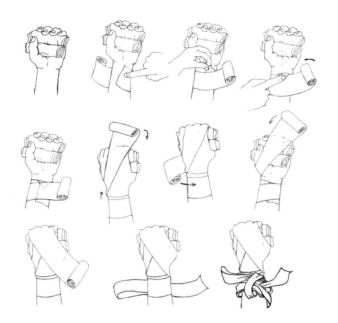

Traction splinting

When a bone is fractured, the muscles around it tend to spasm in reaction to the pain. By tensing around the broken bone, the muscles act like a self-splint. When the femur is fractured, however, the reaction can cause serious damage, because the muscles around the bone of the upper leg are the biggest and strongest in the body. They can drive the broken bone ends into the soft tissues, like spears, cutting blood vessels as well as causing pain. In a closed fracture of the femur, the victim can bleed over two liters of blood internally, which is enough to cause **shock**.

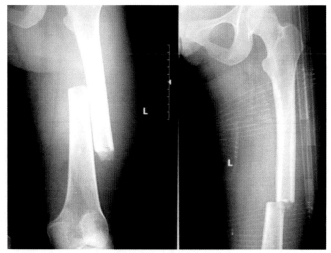

Femur fracture before & after traction splinting.
Photo courtesy of FareTec Inc.

To immobilize a fractured femur and prevent shock, a splint needs to pull **traction** on the leg as well as stabilizing it. Stretching out the leg muscles with traction will also help control bleeding by **tamponading** (compressing) the arteries. While some commercial devices come with tension gauges and recommend traction equal to 10-15% of the patient's body weight, the real measure of adequate traction is **pain control**. When the patient stops screaming and says "Ahh! That feels much better," you know that the traction is adequate.

If it will take more than a minute or so to prepare and apply the splint, or if the splint is the type that fits under the leg, then one rescuer may apply manual traction and elevate the leg. This requires the rescuer to maintain manual traction until it is replaced with mechanical traction and to make a smooth transition without ever letting go. So it is helpful to apply the ankle hitch first – otherwise it is very awkward to work around the first rescuer's hands.

Trained rescuers using commercial splints that fit on one side of the leg (rather than underneath) may omit this step, because they can usually apply mechanical traction within a minute once they have access to the patient. Also, they don't need to elevate the leg to get the splint in position.

Several different types of commercial traction splints are available, and there are several ways to improvise one; but they all work on the same principles. You need:

- A hitch around the ankle to pull traction.
- An anchor at the hip or against the pelvis to hold the other end of the splint.
- Something long and rigid to connect the anchors.
- Something to pull traction on the ankle hitch.

About 84% of all femur fractures are to the proximal third of the bone, but most of these are **hip fractures** in the elderly. In relatively young and athletic people, mid-shaft femur fractures (to the middle third of the bone) are more common.

EMT textbooks recommend traction splints only for mid-shaft femur fractures. This recommendation dates from the years when the only available traction splints (the Thomas and the Hare) had a padded half-ring or curved bar that fit under the crease of the buttock (**ischial pad**). This pad can push the proximal bone segment in a femur fracture upward, causing more damage and pain – especially in a proximal femur fracture, where that bone segment is short. Other traction splints, such as the Sager, do not have an ischial pad, and their developers claim that they work for proximal as well as mid-shaft femur fractures.

Sager does, however, caution against using their splint for a distal femur fracture (near the knee), because of the possibility that the bone could damage the popliteal artery or nerve, if traction caused the bone to rotate. In a wilderness accident, you may not be able to tell where a femur is fractured. But if the application of traction causes (rather than relieves) pain, then you will know that it is not the appropriate treatment, and apply a fixation splint.

Traction splints

The first portable traction splint was designed by a Welsh orthopedic surgeon, **Hugh Owen Thomas**, in 1875. He offered it to the French army during the Franco Prussian War, but they did not adopt it, and it remained almost unknown outside his own practice until World War I. In 1915, Sir Robert Jones (nephew and onetime apprentice of Dr.Thomas) introduced the device to the British and French armies. He called it the **Thomas leg splint**, and by 1918 it had reduced mortality in military femur fractures from 80% to 20% by stretching out the thigh muscles, which tamponaded the blood vessels in the thigh and controlled bleeding. The Thomas splint originally had a full ring that fit around the thigh. Sir Robert Jones made the splint easier to apply with a padded half-ring that fits under the upper leg, right at the crease of the buttocks, and is secured with a strap going over the top of the leg at the groin. A steel rod connected to both ends of the half-ring fits on either side of the leg and forms a notched anchor for the pulley beyond the foot.

In the late 1960's, Glenn Hare developed a nylon ankle harness and ratchet attachment for the Thomas half-ring. The **Hare traction splint** evolved from this hybrid, and retains the same design; but it now has an extendable foot section, a built-in ratchet and cable for applying traction, a flip-down stand at the foot end for elevation, and wide elastic Velcro bands for cradling the leg. The disadvantages of the Hare are that the patient must be supine and it takes two people to apply it properly – one to lift the leg with manual traction while the other positions the splint under the leg.

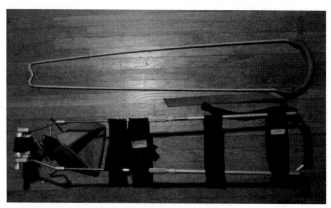

Thomas half ring with the Hare traction splint that evolved from it

In 1972, Joseph Sager and Dr. Anthony Borschneck developed another traction splint, which they patented and began marketing in the 1980's. The **Sager ® splint** (www.sagersplints.com) has a different and more compact design. It looks like a short crutch, and fits inside the leg with the foam-padded cross piece pressing against the **ischial tuberosity** (a bulge on each side of the bone forming the floor of the abdominal cavity). It also has an extendable section at the foot with a hook and cable to pull traction on the ankle hitch; a built-in tension gauge; and wide elastic bands to wrap and support the leg.

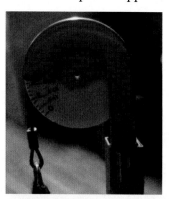

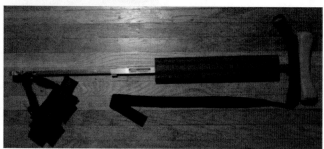

Sager® splints are widely used by ski patrollers at downhill resorts because they are compact and quick to apply. A single person can apply a Sager splint to a patient in almost any position. Sager splints also fit more easily than Hare splints into a helicopter.

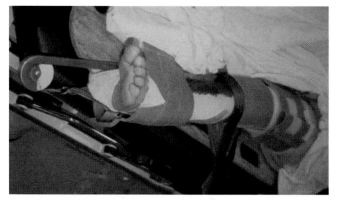

Sager splint for open femur and lower leg fractures
Photo courtesy of Ben Schifrin, MD

In 1986, Richard Kendrick introduced another design for applying traction to the femur, the **Kendrick Traction Device** (KTD), which is much lighter and more compact than the Sager or Hare. It looks like a tent pole with shock-corded sections. Like the Sager, the KTD can be fitted without lifting the leg, but the splint goes on the outer side of the injured leg. (www.medixchhoice.com)

You can adjust the length of the KTD by folding one or more sections at the hip end, which fit into a socket on the hip anchor strap. At the foot end, a nylon strap fits over a projection at the end of the pole to pull traction on the ankle hitch. First, however, an elastic band is wrapped around the knee to prevent too much bending stress on the slender aluminum pole. Then (after applying traction) the other elastic bands are wrapped around the leg. This traction splint is carried by many Nordic ski patrollers and wilderness rescuers, because it weighs only 20 ounces and fits into a zipper pouch that easily goes into a daypack.

The **CT-EMS traction splint** (www.faretec.com) is similar to the KTD, but the segmented pole is carbon fiber rather than aluminum, and it has a pulley system that gives it a 4:1 mechanical advantage, making it easier to apply traction. Traction is applied by pulling a cord that runs through the pulley. The model for EMS has bright orange elastic bands; whereas the version sold to the military (CT-6) is all black. As with the KTD, you must secure the center elastic band over the knee before applying traction; then wrap the other bands around the thigh and lower leg.

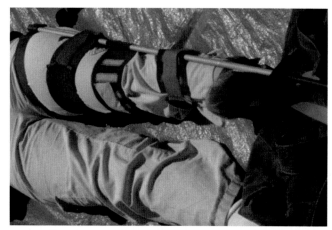

KTD splint in use. *Photo courtesy of Lynn Garcia*

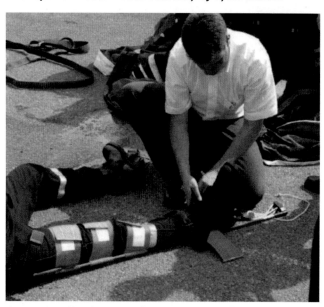

CT-EMS splint in use. *Photo courtesy of FareTec Inc.*

Although EMT textbooks warn against putting the elastic thigh band of any traction splint directly over the fracture, your guide to its placement (without an x-ray to locate the fracture) will be patient comfort.

In splints that use a groin strap to apply counter-traction, the strap may press on the femoral artery and the sciatic nerve, or cause some misalignment in a proximal femur fracture (especially if too much traction is applied). Although there do not seem to be any reports of this problem actually occurring, some padding under the strap (especially above the groin where it crosses the femoral artery) may be helpful.

A splint like the KTD and CT-EMS can be improvised with a long pole, cravats or webbing, and some cord, as shown on the next page.

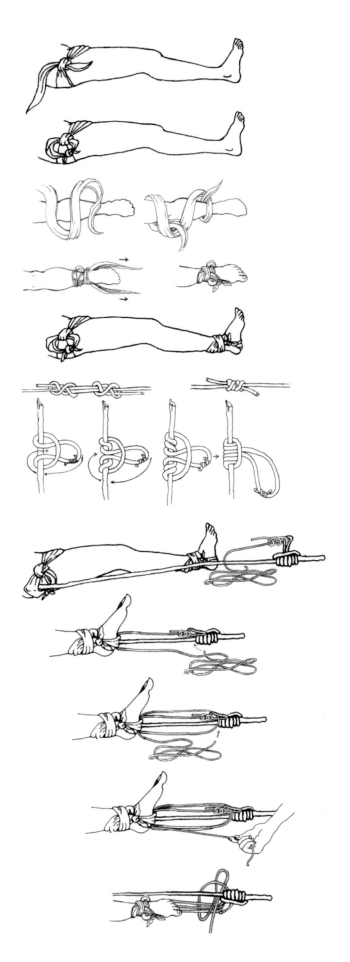

To improvise a splint with one long pole, secure a cravat around the leg at the hip, and either make a loop with the tails to socket the proximal end of the pole, or lash a deep cup with a closed handle to the hip strap as the pole socket. Use a cravat or length of webbing for an ankle hitch. A prusik loop on one end of the pole anchors the pulley system. Tie one end of an 8 foot cord to the prusik loop; pass it through the bottom of the ankle hitch and the prusik loop several times to create a pulley system; pull traction; elevate the splint; and wrap several cravats around the splinted leg to stabilize it.

Dr. Sam Slishman improved on the one-pole design with the light weight **Slishman traction splint**.

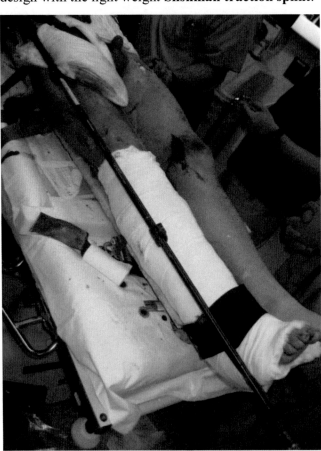

Slishman splint for open femur and lower leg fracture
Photo courtesy of Ben Schifrin, MD

It is a modified Black Diamond adjustable ski pole, but with a pulley mechanism inside the pole for applying traction. (www.geocities.com/slishmansplint/). Like the KTD and CT-EMS, the Slishman splint connects to a groin strap and ankle hitch, which can be improvised or purchased with the splint. But since the modified ski pole is the splint, there is no extra hardware to carry.

Two long paddles (as shown in the photo below) combine features of the Sager and the Thomas half ring – though the blade of the paddle between the legs would have to be well padded.

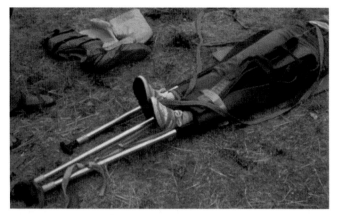

Photo courtesy of Ben Schifrin, MD

You can **improvise a Thomas half-ring** from two cross-country or adjustable-length ski poles.

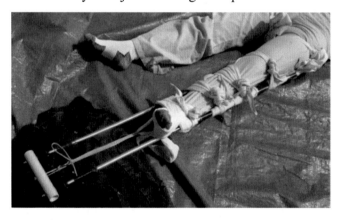

On a winter ski ascent of Mt. Rainier, one skier slid down the icy slope hundreds of yards, fracturing her femur. A former student of the author improvised a traction splint with the patient's ski poles. When a helicopter evacuated the patient, the crew left the improvised splint in place, because it was just as effective as the traction splint they carried.

As shown in the drawings on the next page, interlock the wrist straps of the ski poles by passing each pole tip through the strap of the other pole and sliding the poles past each other until the straps are connected. They will go under the crease of the buttocks, like the half-ring of the Thomas splint. Tie a cravat bandage to the inside ski pole handle to complete the circle and anchor the splint at the hip, as the strap on the Thomas splint does. Secure the cravat to the outside pole handle after the splint is in place.

You can use a cravat bandage or a piece of webbing as an ankle hitch:
- Lay it on the shin in the form of a capital S.
- Bring the tails around the leg and through the opposing loops.
- Slide the tails down to the ankle and adjust them so they are in line with the central axis of the leg.
- Tie them under the bottom of the foot, off-setting the knot so that it won't get in the way.

Connect the two pole tips (which should extend about 12" beyond the foot) with a cross bar. Lash or tape a short stick across the pole tips, or use a ready-made cross-bar – an 8" piece of 1" PVC pipe (shown in the drawing) or 1" aluminum tubing with 2 ½" holes drilled near the ends to socket the pole tips.

Secure an 8-foot length of 1/8" nylon cord through a small hole in the center of the bar - you can also tie in a small metal ring to the cross bar. To pull traction, run the cord back and forth through the ankle hitch and the ring (or around the cross bar) a few times to give a mechanical advantage. Pull it tight until the patient says "Ahh!" then tie it off.

After applying traction, elevate the end of the splint and use cradle hitches (cravat bandages or webbing) to cradle the leg and position it with the knee slightly flexed. Start with the cradle hitch nearest the hip and work down the leg.

To apply a cradle hitch:
- Pass a cravat bandage under the leg and bring the tails up inside the two ski poles.
- Bring both tails down around the poles and under the leg, pulling the tails until the leg is positioned where you want it.
- Then bring the inside tail over the top of the leg and tie it to the other tail above the outside pole.

Conclusion

Assessing bone injuries and aligning them if necessary to improve distal functions or splint effectively are important skills for wilderness emergency care. You should also know how to improvise splints with whatever would be available to you in a wilderness or remote situation, as well as how to use any commercial splints that you carry.

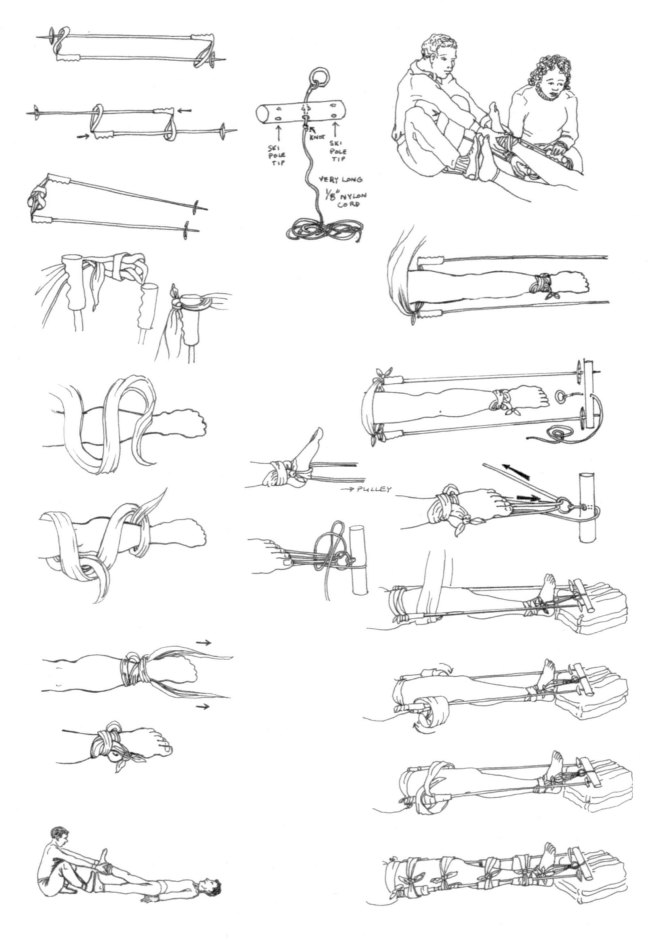

SKI POLE TIP

KNOT

SKI POLE TIP

VERY LONG ⅛" NYLON CORD

→ PULLEY

Chapter 8. Athletic injuries

Photos and x-rays of dislocations courtesy of Ben Schifrin, MD

In a wilderness activity where participants need the full use of their bodies, ligament tears (sprains) or muscle tears (strains) can be disabling. At best, they will interrupt the trip. At worst, they can turn the trip into a survival situation. By knowing how to assess athletic injuries in the field, you can make an informed decision about what to do. Can the patient safely continue after a rest or at a reduced level of activity? Is an evacuation necessary? Will the patient need medical treatment to avoid possible loss of function? If the patient has to walk on an injured joint to get out of a hazardous situation, then you need to know how to support and stabilize the joint (e.g., by taping it).

Assessment of ligament damage is easiest shortly after the injury occurs. As the joint begins to swell, it becomes much more difficult to assess function and integrity. If you reduce the swelling in an injured joint, that will help ease the pain, prevent secondary damage, and speed healing. Putting a dislocation back in joint when you are far from help may save a limb and greatly reduce the difficulties of an evacuation. You should also know how to prevent and rehabilitate athletic injuries in yourself.

Joints and injuries

Joints are joinings of bones, held together by **cartilage** (Latin *cartilago* "gristle"). This cartilage usually forms cables and bands called **ligaments** (from Latin *ligare*, "to bind or tie"). Joints may be immovable, such as the sutures between the cranial bones; slightly movable, such as the joints connecting the vertebrae of the spine; or freely movable, such as the shoulder or knee. Freely movable joints are the most vulnerable to damage. If they are forced beyond their normal range of motion, most of the stress will go onto the connecting ligaments, which will tear. This is a **sprain**. Your first goal with a sprain is to reduce swelling and pain and prevent further damage.

If the knobby end of a bone is forced out of its socket or hinge completely, it is dislocated. You can distinguish a **dislocation** from a fracture because a dislocated joint will have little or no range of motion. Also, the knob of the dislocated bone will usually be an obvious lump. With a dislocation you have two choices: to **stabilize** it in position; or **reduce** it - try to put it back in joint. But if the dislocation is interfering with circulation or nerve function, or causing severe pain, it is urgent to reduce it; and the sooner you reduce a dislocation after the injury, the better your chance of success. When the joint starts swelling and hurting, the muscles can tense in a guarding reaction and lock the bone into its false position.

In urban emergency care, reducing dislocations is a medical procedure done only by physicians. However, wilderness medical experts have been teaching the techniques to lay people for decades, and many people have reduced dislocations successfully in wilderness emergencies. So if you have to deal with a dislocation in the wilderness, you may decide to reduce it, especially if the alternative is that the patient cannot be evacuated or may lose a limb.

Overall, the ankle is the joint most often injured, but in some sports other joints are more at risk. In downhill skiing, for example, the ankle is usually protected by high, rigid boots, so in an accident more bending and twisting force can be transmitted to the knee. In cross-country skiing, less supportive boots make the ankle more vulnerable to injury.

In snowboarding, the knees and ankles are less vulnerable than in skiing because both feet are locked to the same board, so that any bending or twisting stress is distributed over both legs. Snowboarders, however, are more likely to injure their arms when they fall headlong and try to break their falls. In kayaking, the stress of moving or bracing the paddle against the resistance of water is largely transmitted to the shoulder, especially if the paddler holds the bracing arm high. So shoulder injuries are common.

Reconstructing the movements and stresses that caused the injury can give clues to the damage. Athletes are used to analyzing their movements and the effects of stress on their bodies, so they can often describe what happened quite accurately. This information, and the athlete's knowledge of the sport, can help you to assess joint and muscle injuries.

Lubrication and movement

Bone ends and sockets in joints are covered with hyaline cartilage (from the Greek *hyalos* "transparent stone") to reduce friction. Freely moving joints are also called synovial joints, because they are lubricated with **synovial fluid**, so called by Paracelsus because it resembles raw egg white (Greek *syn* "with", *ōon* "egg"). This clear and slippery fluid is secreted by membranes that line joint capsules and tendon sheathes and replenished by the lymph system. It is stored in **bursae** (Latin "sacks" from Greek *bursa* "hide or wineskin"), near the joints.

In a sprain, swelling inside the joint capsule, from accumulating synovial fluid, causes pain. There can also be swelling in the soft tissues around the joint from fluid accumulation. Sometimes a severe sprain will cause **hemarthrosis** - bleeding into the joint (Greek *haima* "blood", *arthros* "joint"). Typically, there will be less swelling but more pain, and the joint will feel warmer than the skin around it. Bleeding in the joint is usually more serious than the puffy swelling caused by synovial fluid, because blood destroys the hyaline cartilage. Once that cartilage is gone, the joint can stiffen and become painful with use.

Some synovial joints move in one plane of motion, like hinges. They are held tightly together by ligaments. Examples of hinge joints are the main joints of the knee (connecting tibia and femur) and elbow (connecting ulna and humerus). Other joints, such as the hip and the main joint of the shoulder, are like a ball and socket. They allow the bone to move in any plane of motion, rotate, and circumduct (spin like a propeller).

The shoulder

The bone of the upper arm, the **humerus** (Latin *ossa umeri* "bones of the shoulder") is held loosely in the shallow socket of the shoulder blade, the scapula, by cartilage. But the four short rotator cuff muscles wrap around the joint and help stabilize it. The **scapula** is attached to the torso only by muscles, so it can move with the arm to give you more range of motion. You can feel the scapula move (with your other hand) as you raise your arm overhead.

The third bone of the shoulder joint, the collarbone or **clavicle** (Latin *clavicula* "tendril" – so called because it is long and narrow), is attached by ligaments to the top of the scapula just above the socket and to the sternum at the other end. When the upper arm is moved in its socket, all of these joints come into play.

Injury to any of the connecting ligaments or muscles of the three shoulder joints can restrict or weaken shoulder movement and cause pain. For example, if any of the ligaments connecting the clavicle with the top of the scapula are torn (**shoulder separation**), it will be difficult or impossible to raise the arm. A patient who does raise the arm will also raise the shoulder. In response to finger pressure, the patient will feel point tenderness where the clavicle attaches to the scapula, and the weight of the arm will pull on the torn ligaments.

Immediate treatment is to support the arm in a sling, then apply ice packs to reduce swelling and pain, as with any sprain. Shoulder separations are most often caused by falling onto the shoulder, though a radiating injury from a fall onto the elbow or outstretched hand is also possible.

Rotator cuff muscles can be torn by activities that put great stress on the shoulders. A serious tear can make the shoulder unstable, as well as causing pain. An athlete will often work through the pain of a minor tear, but compensate with an unbalanced motion that puts more stress on other parts of the shoulder. Inflammation, tendonitis, and further injury may result.

In the back country, activities that require strong, repeated movements of the shoulder, such as paddling, technical climbing and cross-country skiing, can injure the rotator cuff muscles or aggravate the tendons that attach the muscles to bone. The deep, aching pain of rotator cuff tendonitis (which may radiate to the outside of the upper arm) can make it impossible for the patient to continue. A medication such as aspirin may bring some temporary relief from pain and reduce the inflammation, but the patient must stop the activity that is causing the problem, then start rehabilitation.

Shoulder dislocations

When a shoulder is dislocated, the knob of the humerus usually pops out in the front of the socket (anterior dislocation), so you can see and feel a lump there, and the arm will be locked in place. The arm will often be held up or away from the body in an awkward position. There are several techniques for putting it back in joint, but all of the simple ones work by pulling the arm outward (traction) until it clears the rim of the socket and slips back in. You should slowly and steadily increase the traction rather than jerking.

A patient who is alone can use two techniques for **self-reduction**. For the first technique, raise the leg on the injured side, clasp the hands around the knee, and use the strength of the leg to pull the arms forward. A variation is to wrap the arms around both knees, grip the wrist of the injured arm with the other hand, and spread the legs. If the knob of the humerus is pulled far enough out to clear the rim of the socket, it may slip back in place. These techniques are most likely to work for someone who has suffered chronic shoulder dislocations, because the damage makes the shoulder joint easier to both to dislocate and to relocate.

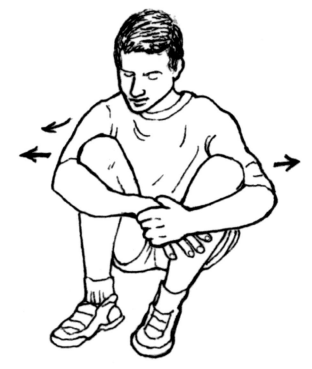

If that doesn't work, the patient can try lying face down on a ledge or large tree trunk with the injured arm dangling and a 15-20 pound weight hanging from the arm. You can strap or tape a day pack to the wrist or elbow and fill it with water bottles or rocks. After 20 minutes or so, the muscles should fatigue enough to pull the knob of the humerus past the rim of the joint and let it slip back in.

If the patient cannot reduce the dislocation with those techniques, an assistant can use either of two other techniques. With the patient sitting or lying face up, pass a loop of cravats or webbing around the patient's flexed arm and your hips. Tie a loop around

the patient's chest for an assistant to pull on from the other side (or secure it to a tree). Hold the wrist with one hand. Then slowly but steadily increase the traction by leaning back until the humerus slips into joint. The other hand can feel the protruding knob of the dislocated bone move back into the socket.

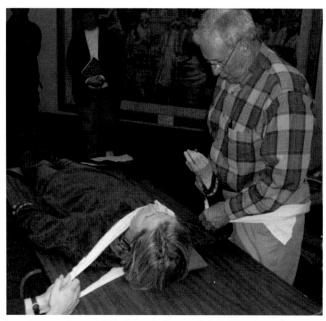

Dr. Serra shows how to reduce a shoulder dislocation. *Photo courtesy of Mark Stinson, MD*

Another way to do the same reduction is to have the patient lie face up with the injured arm outstretched. Sit down where you can grasp the wrist or arm with both hands, plant the ball of your foot (with the shoe off) in the armpit, then apply traction by leaning back.

Elbow injuries

The elbow has two joints: the hinge joint formed by the **ulna** (the bone on the little finger side of the forearm); and the shallow joint formed by the **radius** that enables you to rotate your forearm. You can feel the movement of the radial knob with the fingers of your other hand as you rotate your forearm. Most **elbow dislocations** happen when someone tries to break a fall with an outstretched arm. Another possible mechanism is a forceful pull, for example by stopping a fall from a height by grabbing a hold with one hand If only the radial joint is dislocated, the patient may still be able to flex the elbow, but not rotate the forearm. If the elbow bends the wrong way (hyper-extends), then the knobs of the two forearm bones can tear loose from the ligaments holding them. Usually one or both will be displaced, as the photo below shows. The patient will not be able to move the elbow much.

It is not easy to reduce a dislocation of the hinge joint of the elbow, but if circulation or nerve functions to the hand are impaired, you may decide to make the attempt. Flex the elbow to 70° or 80°; then grip the wrist with one hand to pull while you (or an assistant) apply counter traction with the other hand to the upper arm just above the joint.

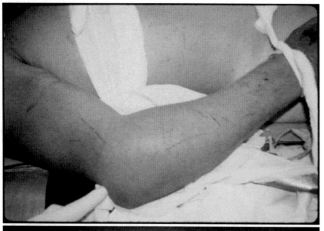

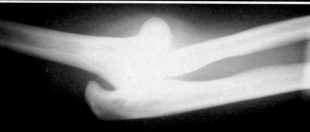

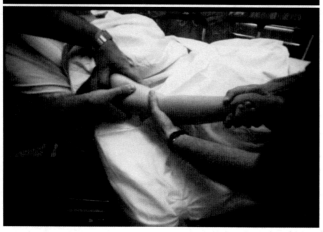

Finger injuries

Sprains of the thumb and fingers are common. In skiing, for example, the second most common joint injury is **skier's thumb**. This is a torn ligament in the thumb joint at the web between thumb and hand. Any

motion that forces the thumb away from the hand can tear the inside ligament. Pushing hard on a ski pole with the thumb looped over the strap or falling on the hand while gripping the pole could cause this injury. The patient will feel tenderness at the torn ligament, and pain when you gently lever the thumb away from the hand with your fingers. A figure-8 wrap of athletic tape, anchored at the wrist, can support the injured thumb joint.

A direct blow to the fingertips can sprain finger joints by either jamming or hyper-extending them. You can immobilize a sprained finger in a slightly flexed position with a flexible splint - a baby SAM splint or a strip of wire mesh wrapped in duct tape. If a finger joint has been dislocated, at least one ligament is probably completely torn. The finger will be crooked and have a bump at the joint. In this case, you can immobilize the entire hand in the position of function (wrist slightly extended, fingers slightly flexed), as well as splinting the injured finger. With a wad of padding in the hollow of the palm, use a gauze roller bandage to wrap the hand in the position of function, as shown in the soft splint for the hand in chapter 7.

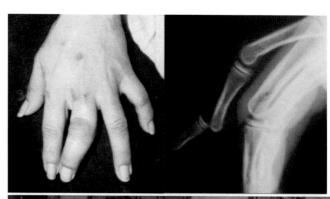

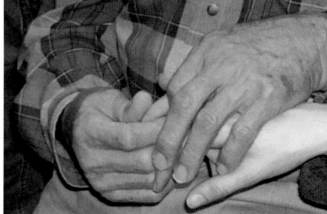

Dr. Serra shows how to reduce a dislocated finger
Photo courtesy of Mark Stinson, MD

72

To put the finger back in joint, flex the finger slightly to relax the tendons; grip it between your two middle fingers; and pull as though you were cracking your knuckles (or the knuckles of your patient). If the finger is slippery from sweat, wrap it in cloth for traction. Gently press the finger back into joint with your thumb as you pull. After putting the finger back in joint, splint it to prevent re-injury, ideally in the relaxed, slightly flexed, position.

The hip

The hip joint, unlike the shoulder, has a deep socket and a strong capsule that thickens into three ligaments. This capsule connects the neck of the femur to the pelvis. Sprains of the hip are rare, because the capsule and joint are so strong. Most athletic injuries around the hip are to muscles or tendons. **Hip pointers**, for example, are tears of the tendons that attach to the bony ridge of the pelvis just below the waist (the iliac crest). These injuries are common in contact sports like football, where a collision can tear some fibers of a tendon loose, but a fall onto the hip can also do it. Pressing on the injury will cause point tenderness, and the patient will feel discomfort when bending away from the injured side. Immediate treatment is to apply ice, just as with a sprain, for two days. But after that, use heat packs, as with a muscle tear, to stimulate circulation. A minor tear of these tendons usually takes two or three weeks to heal.

It takes a lot of force to dislocate the hip. In urban situations, a car collision with the knee hitting the dashboard is the classic mechanism. In the wilderness, a long fall is the most likely mechanism, especially if a climber slams into the rock sideways after being caught by the rope. Usually the femur knob will fracture the rim of the socket as it is pushed out. Evacuation is urgent, because blood supply to the head and neck of the femur is usually reduced or cut off.

A **reduction** takes two people, and (as with other dislocations) should only be considered in a wilderness emergency where help is delayed. With the patient lying face up and the hip and knee flexed 90°, one person holds down the pelvis. The other straddles the patient's lower leg, interlaces his fingers under the calf just distal to the knee, and (with forearms braced on the thighs as a fulcrum) sits down on the lower leg. The

sitting motion provides the leverage to pull the hip back into joint.

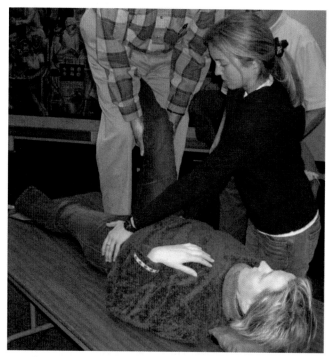

Dr. Serra shows how to reduce a hip dislocation
Photo courtesy of Mark Stinson, MD

The iliotibial band

Athletic people may have problems with a tendon called the iliotibial band (Latin *ilium* "hip", *tibia* "shin bone or flute"). This is a broad band which runs from the iliac crest down the outside of the thigh, past the knee, to the outside knob of the tibia. The main muscle of the buttocks connects with it, and it also serves as a very long tendon for a muscle at the front of the pelvis. Their extended tendon enables these two muscles to act on two joints, the hip and the knee. Friction as the iliotibial band moves over the knee can cause **tendonitis**. Runners and backpackers, as well as dancers and skaters, can suffer from this problem.

Pain on the outside of the knee is the main symptom, which the patient will usually notice after the activity. Moving the leg freely is not painful, but extending the leg and rotating it outward against resistance does cause pain at the knee and sometimes at the hip. Continuing athletic activity will make the tendonitis worse. To relieve the tendonitis, the patient needs to stop the activity that is causing it and do stretching exercises that will gradually restore the flexibility of the muscles attached to the iliotibial band. A doctor can relieve swelling from bursitis by draining excess fluid from the bursa (a sack filled with lubricating fluid that encloses a movable joint) with a hollow needle.

The knee

The hinge joint formed by the tibia and the femur enables the knee to flex and extend. The joint formed by the fibula on the lateral side of the knee enables you to rotate the foot when the knee is flexed, and as it rotates you can feel the fibula knob moving.

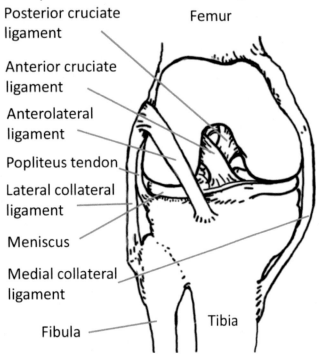

Posterior cruciate ligament
Femur
Anterior cruciate ligament
Anterolateral ligament
Popliteus tendon
Lateral collateral ligament
Meniscus
Medial collateral ligament
Fibula
Tibia

Knee injuries

The **medial collateral ligament** connects the femur to the tibia on the medial (inside) of the knee; the **lateral collateral ligament** connects the femur to knob of the fibula on the lateral (outside) of the knee; and the recently rediscovered **anterolateral ligament** connects the femur to the tibial knob on the lateral side of the knee. These ligaments prevent the knee from being bent sideways and help prevent it from extending the wrong way (**hyperextension**), so any impact or stress that forces the knee in those directions can tear the ligaments. An impact or force on the medial side of the knee is rare except in sports like wrestling, where an opponent may attack from inside the legs. In most activities, the medial side of the knee is sheltered by the other leg. So the lateral collateral ligament, a pencil-thick cord, is seldom injured.

The medial collateral ligament is often injured because impacts to the lateral side of the knee are common. In sports that involve blocking and tackling, if the foot is locked to the turf by cleats, it cannot relieve the stress by sliding. Falls in skiing can also tear the medial collateral ligament by bending the knee inward or twisting it. A slow, twisting fall is especially dangerous in downhill skiing, because it may not release the bindings. High and rigid ski boots transmit most of the stress to the knee. Any other activity that involves sudden deceleration or change of direction can also injure the medial collateral ligament.

Twisting stress on the knee can also injure the **anterior cruciate** ("crossing") ligament, which is anchored to the front of the knob of the tibia, angling up and back through the joint to the rear of the knob of the femur. It can also be torn by a frontal blow to the femur or by hyper-flexing the knee (doubling it up forcefully). The **posterior cruciate** ligament, which crosses up and forward from the rear of the tibial knob to the front of the femoral knob, is seldom injured because it is less likely to be stressed in an accident.

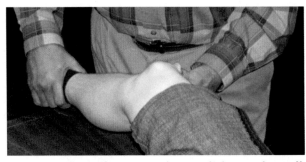

Dr. Serra shows how to reduce a dislocated patella
Photo courtesy of Mark Stinson, MD

If the **kneecap** (Latin *patella* "a small dish or pan") slides out of position, usually to the outside, it can lock the knee joint. To put it back in place, hold the leg up with one hand under the knee and the other hand gripping the leg near the ankle. Slowly straighten the leg while pushing the kneecap back in place with your thumb.

Dislocations of the knee joint itself are rare, but easy to align for splinting because the ligaments will be badly torn. You should splint the knee in a slightly flexed position. Rapid evacuation is important because there is often artery damage.

Assessing knee injuries

Before testing the knee for ligament damage, check it for deformity. If there is any sign of a fracture, the knee should be immobilized. If the injury appears to be a sprain, however, you can do some quick tests to assess the damage to ligaments. You should test the knee as soon as possible after the injury, because too much swelling, tension, and guarding can mask ligament damage. In each test, you position the knee so that you can isolate and pull on a specific ligament. Watch the patient's face, and stop the movement at the first sign of pain. A complete tear may allow much more movement, with little or no pain. Another sign of ligament damage is the lack of a definite end point to the motion, because it feels as though you are pulling on a rubber band.

With the knee flexed 90°, you can do the **anterior drawer test**: press on the femoral knob (to either side of the patella) with both thumbs, wrapping your fingers around the calf just below the knee. Knee laxity shows a damaged anterior cruciate ligament; and a mushy end point to the motion with no pain suggests a complete tear of the ligament.

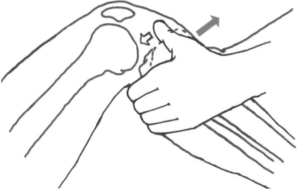

Pushing the tibia backwards tests the posterior cruciate ligament (which is seldom injured).

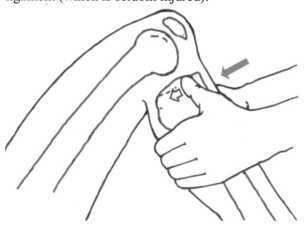

You can also test the anterior cruciate ligament with the **Lachman test**. Have the patient lie face up with the knee flexed about 30°. Make sure that the leg is relaxed. Support the thigh with one hand or have an assistant do it. Grip the calf just below the knee and try to pull the head of the tibia forward..

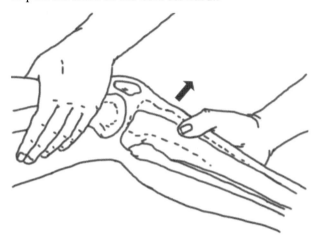

To test the collateral ligaments on either side of the knee, have the patient lie face up and relax the injured leg. With one hand, support and flex the knee slightly. Press the knee gently inward as you press the ankle outward with the other hand. This will test the medial collateral ligament.

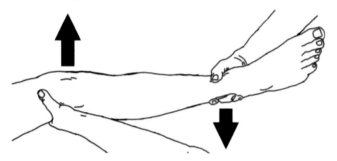

To test the lateral collateral ligament (which is seldom injured), move the hand on the ankle to the knee and the hand on the knee to the ankle. Then push the knee gently outward.

Compare the injured knee to the other one and ask about what is normal for the patient. Some people have looser joints than others, and women generally have looser joints than men. Also ask questions to reconstruct the mechanism of injury. Was there a direct impact to the knee or leg? If so, from which direction, and which way was the patient moving? Was it a twisting stress, with the foot trapped? Did the patient hear a snap? Did the knee give way immediately (suggesting an anterior cruciate tear), or gradually stiffen up? Was there a previous injury? Answers to questions like these, together with the results of the knee laxity tests, will help you to assess knee injuries and decide what to do in the backcountry.

Knee trauma can also damage the **menisci** (Greek *meniskos* "crescent-shaped"), the shock-absorbing pads in the knee joint. Once grown, menisci heal poorly if injured, because the inner parts have no blood supply. Torn cartilage from the menisci can lock the knee joint, usually preventing full extension of the leg. The effect is sudden, which distinguishes it from the gradual stiffening that can follow ligament damage. In a backcountry emergency where the patient must walk out, a locked knee joint can sometimes be opened by flexing it over a rolled foam pad behind the knee.

The ankle

The two lower leg bones, the tibia and fibula, have conspicuous knobs on the medial (inside) and lateral sides of the ankle. These knobs form a mortise over the ankle bone (talus), which allows the foot to flex upwards (**dorsiflex**) and downwards (**plantarflex**). Because the fibula knob on the lateral side of the ankle is closer to the foot than the tibial knob, the foot cannot roll outward (**evert**) nearly as far as it can roll inward (**invert**). Inverting the foot enables us to stand with our legs spread and feet planted; and to change direction when walking or running. But we seldom need to evert a foot strongly except when using the inside edge of a downhill ski to turn.

When the foot is angled up (dorsiflexed), the ankle joint is locked tightly, allowing little rotation or rolling of the foot. This gives the ankle maximum stability when the weight is on it and the muscles of the leg are pushing off from the ground. When the foot is angled down (plantarflexed), the joint opens up somewhat, allowing more play.

This motion is restrained by ligaments. Tears to these ligaments (ankle sprains) are the most common athletic injuries. About 85% of these sprains damage only ligaments on the lateral side of the ankle, when the foot inverts (rolls inward). Skiing is one of the few sports likely to tear the ligaments on the medial side of the ankle, when the turning skier catches the outside ski so that the leg is pulled and rotated away from the body with the ski tip buried.

Every time that a running or walking athlete changes direction by turning inward from the planted foot, the ankle must invert. If the ankle is forced to invert beyond its natural range of motion, the ligaments on the lateral side will be torn. This can happen when cutting or turning too sharply, landing badly after jumping, or just running on an uneven surface.

Two ligaments connect the knob of the fibula, on the outside of the ankle, with the talus: the **anterior** and **posterior talofibular** ligaments. The anterior ligament angles forward and is the first to be stressed and torn in an ankle sprain. The posterior ligament angles backwards and is very seldom injured, because ankle inversion puts little stress on it. Between these two ligaments, the **calcanofibular** connects to the heel bone (**calcaneus**). If the anterior talofibular ligament tears, the calcanofibular is next in line for damage.

Ankle sprains & fractures

Mild ankle sprains are slight tears of one ligament. Inverting the foot may be painful, but the patient will have full range of motion. Also, the joint will be stable enough to bear weight. In the uncommon injury of the deltoid ligament on the medial (inside) of the ankle, everting the foot may be painful. Mild sprains may heal in a week or less if the swelling is controlled, and the joint rehabilitated.

Moderate sprains are partial tears of one ligament. Range of motion may be limited, especially inversion, and putting weight on the ankle will be painful, but the joint will still be stable. Moderate sprains may take several weeks to heal.

Severe sprains tear one ligament completely and may tear others as well. Usually the patient will not be able to move the ankle at all within thirty minutes of the injury, because of the swelling and pain. The joint will feel unstable to the patient, and it will be difficult to put weight on it. Severe sprains may take months to heal and may require surgical repair.

If the mechanism of injury included rotation of the foot, one or both of the ligaments that connect the tibia to the fibula (tibiofibular) may also be torn. The patient will feel pain in that area when the foot is rotated outward with the knee flexed 90°. Sprains that damage the tibiofibular ligaments usually take longer to heal than sprains that damage only the ankle ligaments.

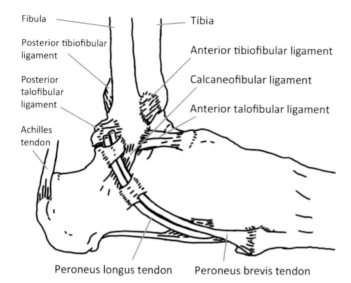

Fibula
Tibia
Posterior tibiofibular ligament
Anterior tibiofibular ligament
Posterior talofibular ligament
Calcaneofibular ligament
Anterior talofibular ligament
Achilles tendon
Peroneus longus tendon
Peroneus brevis tendon

When an ankle ligament is torn, the patient may hear or feel it. Within a few minutes, after the pain of the tear subsides, the ankle will usually feel better until swelling begins to compress nerves. This relatively pain-free interval of half an hour or so is the best time to examine the ankle in the field. If the cartilage holding the peroneal tendons in place tears, they may be pulled out of their groove. In an ankle fracture, usually one or both ankle knobs crack, and you will probably find point tenderness on the proximal part of the knob. Pain from a fracture is usually more severe and does not subside.

A patient with bone tenderness (especially on the proximal part of the ankle knob) who cannot bear weight probably has an ankle fracture and should get an x-ray. A patient with no bone tenderness who can bear weight probably does not have an ankle fracture. These are the **Ottawa ankle rules**.

Ankle dislocations

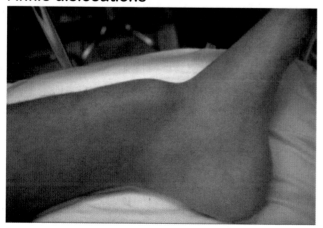

If the ankle is dislocated, it will be deformed, and the patient will not be able to move it much. To reduce the dislocation, flex the patient's knee 90° to relax the tendons. Grip the ball of the foot with one hand and lift the foot; let the weight of the leg shift the bones back into place, using the other hand to guide them.

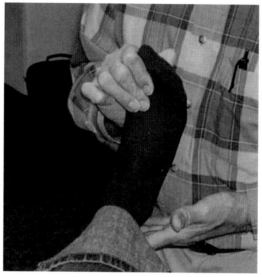

Dr. Serra shows how to reduce an ankle dislocation
Photo courtesy of Mark Stinson, MD

Tendon injuries

Tendon injuries in the ankle may be mistaken for sprains. For example, the two **peroneal tendons** hook around the back of the outside ankle knob for leverage. They can be felt there when you roll the foot outward (evert it). Skiers use the peroneal muscle to set the inside edge of the turning ski. If they catch a ski, however, and bend the leg forward to recover, the peroneal tendons may pull out of their groove, which is a disabling injury. If swelling is not too severe, you may be able to feel the tendons stretched over the ankle knob, and push them back into their groove. Treatment, however, may include surgical repair of the cartilage that holds the tendons in place.

The **Achilles tendon** connects the big calf muscle to the heel bone. When you stress it by springing forward forcefully off your foot, you can tear it. Most Achilles tendon ruptures are in athletes over thirty. The patient will be limping and may report that something popped in the ankle. Some patients say the injury felt like being kicked in the back of the calf. To check the tendon, have the patient lie face down, flex the lower leg 90°, and squeeze the calf muscle (Thompson test).

If the foot does not move away from the shin, the Achilles tendon is ruptured.

Emergency treatment of sprains

Swelling impairs circulation and causes pain in an injured joint by compressing blood vessels and nerves. With a mild to moderate sprain, swelling can cause more damage and loss of function than the original injury. The first goal in treating a sprain, therefore, is to reduce the swelling.

The traditional mnemonic is **RICE**: Rest, Ice, Compression, Elevation. Elevating the joint helps drainage, along with compression, and avoids pumping too much blood to an area where it may accumulate and seep into tissues from damaged vessels. Cooling the joint constricts blood vessels and slows the release of synovial fluid. Some orthopedists and athletic coaches, however, question whether icing actually helps to reduce the swelling from a sprain.

Wilderness rescuers may not have access to ice. **Chemical (endothermic) cold packs** are of limited use. They do not get very cold, and they warm up in 10 minutes or less. If **ice** is available, crush it and seal it in a plastic bag. Apply the ice for 20 minutes every two hours, or at most 20 minutes every hour. In between the ice packs, apply **compression** with a wide **elastic bandage**. If no ice is available, wet the bandage and loosen it between periods of compression.

To secure the ice pack, first wrap the elastic bandage loosely around the joint until it is covered. Then apply the ice pack, and continue wrapping the bandage around it until it is secure. **Chemical gels** are also used to reduce swelling, but they get as cold as the temperature of the freezer, which may be well below the freezing point of water. Also, gel packs stay cold a long time. You must be careful to wrap the ankle well under the gel pack, to avoid giving the patient frostbite.

You can make an ice pack by adding one part rubbing alcohol to two parts crushed ice in a plastic bag and freezing it. The result will be more malleable than ice alone, so that it will conform to the shape of the ankle, but it will not be as cold as a gel can get. A bag of frozen peas also makes a good ice pack, because it conforms to the shape of the joint.

Compression works on a sprain only if it is applied to the swelling. Simply wrapping the joint with an elastic bandage would put most of the pressure on the bony knobs. So cut a **horseshoe** from a cotton or felt **pad** (at least 1" thick) to fit around the kneecap or ankle knob. APB pads are good, and several folds of disposable diaper also work. Fit the horseshoe around the outside ankle knob so that the open side is towards the heart.

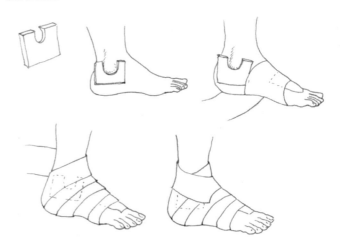

Then wrap the joint with an elastic bandage. Elastic bandages should be at least 4" wide, because it is easy to cut off circulation or compress nerves with a narrower bandage. When applying compression, check distal circulation and sensation at regular intervals. Test capillary refill in the toenails (or the skin of the toes if the patient is wearing nail polish), and compare nerve function with the other limb. If distal functions are impaired, loosen the bandage.

Rehabilitating joint Injuries

If a sprain is not so severe that it requires surgery, you should begin rehabilitation as soon as the swelling goes down. Immobilized muscles lose strength twice as fast as they regain it after an injury, which delays recovery of full function and increases the chance of re-injury. Physical therapists have a saying about sprains: for every day in the cast, two more days of rehabilitation.

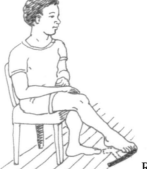

Rehabilitation begins with **range of motion exercises**. For a sprained ankle, sitting with the leg dangling and writing alphabets with the big toe simulates the joint's natural movements. This exercise can be combined with contrast baths: immersing the ankle alternately in basins of warm and ice-cold water, for a few minutes at a time, as you exercise.

When you can easily do range of motion exercises, begin **resistance exercises**, using a strip of surgical tubing or bicycle inner tube. For the ankle, pull the toes up, down and to either side. Tubing also works for knee and shoulder exercises, though exercise machines in a gym are more convenient. It is important, however, to keep weight off a sprained ankle or knee until they can bear weight painlessly. Days on crutches can save weeks or months of limping.

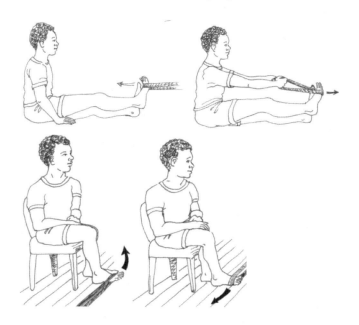

Balance exercises are the last stage of rehabilitating a knee or ankle injury.

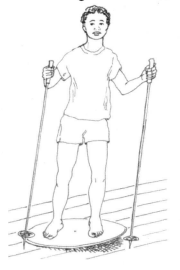

If you can stand on one foot for 30 seconds, you are ready to begin. You can make a balance board by cutting an 18" circle from plywood, then screwing one-half of a wooden ball to the center. Plant your feet on either side of the center and try to balance the board on the ball. If you feel unstable, you can hold a pair of ski or hiking poles for safety, planting them when you are in danger of losing your balance.

Athletes with unstable ankles often tape them before competition. Athletic tape is porous, so that it does not trap moisture on the skin. **Taping** is designed to limit motions that would pull on loose and weakened ligaments. Usually these are the ligaments on the lateral side of the ankle. Apply vertical and horizontal strips of tape alternately, so that they interlock. Begin with vertical strips on the inside (medial side) of the leg and pull them strongly before sticking them to the outside (lateral side). This will evert the ankle as much as possible. Finish the taping with some diagonal strips. If the tape does not stick well, try wiping tincture of benzoin on the skin first.

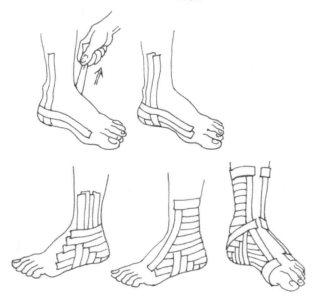

Taping a sprained ankle, when the patient must walk, follows the same principles, but the tape must not circle the ankle or leg completely. Otherwise, it will inhibit circulation as the ankle swells. A strip of bare skin should be on the front of the shin and the top of the foot. This technique is called the **Gibney wrap**.

Several types of sprained ankle braces are available, including one that that can be inflated. Elastic wraps can help stabilize a knee, but do little to support a sprained ankle for walking.

Muscle tears (strains)

Skeletal muscles are bundles of long cells called fibers. Each fiber is in turn a bundle of filaments called **myofibrils**, which contract or lengthen the muscle fiber by sliding past each other. Like most other cells in the body, muscle fibers work best when they are suffused with blood. Blood warms them and supplies oxygen and nutrients while carrying away waste products. The optimum working temperature for skeletal muscles is 102°F.

Muscles merge into tendons at each end, which connect the muscles to bones. Tendons are white, glossy cords or bands that do not contract or stretch. When a muscle is overstressed, it may tear. This happens about 40% of the time. About as often, the junction between muscle and tendon tears, especially in young athletes. Less commonly, the tendon may tear, or uproot itself, pulling out the piece of bone to which it is attached. This last injury, an **avulsion** ("pulling") **fracture**, is most common in immature athletes, because many of their tendons attach to **growth plates**, which are not as strong as mature bone.

Muscles and tendons can be overstressed by strenuous effort, as when lifting a heavy weight or by a sudden motion (starting, stopping or changing direction). Muscles are more likely to tear when they are cold, because cold makes them stiff. They are also more vulnerable when weakened by fatigue or lack of exercise, because they respond to a demand that is beyond their strength by tightening up.

A slight strain (grade I) tears only a few fibers. The athlete will feel the muscle tighten up over several moves, and it will probably be stiff the next day. A grade II strain is a partial tear which the athlete will feel when it happens and often hear as a pop or snap. Pain is usually intense, and the muscle will often spasm. Immediately after the injury, before swelling begins, the rupture can often be felt by the fingers as a break in the muscle. Grade III strains are disabling injuries that tear a muscle extensively, sometimes completely. Others may hear the snap or pop, and the rupture is usually easy to feel with the fingers.

Treatment of a strain begins by preventing or reducing swelling. Just as with a sprain, use the RICE treatment. Resting length for the muscle is in a partially stretched position. For a grade III strain, a splint may be needed to maintain that position. Apply ice packs, 20 minutes every two hours, until the swelling subsides. This may take from one to three days, depending on the severity of the injury.

To apply **compression**, put a pad over the muscle tear and secure it with an elastic bandage. When the tear is healed, **rehabilitation** begins with range of motion and stretching exercises. Stretch slowly and hold each stretch for 20 seconds before relaxing. When range of motion is restored, do progressive resistance exercises until the muscle is back to full strength. For a slight strain, this may take a few days. For a grade III strain, recovery may take weeks or even months.

Lower back injuries and pain

Injuries to the spine that can endanger or damage the spinal cord are described in chapter 11. But even if the vertebrae and spinal cord are intact, stress to the lower back from an awkward movement or improper lifting technique can cause lower back injuries and chronic pain. Poor posture and sedentary habits weaken the muscles that support and stabilize the lower back, and can make injury more likely.

Each pair of vertebrae are separated and cushioned by a tough sack of cartilage with a gel-like core, misleadingly called a disc. Between each pair of vertebrae, towards the posterior of the spinal column, a pair of nerve roots branch out to each side. Uneven stress on a disc can cause part of the cartilage to herniate - bulge like a weak spot on a tire. If the bulge presses against a nerve root, it will cause chronic lower back pain (which may also radiate down one leg), and possibly tingling and numbness as well.

You can help restore good posture and prevent lower back injuries with a simple exercise when you are seated. Sit up straight and raise both feet about an inch from the floor. Feel how that makes you arch your back and tense the abdominal muscles. Maintain that posture until the muscles tire, rest, and do it again. This exercise can be done sitting at a desk or computer, and can also help relieve boredom at a dull meeting.

Preventing athletic injuries

Muscles need to be both strong and flexible to avoid tearing from the stress of extreme or sudden effort. Before a workout, it is important to induce more blood into the muscles you will be using. This warms the muscles up and makes them more elastic. Before lifting heavy weights, do the exercise with a light weight. Before running or other aerobics, do the motions slowly and easily. **Stretching** should be done **after** a strenuous workout (not before). Otherwise, muscles that have been strongly contracting may not regain all their elasticity.

Although most freely moving joints are held together by ligaments, adjacent muscles help prevent joint injury because they control joint motion during activity. If these muscles are weak, there is a greater risk of losing control, and forcing the joint beyond its normal range of motion. Also, weak or injured muscles can imbalance movement as the athlete compensates. This can cause chronic joint injury or tendonitis.

Aerobic exercise is important for injury prevention, because fatigue causes many athletic injuries; but perhaps the most neglected conditioning for wilderness activities is balance exercise. Whenever we are on our feet, we are continually overbalancing and correcting. When we are moving fast, as in skiing or scrambling over rough terrain, our corrective movements must be stronger, faster and more accurate.

Carrying a load makes it more difficult to regain balance and more dangerous to lose it. A violent, wrenching movement to avoid a fall can strain a muscle, and falling is probably the most common way to injure a joint. Balance exercises speed up the corrective movements that enable us to control our motion and reduce the chance of accidents.

Conclusion

Injuries to joints and muscles are common in wilderness activities, especially sprains. Immediate first aid for a sprain is to minimize the swelling. You also need to know how to assess a sprain, and how to tape or wrap a sprained ankle or knee if the patient must walk out to escape a hazardous situation. Rehabilitating a sprain with range of motion, strength, and balance exercises is important so as to regain function and prevent further injury. For muscle tears (strains), first aid is to reduce the swelling with ice or cold packs, then stimulate circulation with heat. Reducing dislocations is technically a medical procedure, but wilderness medicine experts have been teaching the techniques to lay people for many years, so that they will have the option of using them in wilderness emergencies.

Chapter 9. Head injuries and brain function

Under the skin of the scalp is a network of blood vessels which can bleed copiously from a wound. Inside the skull, the brain is enclosed in three membranes. The thick, tough outer layer is called the dura mater (Latin "strong mother"). There are arteries between the dura mater and the skull, and if any of them are ruptured by an impact to the head, any blood accumulating inside the skull will press in on the brain. As **intracranial pressure** (ICP) increases, the patient's level of responsiveness will decline, and other vital functions (breathing, pulse, and blood pressure) may change, especially in a fracture at the base of the skull, near the cerebellum and brain stem.

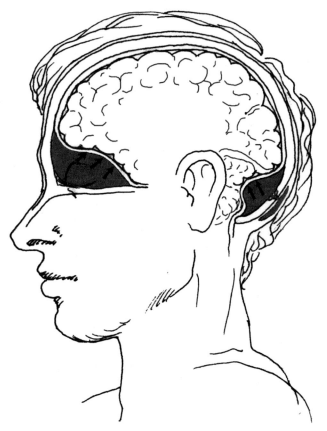

Inside the dura mater is a thin membrane called the arachnoid ("spider-like") because it is a web-like array of blood vessels. The inner layer is called the pia mater (Latin "tender mother"). In the space between the arachnoid and the pia mater, **cerebrospinal fluid** (CSF) cushions the brain against impact. If CSF is leaking out of the ears or nose, then the skull is fractured, and the membranes ruptured.

In a wilderness accident, you need to assess patients for head injuries, recognize the physical signs of skull fracture or concussion, and evaluate and record the symptoms of brain injury. You also need to protect the patient against further injury and make evacuation decisions.

Scalp wounds

If there are no signs of a skull fracture, you can use direct pressure on the wound to control bleeding. If there are signs of a skull fracture, you can pull the wound edges together by grasping tufts of hair (if it is long enough) on either side, then tie the tufts together over a dressing. For someone with short or no hair, you can pull the edges of the wound together with tape. Unless the bleeding is copious, however, you should clean the wound by irrigating it (provided that there is no sign of a fracture) and protect it with a sterile dressing, just as with any other wound.

Skull fracture

When you examine the head (see chapter 2 on patient assessment) look for any open wound, blood, or deformity. Then feel the skull, gently, for any deformity. Check the eyes and behind the ears. If an artery between the dura mater and the skull is ruptured by a skull fracture, blood can seep into the tissues around the eyes (raccoon eyes) or behind the ears (Battle's sign), giving them a bruised appearance.

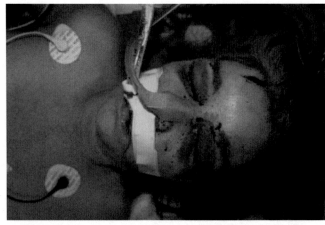

Fallen climber with a skull fracture & raccoon eyes
Photo courtesy of Ben Schifrin, MD

Cerebrospinal fluid (CSF) may leak out of the ears or nose. It is a clear fluid, like raw egg white. If blood is coming out of the nose or ears, capture some on a gauze pad or piece of cloth. Blood alone will spread into a uniform, dark red patch. Any CSF mixed in the blood will separate, forming a yellow ring around the patch (ring test). Leaking CSF means that the patient has a skull fracture which has also torn the protective membranes, opening a path for infection of the brain.

Assessing brain functions

Always ask anyone who has had a fall or collision:
- Did you hit your head?
- Did you lose consciousness?
- Do you have any pain in your head or neck?

If the patient is not sure, try to reconstruct the sequence of events. Any gap in the story suggests temporarily altered consciousness, amnesia, or both. After checking the skull for blood and deformity, check the eyes for:
- Pupil size (Unequal? Both dilated?)
- Light response (Slow? Absent?)
- Vision ("How many fingers?")
- Motion ("Without moving your head, follow my fingers with your eyes.")

Some people have naturally unequal pupils, but if one pupil is completely dilated, then there is an injury on that side of the brain putting pressure on the cranial nerve. Dilation is the relaxed position of the iris muscle, and the motor nerves to the eye, including the pupil, are the only ones that do not cross. You may also find loss of function on the opposite side of the face and body, as with a stroke. Does the patient feel any tingling or numbness? Check and compare sensation ("Which finger am I touching?"), movement, and strength on both sides of the body. Record the results and note the time.

Also keep checking responsiveness by talking to the patient and record the results regularly. A simple mnemonic for level of responsiveness is **AVPU**:
- Alert
- Responds to Vocal stimulus
- Responds to Pain stimulus (e.g., a pinch)
- Unresponsive

Alert patients are already aware of their surroundings as you approach, and give clear answers to your questions. An alert patient may or may not be fully oriented to identity, time, place, and event. A patient who is not fully alert and oriented, but at least responds to your voice by looking at you and answering you, is still showing a fair level of responsiveness. A patient who responds only to pain is lower on the scale.

For a more detailed assessment, use the **Glasgow Coma Scale** (GCS), which is described in the chapter on patient assessment. A patient with a perfect score of 15, no loss of consciousness and minimal symptoms, may be all right but should be watched carefully for the next day or so. Watching is important, because there could be a slow bleed in the brain that gradually affects function. Anyone who scores less than 15 after a blow to the head should be evacuated; and anyone who scores less than 13 is at high risk. A score of 8 or less is generally considered a **coma** (Greek *koma* "a deep sleep"), and the longer the patient remains in a coma, the poorer the chance of survival. If you check the GCS repeatedly and the score is going down, then pressure inside the brain is increasing. The only way to save the patient is by rapid evacuation to a hospital where brain surgery can relieve the pressure.

Cushing's Triad

A patient may rouse briefly after a head injury (lucid interval) then become unresponsive as pressure on the brain increases. Increasing pressure on the brain causes a set of signs called Cushing's triad:
- **Pulse pressure** (difference between systolic and diastolic pressure) widens.
- Heart rate slows down (**bradycardia**).
- Breathing becomes irregular.

Pressure inside the skull is called intracranial ("within the skull"). As increasing intracranial pressure (ICP) interferes with circulation and reduces the supply of oxygen to the brain, systolic blood pressure goes up. This increases circulation to the brain, but also increases ICP even more.

The pressure also interferes with sympathetic nerve impulses that normally trigger release of **epinephrine** from the adrenal glands signaling the heart to speed up; whereas **acetylcholine** (which signals the heart to slow down) is delivered directly from the nerve endings to the heart's pacemaker.

Breathing becomes irregular. The patient may hyperventilate; breathe irregularly; or stop breathing. Other signs and symptoms include severe headache, nausea and vomiting as well as gradual loss of responsiveness. There are many other possible causes for increased systolic blood pressure or irregular breathing, but these two signs combined with bradycardia suggest intracranial bleeding.

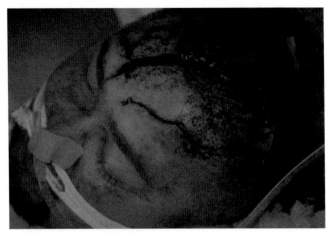

Unresponsive fallen climber with a skull fracture.
Photo courtesy of Ben Schifrin, MD

Concussion

Even if the skull is not fractured, a blow to the head can bounce the brain inside and rupture blood vessels. This injury is called a concussion (Latin *concussus* "shaken violently"). Effects of a concussion may include loss of consciousness, amnesia, and blurred or double vision as well as dizziness, balance problems, and nausea. Many attempts have been made to grade concussions on a scale going from mild to severe. These are based mainly on whether the patient lost consciousness or had amnesia and for how long. But any blow to the head that causes changes in brain functions is serious, and if brain functions are deteriorating, then the patient's condition is critical. It is especially dangerous for someone who has had one blow to the head to risk another impact.

A concussion that causes a slow bleed inside the skull can have delayed effects, days or weeks after the patient seems to have recovered. Headache is the most common symptom a (50% of cases). Other symptoms may include neck pain, ringing in the ears, dizziness, or drowsiness. Behavioral effects may include depression, loss of emotional control, anxiety, irritability, sleep disturbances and hypersensitivity to noise or light. The patient can also have cognitive problems including loss of memory, concentration or attention.

Recent studies of concussions in contact sports like football have used brain scans to reveal neurological damage. Researchers thought that the scans would show a difference between players who had been diagnosed with concussions, and those who had not. But the scans showed damage in the brains of all the players. So impacts to the head can have lasting effects even if there have been no obvious signs of concussion or intracranial bleeding.

What can you do?

Recognizing head injuries and assessing the damage are important skills for wilderness responders, because they enable you to make prompt decisions about evacuation. You also need to watch and guard the patient's airway, because head injury patients often vomit. Be ready to clear out the vomitus before it can be sucked into the lungs, using a suction device or cloth. If you are trained to do so, you can insert a plastic airway to protect an unresponsive patient. After taking spinal precautions, put the patient in a head-up position if possible, with the body elevated about 30° to help relieve pressure inside the skull. If there is an open wound on the head, clean it by irrigation and cover it with a sterile dressing. But if there is any sign of skull fracture, be careful not to put direct pressure on the skull.

Prevention

In the United States, there are 2,000,000 head injuries per year that require a visit to an emergency department, and 200,000 of them cause death or permanent disability. What can you do to prevent them in your wilderness activities? In mountaineering:

- Watch for rock-fall.
- Position climbing ropes so that they do not drag and knock off loose rocks.
- Make sure that everyone in your group knows the signal "Rock!" and how to react to it.
- When one person is climbing or scrambling over loose rock, keep the group out of the fall line.
- Pick routes that minimize the possibility of serious falls and rock-fall.

For climbing and other sports with a serious potential for falls or collisions, such as bicycling (especially mountain biking), downhill skiing and boarding, and swift water boating, you can reduce the risk of head injury by wearing helmets designed for the sport.

Chapter 10 Eye, facial, and dental injuries

Photos courtesy of Ben Schifrin, MD

Tears secreted from ducts in the inside corners of the eyes keep the sensitive surfaces moist, and the lids spread the moisture over the surface as we blink. Light comes into the eye through the transparent cornea (Latin "horny," i.e., thin and tough). The anterior chamber of the eye behind the cornea is filled with an alkaline solution called the aqueous humour (Latin *aqua* "water"), which is slowly secreted from glands under the iris, circulates out through the pupil and is reabsorbed.

The shutter-like iris muscle controls the amount of light coming in through the pupil, and the lens can be pulled flatter or relax into a more spherical shape to focus a distant or near image on the retina. Inside the eyeball, the optic nerve spreads out into the retina, a layer of light sensitive cells covering much of the inner surface. So much processing of visual information takes place in the retina that it could almost be considered an extension of the brain. A transparent gelatin-like substance called the vitreous ("glassy") body fills the main (posterior) chamber of the eyeball.

The word "humour" is a vestige of the ancient idea that the balance of four humours (Latin *humorem*, "fluid") in our bodies determines our health and temperament. The word "iris" was borrowed from the Greek for "rainbow" by a fanciful anatomist. The word "pupil" comes from the Latin for "doll," because you can see a doll-like image of yourself if you peer closely into someone's pupil.

How can these structures be impaired or damaged and what can you do about it? The most common (and least serious) problem is a foreign body on the surface of the eye. Even a tiny speck is very irritating because the cornea is so sensitive.

Foreign bodies on the surface

If blinking doesn't remove the irritant, you can try irrigating the eye with wetting solution (artificial tears), sterile saline, or disinfected water. You should squirt from the inside corner with the head tilted to let fluid drain downward. Another technique is to grasp the lashes of the upper lid and pull it outward and down over the lower lid. If the speck sticks to the inside of the upper lid, it may then adhere to the outside of the lower lid. You can also roll up the upper lid on the shaft of a cotton swab and (looking in a mirror if you are doing it on yourself) use another, well-moistened swab to dab the speck off the inner lid if you see it. Never use a dry swab or cloth on the eye or lid because it will leave lint on the surface.

A foreign body that will not come off the eye's surface or is embedded is much more serious. Paramedics may carry a pen-like device with a small magnet on one end to remove bits of metal from the surface of eye, and a loop of fine wire on the other end to capture non-metallic foreign bodies. However, if you have not been trained at that level, you should protect the eye and evacuate the patient. An eye patch should cover the eye without touching it. For wilderness situations, the patch should have a pinhole in the center, which will admit light and help to keep the eye focused straight ahead.

Eye infections

Eye irritation may be caused by allergies that are known to the patient. But an eye infection requires medical care. Signs and symptoms may include a pink or red appearance of the white of the eye caused by inflammation, itching, tearing, pus, crusted eyelashes, or lids stuck together in the morning. Rinsing the eye several times a day with sterile saline or disinfected water may help. Yellowish pus suggests a bacterial infection, and antibiotic eye drops may help. But you should never use eye drops containing steroids, unless they are specifically prescribed by an eye doctor, because if the infection is viral, they can cause ulcers (open sores) in the cornea.

Penetrating injuries to the eye

If the cornea is pierced, you will probably see watery fluid leaking out, perhaps forming a small droplet on the surface. If the main chamber of the eye is pierced, a thicker (vitreous) substance may be oozing out. If something is still embedded in the eye, you should not try to remove it unless you have the necessary medical training. For any penetrating injury of the eye, you should try to prevent eye movement and evacuate immediately.

Put shields over both eyes that block out light (except for pinholes in the centers) and are held clear of the eyes. You can improvise patches from cardboard and duct tape, and hold them clear of the eyes with donuts twisted from small cravats or other pieces of cloth. Or you can use the inverted bottoms cut from paper or plastic cups, taped in place.

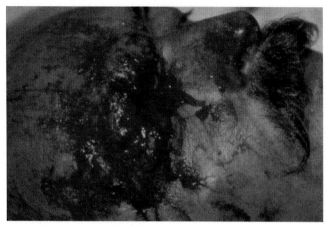
Eye injury

Blunt trauma and lid lacerations

A blow to the eyeball can rupture blood vessels inside and cause bleeding into the anterior chamber. This is called hyphema ("suffused with blood"). The blood may tinge the fluid pink or show a distinct layer from the bottom of the chamber. You need to protect the injured eye with an eye patch or sunglasses, and evacuate the patient to an eye doctor. An eyelid injury that interferes with its functions of covering and lubricating the eye also requires patching and evacuation. A layer of bacitracin ointment can help keep the surface of the eye and the lid from drying out.

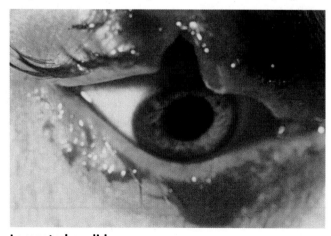
Lacerated eyelid

Retina damage

The retina can be accidentally damaged in two ways: first, by an impact that detaches it, and secondly, by solar radiation. Damage from solar radiation is most common when someone stares directly at the sun without eye protections (e.g., during an eclipse). While the cornea and lens absorb the high-energy ultraviolet, visible light and near-infrared of enough intensity can damage the retina. The patient will have blurred vision, a possible blank spot in the center of the visual field, and sometimes a headache. The visual problems may clear up within a few months, depending on how serious the damage is. Treatment is to protect the eye with a patch or dark sunglasses.

If the retina is detached by an impact, the patient will see flashes of light or floating spots, and vision will painlessly fade as the retina continues to detach. This is an urgent problem that requires rapid evacuation and eye surgery. An impact to one eye may cause temporary loss of vision in both eyes, but if the patient has adequate vision in the good eye to negotiate the terrain safely, and walking is the fastest way to get out, you can put a patch over the injured eye and hike to the trailhead.

Problems with eye movement

Whenever an impact occurs to the face or head, one of the functions that you check during assessment is eye movement. If the eyes cannot move in one or more directions, there may be a fracture to the bony orbit of the eye which anchors the eye muscles. Probably other signs and symptoms of skull fracture will be evident as well (see the chapter on head injuries).

Contact lenses

Any injury or medical problem that interferes with circulation or dehydrates the patient can dry out the eye and cause the contact lens to adhere. So you may have to remove the lenses as a precaution. You should certainly remove lenses in an unconscious patient. A contact lens container and a small sealed bottle of sterile saline in your first aid kit will enable you to store and safeguard the lenses, though the patient may have these. In winter weather, you may have to keep them close to your body to prevent them from freezing.

Hard lenses are not intended for long-term wear, so it is especially important to remove them. They are smaller than the iris, so you can see circles of their rims within the iris. Contact lens wearers know several techniques for removing hard lenses. For example, you can slide the lens gently to the outside corner of the eye pull down and out on the skin near the corner, stretching out the lids. This may pop out the lens. To remove a soft lens, however (which is larger than the iris, extending into the white of the eye), you usually have to pinch it between your fingers and pull it out. Another technique that works for both hard and soft lenses is to use a mini-marshmallow. Pull it in half to create a sticky surface, and use it to capture and slide out the lens. The sugar in the marshmallow will not harm the lens or the eye.

Nose

Minor bleeding from the nose, whether it is from an impact or spontaneous, can usually be controlled by pinching the narrow part of the nose, which puts pressure on the small arteries of the septum (the cartilage that divides the 2 nostrils). Keep up the pressure for 10-15 minutes. A binder clip (with padding underneath) can replace finger pressure. For more serious bleeding, you should usually have the patient sit leaning forward and spitting out blood in order to prevent the blood from trickling into the air passages or making the patient nauseated. Applying ice to the nose, forehead or back of the neck, however, is not effective.

If pinching the nose does not stop the bleeding, you can consider using an over-the counter spray or drops that constrict blood vessels when applied to the inside of the nose. For bleeding from blood vessels in the cavity behind the nose, you can insert a Foley catheter (a long plastic tube with an inflatable bulb on the end) into the sinus through the nostril, then inflate the bulb to apply pressure in the sinus. But a patient with a nosebleed that will not stop should be evacuated.

Conclusion

The cornea of the eye is very sensitive, so even a small speck on the surface will be irritating. An injury to the eye needs to be protected with an eye patch during evacuation, and if the lid is injured, the eye must be kept moist. Nose bleeds that you cannot control also require evacuation.

Dental emergencies
With the technical assistance of J.M. Yee, DDS, & J.F. Vincek, DDS

Dental emergencies may seem relatively minor compared to other injuries and illnesses, but they can have serious consequences, especially on a long wilderness trip. Pain from a dental injury or infection can be so excruciating that it will incapacitate the patient. Infection can spread to other parts of the body. By learning to recognize and cope with dental emergencies in the wilderness, you may be able to save a trip, a tooth or even someone's life.

Associated injuries

Any trauma that damages teeth can also damage the head or face. It is important, therefore, to check for associated injuries which may be more dangerous, no matter how distracting the dental pain is. Did the patient lose consciousness during or after the accident? Are vision and eye movement normal? If there is bleeding inside the mouth, you may have to pack the wound with gauze to protect the airway. Bleeding injuries to the mouth can cause airway problems, especially if the patient's level of responsiveness is depressed from an associated head injury. Is the patient positioned so that blood or saliva will drain rather than being aspirated?

Injury to the orbit (the eye's bony socket) can cause the eye to droop down. Are there signs of skull fracture, such as blood or cerebrospinal fluid coming out of the ears or nose, raccoon eyes, or a bruised appearance behind the ears? If there is pain, how long has it lasted? Is it steady or intermittent? Does anything make it better or worse?

Check whether the soft tissues of the mouth are moist, smooth, and pink. If not, an injury may be disrupting their blood supply. Sometimes an impact to the jaw makes the patient bite the tongue. This injury usually heals within a week after suturing, because of the tongue's rich blood supply. However, it can make eating all but impossible.

If the lower jaw is fractured, you may feel a step deformity in the bone. You may also notice that the teeth on that side are misaligned. If the jaw hinge fractures, it will be difficult and painful for the patient to move the jaw. The upper jaw can also fracture, most commonly toward the front. Check for misalignment of the upper teeth as well as deformity and point tenderness in the jaw. Stabilize a fractured jaw with a cravat jaw bandage. Tie a half-bow for quick release, in case the patient becomes nauseated.

Medical history

Medical history is also important. In a patient with a heart murmur or prosthetic heart valve, severe bacterial infection from dental injury or disease can cause heart failure within seven days. Dental history may give you clues to damage caused by trauma. Teeth which have had root canal work, for example, are more likely to break. After getting the medical and dental histories and checking for associated injuries, examine the teeth, which may be cracked, broken, displaced, impacted, loosened, or knocked out.

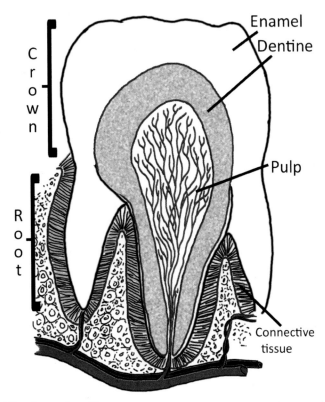

Broken teeth

If only the tooth's outside layer of hard white enamel is broken, the damage is minor. Pieces of a broken tooth, however, may be embedded in the lip. If the yellow dentine under the enamel is broken, the patient may feel considerable pain. If the red pulp is damaged, the patient will feel intense pain, and the tooth may become infected. The patient may also have trouble focusing the eyes. In a severe case, the patient may have a swollen face and may have trouble breathing. Occasionally an infection may spread through the sinuses to the eye or brain. So any fractured tooth that exposes the pulp requires rapid evacuation and dental surgery. Exposed dentin as well as pulp is very sensitive. Air and temperature change can both cause pain. You can protect the broken surface from exposure by painting it with Copalite, a liquid sealant that you can buy from your dentist.

Temporary filling

If the patient loses a filling or cracks the tooth without exposing the pulp, a temporary filling will protect it and possibly reduce the pain. It will also round off any jagged edges left by the break, preventing lacerations of the tongue and mouth. A lost filling may only leave a shallow hole or may go down to the pulp. If you are not sure which tooth is hurting, you can locate the pain by tapping on teeth in the affected area.

First, apply a topical anesthetic such as Hurricaine or a topical sedative such as Eugenol with a cotton pellet gripped in tweezers. Zinc oxide powder mixed with Eugenol forms a paste with a sedative, which hardens into a temporary filling. The disadvantage is that you must mix it on a clean surface and to the right consistency. Cavit dental filling paste is ready to use, but has no sedative in it. If you have neither of these, you can use sugar-free gum.

Mix or squeeze out enough paste to do the job in a thimble-sized dental mixing dish. Use a dental spatula and toothpick to roll the paste into a ball. Apply the paste to the cavity or broken surface with the spatula and quickly smooth it into shape. Have the patient bite down on a clean piece of gauze. Remove the gauze and any excess filling. The paste hardens within 10 minutes when exposed to saliva or other moisture.

Displaced teeth

A tooth may be displaced by a blow that forces it deeper into its socket (intrusion). A hard blow to the bottom of the jaw, for example, can drive the teeth together forcefully enough to cause an intrusion. This could occur in a forward fall. An intruded tooth may penetrate through the bone to a sinus. Teeth may also be forced outward or to the side (extrusion). To stabilize extruded teeth, have the patient bite down on a clean piece of gauze or cloth.

Knocked out teeth

This accident happens to 5,000,000 people per year in the U.S. If a tooth is knocked out, you should try to re-implant it. The only exception might be a known baby tooth in a child, which would just impede the emergence of the adult tooth. A tooth properly re-implanted within 30 minutes has a 50% chance of survival. After two hours out of the socket, however, its chances drop below 10%.

When you find the tooth, hold it only by the crown (the part that is normally visible when the tooth is in its socket). Use sterile gloves, if you have them. Do not touch the root. If the tooth is dirty, rinse it with sterile saline solution (not plain water). If you don't have saline, use milk or the patient's saliva. Never scrub the tooth, however, because it would damage the cells on the root's surface.

If you have trouble inserting the tooth, rinse the socket with saline. Once the tooth is in, have the patient hold it in place by biting down on clean gauze or cloth. A dentist will splint the loose tooth to the adjacent teeth with fishing line, which will allow slight tooth movement. This is important to prevent the bone from growing into the tooth, which would kill it.

If the tooth will not go in, try to preserve it. Hank's Balanced Salt Solution (HBSS) is recommended by the American Association of Endodontists. It includes sodium chloride, glucose, potassium chloride, sodium bicarbonate, sodium phosphate, potassium phosphate, calcium chloride, magnesium chloride, and magnesium sulfate. This combination has a 90% chance of preserving the cells on the tooth root for up to two hours. HBSS also makes Save-A-Tooth, which comes in a protective container. They claim that it can keep a tooth viable for up to 24 hours.

What if you don't have either of these products with you? Milk is the next best choice to keep the tooth alive, and sterile saline is better than nothing, although they are unlikely to keep the tooth viable for more than about 20 minutes. Holding the tooth under the tongue will supply it with nutrients, but also expose it to oral bacteria. It could also cause the patient to aspirate or swallow it.

A blow that knocked out a tooth may have caused a head injury as well. A patient whose level of responsiveness is deteriorating may swallow or even aspirate a loose tooth. If you cannot find the tooth, assume that it was aspirated until proven otherwise.

Medications

Eugenol (oil of clove) on the damaged tooth will sedate it. Hurricaine and Dibucaine ointment are topical anesthetics. Hurricaine is available over the counter as a spray, liquid, or gel. The gel is probably best, because it clings to soft tissues and doesn't wash away as easily as the liquid. Eugenol (oil of cloves) is included in over-the-counter emergency dental kits. Ibuprofen (two tabs every four hours) will help reduce the pain. Medically qualified rescuers can prescribe Tylenol #3 (acetaminophen plus codeine) or Demerol or inject a local anesthetic such as Lidocane. If there is bleeding, however, do not give aspirin, because it slows the clotting of blood. A cold pack to the jaw may also help, but do not let the patient suck ice, because the sucking action may loosen the damaged tooth or pull out blood clots.

Dental disease and infection

Dental disease can also cause emergencies on a wilderness trip. Cavities form when bacteria absorb sugar that is left on the teeth and produce acid as a waste product. A deep cavity, like a dental injury, can open the way to infection of the pulp (pulpitis). This infection can produce gas inside the tooth or the surrounding bone. Going to higher altitude will increase the pressure of the gas trapped in the tooth, which may greatly increase the pain. Applying a cold pack to the jaw or cold water to the infected tooth will reduce the pressure and help reduce the pain.

On a long trip, each participant should have a personally prescribed antibiotic such as penicillin or erythromycin. A 500 mg. tablet four times per day will help to control infection, but the pain will continue until a dentist opens the tooth and relieves the pressure.

Emergency dental kit

Assemble or buy a kit suitable for the length of your trip, distance from dental help, and level of your training. Your dentist may be willing to prescribe medications for your own use. Items in boldface might be all that you would want to carry in a small kit, but for a group kit you could add other items on the list.

Tools

- Large plastic tweezers
- Dental spatula and **toothpicks**
- Dental-sized mixing dishes or pads (2)
- Dental mirror (plastic)

Materials

- Cotton balls (to roll into pellets)
- Gauze pads (2" x 2")
- Hemotrol patient bite sponges (2" x 2")
- Sterile saline: 1/4 t. salt per cup disinfected water
- Save-A-Tooth
- **Temporary filling**:
- Copalite to cover and seal broken tooth surface
- Temporary cement with methyl and propyl paraben (for re-cementing a loose crown or bridge)

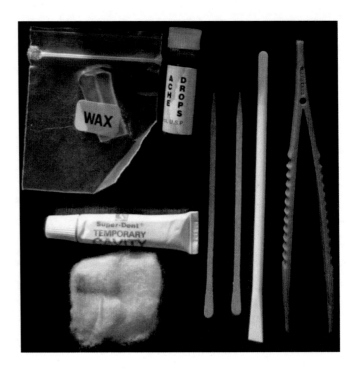

Medications

- Ibuprofen
- Or Tylenol #3 Rx (acetaminophen plus codeine)
- Demerol Rx
- Hurricaine (topical anesthetic)
- **Eugenol** (oil of cloves)
- Dibucaine ointment, 1% (topical anesthetic)
- Lidocaine Rx (injectable)

Conclusion

Dental emergencies can cause excruciating pain, and in some cases, may lead to dangerous infections. A backcountry dental kit should contain materials to ease the pain of a damaged tooth and temporarily plug a hole or break which exposes the sensitive pulp. An expedition kit should have materials for doing more durable repairs. Rescuers should be able to assess not only dental damage, but also associated injuries, which may be far more dangerous.

Chapter 11. Managing spinal injuries

Spinal anatomy and spinal injury

The seven cervical vertebrae are the most vulnerable to injury because the neck gives them little support or protection. Any vertebra can be injured by a direct blow, but cervical vertebrae can be injured by a blow to the top of the head as well. Cervical vertebrae are also vulnerable to bending and twisting forces, which can tear the ligaments that hold the vertebrae together. If enough of these ligaments are torn, the vertebrae become unstable. If a vertebra shifts sideways by one-third of its diameter, it will sever the spinal cord.

The twelve thoracic vertebrae are attached to the ribs, so that the rib cage helps to stabilize them. The lumbar spine in the lower back, with five vertebrae, is more flexible, but it is stabilized by the strong muscles of the abdomen and lower back. It can be injured by a radiating force from a hard fall on the tail bone as well as by a direct blow. The five sacral vertebrae are fused together in the pelvis.

The spinal cord is a continuation of the lower brain (the medulla oblongata). It is bathed in and cushioned by the same cerebrospinal fluid as the brain and sealed in protective membranes (dura), which are contiguous with the membranes around the brain. Nerve roots branch out from the spinal cord to either side, between each pair of vertebrae. Sensory and motor nerves proliferate from the nerve roots.

In the fetus, the spinal cord fills the vertebral canal of the spinal column for its entire length. Since the spinal cord grows more slowly than the spinal column, however, it only reaches the first lumbar vertebra in an adult. From the base of the spinal cord, a bundle of nerves, the cauda equina (Latin "horse's tail"), continues down the vertebral canal into the sacrum.

If the spinal cord is pinched, bruised, or cut by an injury, its functions will be impaired below that point. The patient may feel tingling and numbness or have complete loss of sensation. Loss of motor function may range from weakness to complete paralysis. Even if the patient is paralyzed, however, the damage may not be permanent. If the spinal cord is bruised or pinched rather than cut, the patient may recover, provided that rescuers protect the spine from further injury.

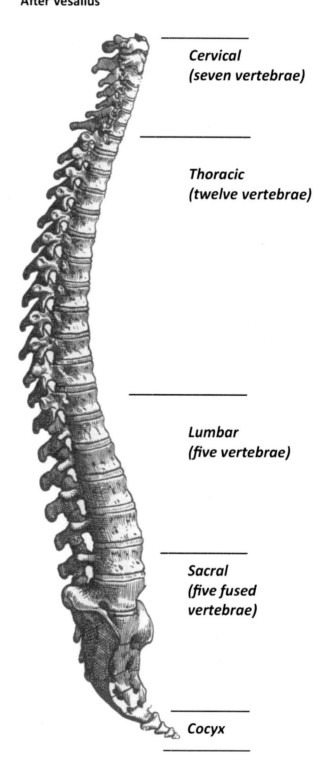

Five Regions of the Spine
After Vesalius

Cervical
(seven vertebrae)

Thoracic
(twelve vertebrae)

Lumbar
(five vertebrae)

Sacral
(five fused
vertebrae)

Cocyx

Spinal assessment

Patient assessment includes head-to-toe exam, vital signs, and medical history. When doing the head-to-toe exam, you may be able to feel **deformity** in the vertebrae with your fingertips or elicit **point tenderness** with gentle pressure, as with any bone injury. Also, the patient may have a stiff neck. The absence of these signs and symptoms, however, does not rule out a spinal injury, especially if there are signs or symptoms of serious head or face injury.

As with any possible injury, try to reconstruct and visualize the mechanism – could it have caused a spinal injury? Was there a direct impact to the spine, caused by a fall or collision? An impact to the head or the tailbone that could have compressed and cracked vertebrae? Bending or twisting of the neck that could have sheared ligaments holding the vertebrae together? Also ask if there is any pain or discomfort in the neck or the rest of the spine, and if so can the patient tell you where it hurts.

Check neurological function in the fingers and toes: sensation, movement and strength. To test sensation, ask: "Which finger (or toe) am I touching?" and block the patient's view to make sure that you get an honest response. Try a soft touch first, with your fingertip. If that gets no response, try a sharp touch with your fingernail or a pin. Then ask the patient to wiggle the fingers (or toes) in both hands or feet. To test and compare strength in the hands, have the patient grip your two crossed fingers with each hand and squeeze. With each foot, have the patient push down, then up, against your hand. Check sensation in one limb at a time, but always test and compare motor functions (movement and strength) on both sides simultaneously.

Loss of function on one side of the body only may be from a brain injury or stroke. If it is only on one leg or arm, it may be from an injury to that limb. Spinal injuries affect both sides of the body equally. In cold weather, however, hypothermia or frostbite may be interfering with neurological functions and masking the effects of a possible spinal injury.

Visualize the patient standing in the anatomical position, with palms forward. Nerve roots branching out through the cervical vertebrae supply the head, neck and shoulders with sensory nerves. They also supply the back down to armpit level, the arms (except for a strip on the front) and the hands. Nerve roots branch out from the thoracic spine almost horizontally, so that the level at which loss of function begins will be close to the level of spinal injury. Nerves from the lumbar spine serve the lower back, abdomen, the fronts and sides of the legs, and the feet except for the outside edge including the little toes. Nerves to the little toes, backs of the legs, buttocks, and genital organs come from the sacral spine. Loss of sensation to these areas alone would suggest an injury to the pelvis.

Watch for abnormal breathing. If motion is not visible, feel the chest and diaphragm with your hand. If breathing in an adult or older child is from the diaphragm alone, with only the abdomen moving, a neck injury may have damaged the spinal cord. This could be interrupting signals from the brain to the muscles which expand the rib cage. If, however, only the upper chest is moving, a neck injury may have damaged the nerves that carry signals to the diaphragm. These nerves branch out from the spinal cord high in the neck, so they are seldom cut off from the brain by spinal injury.

Although a spinal injury may cause loss of voluntary movement to some parts of the body, they may still move reflexively in response to a stimulus. Normally the nervous signal would pass through the brain, which would moderate the response. If the reflex is exaggerated, and uncontrolled, this suggests spinal injury. For example, a tap below the kneecap may cause the leg to jerk up violently. Or the patient may show priapism (uncontrolled erection).

Before moving a patient, you should usually splint any fractures or joint injuries and dress any open wounds. In an outdoor rescue, however, you also need to protect the patient against cold, wind, and wet. If the patient has a spinal injury, therefore, you should do only what is necessary to protect against further injury before backboarding. Get the patient off the snow or cold ground as soon as you safely can.

Clearing the spine

Studies of EMS responses in urban situations have found that most backboarding was unnecessary. So emergency medical systems in the U.S. are now training EMTs to rule out spinal injury (clear the spine) if possible. In a wilderness accident, you are unlikely to have the equipment to stabilize the spine effectively during evacuation. You also may not be in a place where you can bivouac and wait for rescue. Moreover, you should not backboard a patient unless it is necessary because:

- Backboarding is uncomfortable, and on a long wilderness evacuation, it will be excruciating.
- Backboarding impairs breathing, and a patient who vomits will aspirate (suck the vomit into the lungs) unless the rescuers instantly turn the backboard onto the side and clear the airway.
- Prolonged backoarding can cause pressure sores and nerve damage.
- Even with the right equipment, backboarding does not completely immobilize the spine.
- Backboarding will make a rescue more difficult, delay evacuation and increase the risk for rescuers.

So it is important to be able to rule out spinal injury (clear the spine), if possible, in a wilderness accident. What do you need to clear the spine after an accident that could have caused spinal injury? The mnemonic for the pre-test is PASS. You need:

- A reasonably **pain-free** patient. Any painful injury, such as a fracture, deep laceration, or serious burn, may mask the pain of a spinal injury.
- An **alert** and fully responsive patient who can give reliable answers to your questions, and has **good motor functions**, e.g. can show you two fingers on request. If the patient is not fully responsive because of a head injury, heat illness, hypothermia, altitude illness, or a medical problem, then you cannot clear the spine.
- A **sober** patient. Alcohol, recreational drugs and some medications can alter mental functions or suppress pain. If the patient is experiencing such effects, you cannot clear the spine.
- A **sane** patient. Patients who are mentally disturbed may not give reliable answers. Psychotics, in particular, may be disconnected from reality, including their own pain.

Once the patient passes the pre-test, feel the spine for deformity or point tenderness, and check spinal functions: sensation, movement, and strength. If you find no signs or symptoms of spinal injury, caution the patient to stop if it hurts, and:

- Turn the head from side to side (rotate).
- Put the chin on one shoulder, then the other.

- Lift chin and look up (extend).
- Put the chin down on the chest (flex).

To rule out a possible injury to the lumbar spine, have the patient twist from side to side, stretch sideways in both directions, bend backwards, and then bend forwards from the waist – again cautioning the patient to stop if it hurts.

Impaired distal nerve functions on both sides, (tingling, numbness, weakness, paralysis) or **deformity of the spine** are signs of spinal injury that would require some means of **spinal motion restriction** during evacuation to prevent further injury. In a wilderness situation, that usually means bivouacking and sending out for help.

Applying a **cervical collar** (or improvising one with a SAM splint) can help stabilize the neck and remind the patient not to move it. With a cervical collar on, an **alert patient** can usually move him or herself to a safe and comfortable position with much less spinal motion than rescuers will cause by extricating the patient. But extrication techniques are still needed for patients who are unresponsive or unable to extricate themselves because of injuries or entrapment.

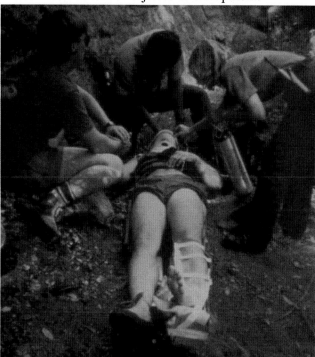

This fallen rock climber may have a spinal injury. Rescuers have applied a cervical collar, splinted the fractured leg, and administered oxygen while waiting for a backboard. *Photo courtesy of Ben Schifrin, MD*

Going Into neutral

If the neck is bent or twisted, you must move it into neutral position to open the airway and stabilize the cervical spine.

- Apply gentle inline tension (pull).
- If the neck is bent to the side, move the head to the center line without rotating it. Then rotate it if necessary until the face is forward.
- If the neck is straight but the head is turned to the side, rotate it until the face is forward.

To control the cervical spine, you need to grip the bony parts of the head. One way is to hook the fingertips under the base of the patient's jaw and skull, while pressing in gently with the heels of the hands. This technique gives good control when moving the neck into neutral position or doing a logroll.

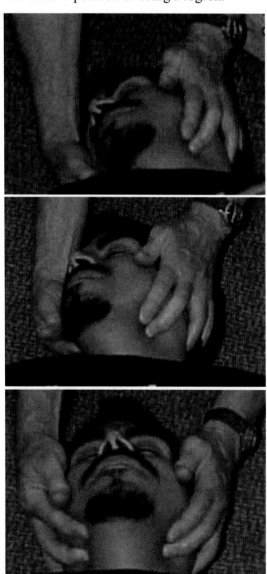

Another technique is to wrap one hand around the base of the jaw and the other around the base of the skull. This may be easier for rescuers with small hands.

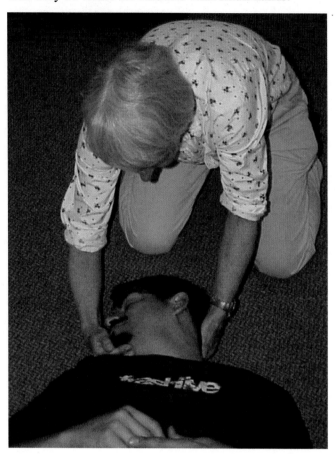

If the patient is not breathing, and you suspect cervical spine injury, try opening the airway with the jaw thrust maneuver. If the patient is still not breathing, however, and you cannot get air in, you must use the head tilt chin lift maneuver.

Position a patient who begins retching or vomiting so that the vomit will drain out and not be inhaled. Also, if bleeding is in the mouth or nose, make sure that blood does not go down the airway. For example, if the patient is lying face up, logroll onto the left side. On an unresponsive victim, use a suction device, if you have one, to help keep the airway clear. If you suspect a spinal injury, try to keep the neck lined up with the body and roll the body as a unit. But keeping the airway open is your first priority.

Straightening the pretzel

To be stabilized on a backboard or gurney, the patient's body needs to be straight. Any bend or twist in the neck or torso will stress the spine and make the patient unstable on the backboard. Therefore if the patient who cannot safely move herself is found in a bent or twisted position (a pretzel), you need to straighten the body and limbs in a way that will minimize the possibility of spinal damage. You should have four rescuers.

The patient is prone (face down), body twisted and legs bent. A team of four is best for bringing her body into alignment.

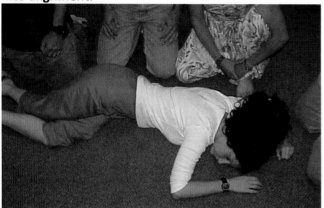

Begin by having each rescuer stabilize one part of the patient's body: head and neck; shoulders and upper torso; pelvis; and legs.

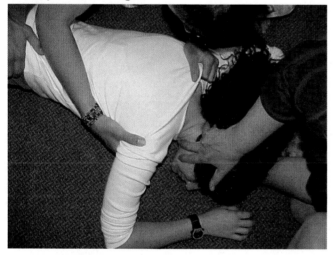

The lead rescuer gives directions to the rest of the team. This rescuer must control the head and neck, without ever letting go, until another rescuer takes over or the patient is completely backboarded. The second rescuer controls the upper torso by the shoulders, and the third controls the pelvis. These rescuers keep the torso in alignment with the head until the patient is backboarded. The fourth rescuer straightens the patient's arms and legs.

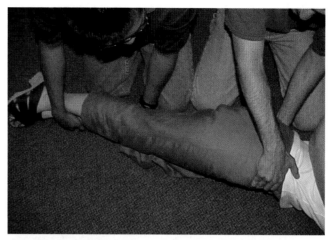

Straightening the legs

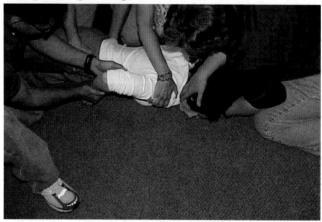

Lifting the elbow to align the arm with the body

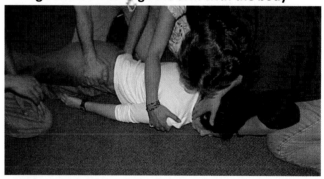

Aligning the plane of the chest and shoulders with the plane of pelvis and bringing the neck into neutral

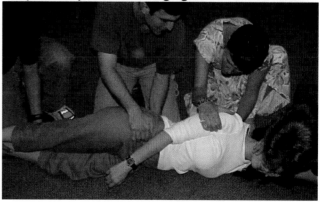

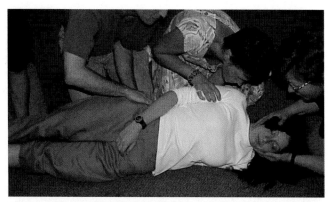

The patient is aligned and on her side.

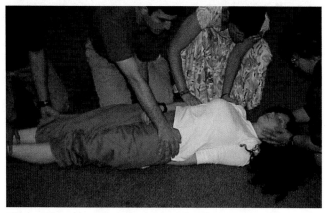

The patient is aligned and supine (on her back).

Photos courtesy of Ruth McConnell

If the patient is already supine (face up), the fourth rescuer straightens the arms so that they are alongside, then straightens the legs, moving slowly and in one plane of motion at a time. If the patient is on her side, first straighten the limbs and torso (starting with the neck), then logroll onto the backboard. When logrolling, keep the head facing forward and the plane of the shoulders at the same angle as the plane of the pelvis. If the patient is prone (face down), align as well as possible before logrolling onto the side, keeping everything in the same relative position, then move the neck into neutral position. Finish aligning the body and limbs, then logroll onto the backboard. If the patient is jammed into or around something, you may not be able to align in place. Instead, you may have to maintain at least part of the pretzel as you move the patient away from the obstacle. Then finish aligning.

If you find someone lying face down with no signs of breathing, and you are alone, you should keep the spine as straight as possible while doing a logroll. Kneel behind the patient's head, so as to minimize rotation of the neck when you logroll. With the patient's arms at his side, cross the ankles, then with

one hand controlling the head, grip the far arm at the elbow, clamp it against the patient's side, and roll the patient towards you. Then check for breathing and circulation.

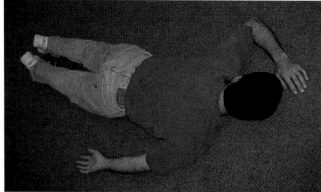

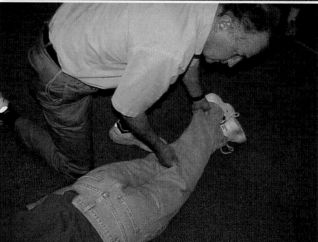

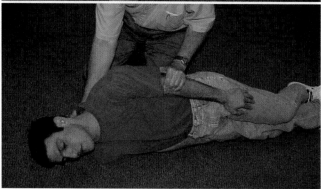

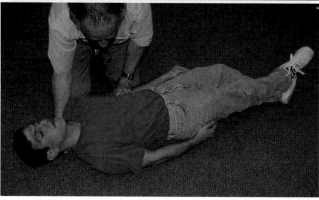

Securing the patient

One way to get a patient onto a backboard is by logrolling onto the side of the board, after applying a cervical collar. Open the shirt if necessary so that the collar is on skin, not cloth. Logrolling requires the same teamwork as straightening the pretzel, with one addition. As the team logrolls the patient's body onto the side, one rescuer wedges the board alongside and tilts it up slightly. The head of the board should be about a foot beyond the patient's head. Then the team logrolls the patient as a unit onto the board, after the rescuer holding the board checks the patient's back (if this has not already been done). Next, the team slides the patient diagonally towards the head of the board (at the leader's signal) until the whole body is straight and centered on the board.

Another technique is to lift the patient and slide the board underneath, but this is more strenuous especially with a heavy patient. Both techniques require clear directions from the leader and coordination of the rescuers' movements. When logrolling, each rescuer needs to watch the head and keep the body aligned with it as the patient is moved.

You can secure the patient to the board with cravat bandages or webbing. Pre-sewn sets of straps that are secured with Velcro make the task easier, but the principles are the same. For a small patient, you may also want to prepare long, thin blanket rolls or pads secured by tape. A roll should just fill the space between the patient's side and the edge of the board, so as to prevent sideways slippage. Pads under the knees, small of the back, and neck will make the patient more comfortable and secure on the backboard. A half-inch pad under the head cushions it and prevents hyper-extension of the neck. Be careful not to bend the neck forward, however, while easing the head onto the pad. You can position these pads in advance and tape them to the board. A pad between the legs will also help to keep the patient more comfortable and secure. If you are administering oxygen, however, the tank usually goes between the patient's legs.

Begin by securing the chest and pelvis to the board. Then secure the legs. If the patient moves on the board before being secured, the rescuer controlling the head can keep the neck aligned with the body. If two rescuers have opposite ends of the same cravat, they need to coordinate their movements. Otherwise, they may rock the patient's body back and forth as they try to pull the cravat tight. Always pass the cravat or webbing down through the top of the slot in the board so that it is as close to the patient's body as possible.

When directing the tie-down, the team leader should think about how the backboard may be tilted during transport. Ties going straight across, together with padding, keep the patient from sliding to the side. Diagonal ties across the shoulders and groin, and stirrup ties around the feet, help prevent sliding towards the head or foot. A very effective way to secure the chest with cravats is to tie a short loop at each hip (about 1' long), bring two cravats down over the tops of the shoulders and diagonally across the chest, and pass them through the opposing loops. Then two rescuers (one on either side) pull the cravats tight as the patient exhales and tie them to the backboard or to the taut length of cravat with half-hitches.

You can prevent the patient from sliding down the board with stirrup ties around the hips and feet. For each hip, tie a cravat at the waist, pass it around the thigh, and bring it back to tie at the same slot. For each foot, tie a cravat to a slot at knee level, pass it diagonally across the shins, around the instep, and back to the same slot.

Secure the head last. One technique is to fold a blanket into a 12" strip and lay the strip across the board, easing it under the patient's head without lifting the head more than about ½". Then roll the two ends of the blanket strip in until they stabilize the head from either side. Finally, secure the forehead to the board. In practice sessions, use two cravats, twisted around each other to form an "X" on the forehead, with cushioning pads on the forehead and under the head. The four tails of the cravats are secured far apart, for leverage. In a real backboarding, you can use wide strips of duct tape across the forehead instead of cravats. Some commercial devices for securing the head have straps secured with Velcro, and others require tape, but they work on the same principles.

If you are using a commercial set of nylon webbing, or a backboard with attached straps, and they are not sufficient to stabilize the patient during evacuation (or have broken buckles), you will have to supplement them with cravats or webbing.

Backboarding

Photos courtesy of Ruth McConnell

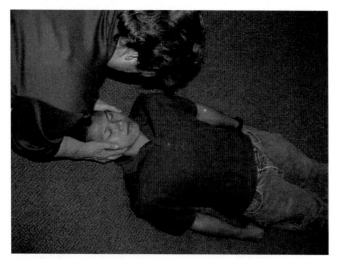

The patient leader stabilizes the neck until the patient is completely secured to the backboard.

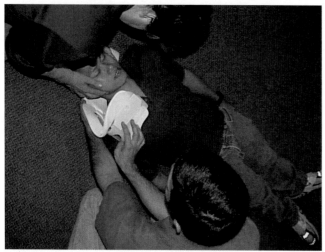

Another rescuer applies a cervical collar.

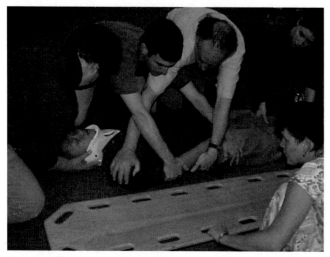

Two or three team members get a grip on the patient - note the crossed arms... -

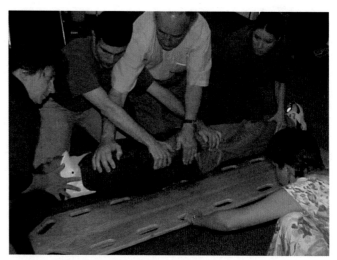

...and roll him towards themselves as a unit. The patient leader gives the signal. The rescuer holding the backboard checks the patient's back; then she reaches across the patient with one hand to grip the pelvis and assist the log roll onto the board.

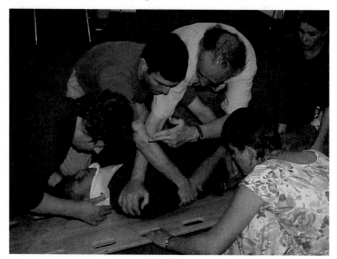

The team slides the patient diagonally upward until he is centered on the board.

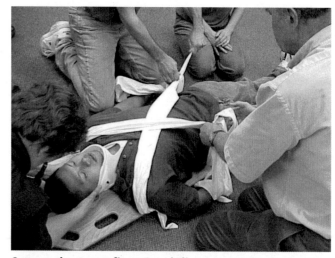

Secure the torso first. Bandolier straps also keep the patient from sliding upwards on the board.

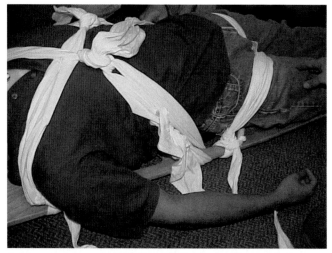

Stirrup straps around the thighs keep the patient from sliding down on the board.

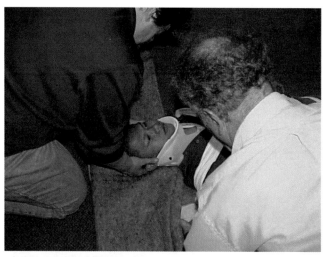

Slide a blanket (folded into a long strip) under the patient's head.

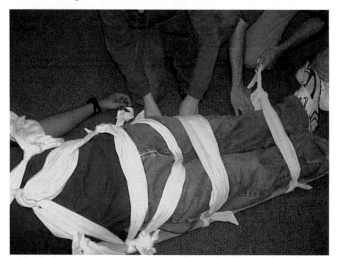

Secure the pelvis and legs with cross ties.

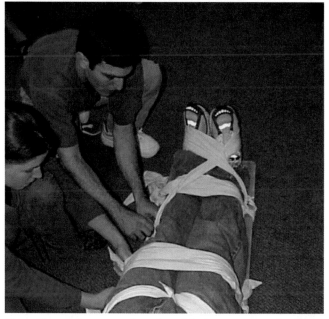

Use stirrup ties, crossing the shins, to secure the feet.

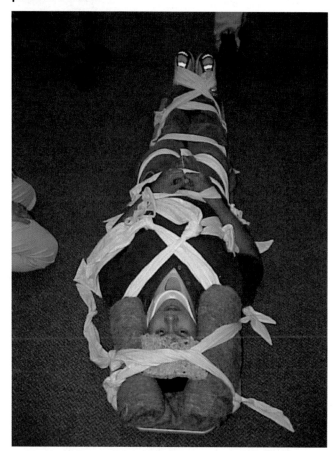

Roll the blanket up on either side of the head, and have another rescuer hold the rolls against the head as the patient leader withdraws her hands. Secure the head with two cravats tied down in an "X", which also hold the blanket rolls against the head. With a real injury, it would be better to tape the head down. Most commercial immobilization devices for the head use tape or Velcro straps, and foam blocks sealed in plastic.

Testing the ties

In a practice session, the rescue team should test the ties that secure the patient before harnessing themselves for the carry. After lifting the backboard, rotate it 90° so that the patient is sideways and check for slippage. This maneuver can also be used for going through a narrow opening, or if the patient becomes nauseated and needs to be positioned for vomiting.

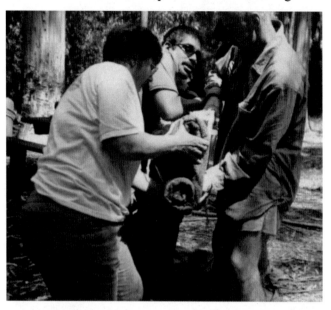

Tilting the board sideways 90°, then 45° downward

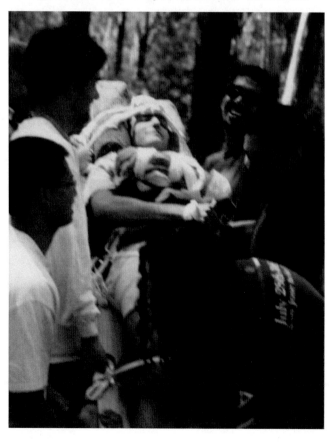

The second test is to lower the feet until the board is tilted 45°. This simulates going up or down a hill or stairs. Usually, the patient's feet should be downhill when traversing a slope or on stairs.

Lifting and carrying the backboard

Before letting a team lift the backboard, the leader should position rescuers according to their size and strength. Usually six to eight rescuers are needed to carry a backboard comfortably for more than a short distance, especially if the team must go up or down stairs or over rough terrain. The largest rescuers should be toward the patient's head, and the smallest rescuers toward the patient's feet. Rescuers on opposite sides of the board should be of similar height, so far as possible. All of the team members should know their places before putting the patient on the backboard.

Only one leader should be giving directions, answering team members' questions, and evaluating their suggestions. A rescue operation is not the place for a discussion session. Lack of leadership not only handicaps the operation, it also shakes the patient's confidence in the ability of the rescuers. The rescuer who controlled the patient's head during backboarding, however, should continue talking with the patient, maintaining rapport and explaining what is happening.

If the board must be carried more than a short distance, and has no carrying straps, these can be improvised from cravats or webbing. Pass a cravat or piece of webbing through each slot of the backboard, and tie them into loops of equal length. Then give each carrier a cravat or sling to use as a bandolier and pass through the loops, adjusting the length to equalize height differences. These carrying straps will support most of the weight of the backboard from the rescuers' shoulders, so that they can use the handgrips to stabilize and control the load.

When carrying the backboard up or down a steep slope or stairs, pass it from hand to hand with the feet planted. Rescuers should never move their feet while supporting the board on a steep or slippery slope or on stairs. The pair of rescuers in the rear pass the board to the other four, walk to the front, and take their positions. Then the board is passed forward, and the operation repeated until the team is on level ground again. If the team is not used to this exercise, they should practice it first with an empty backboard.

If there is not enough space to walk around the team on stairs or a steep slope, rescuers can crouch and move under the board to get to their new positions while the rest of the team supports the board without moving their feet.

Other spinal management equipment

A portable stretcher of strong nylon fabric with a frame of aluminum tubing is less bulky and easier to transport in the wilderness than a backboard, and a patient can be secured to it in the same way. A vacuum mattress (along with a supporting stretcher) is the most comfortable way to restrict spinal motion, but it is more expensive than the alternatives. It is filled with thousands of polystyrene balls, which mold themselves to the body when the mattress is evacuated with a vacuum pump. It also curls around and supports the head, eliminating the need for a cervical collar.

If you lack equipment to stabilize the spine effectively in a wilderness accident where you suspect spinal injury, usually the best choice is to bivouac and send people out to get help.

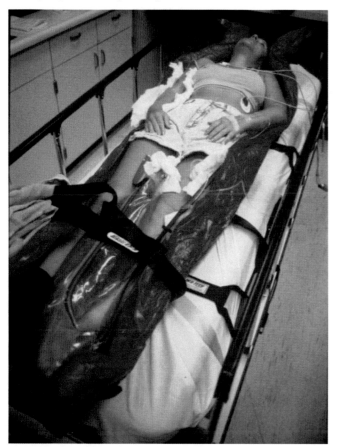

A vacuum splint molds to the body.
Photo courtesy of Ben Schifrin, MD

Spider straps

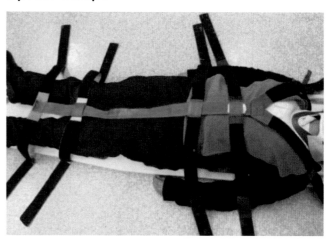

Spider straps have one set of diagonal straps that go over the shoulders of the patient, and four sets of straps that can be slid along the central strap to the correct positions for the patient. They fasten to themselves, after being passed through the holes in the backboard, with Velcro. Shoulder straps go over the top of the shoulders, then down through the holes that are under the shoulders. They prevent the patient from sliding upward during transport. Ask the patient to take a deep breath, and hold the central strap with one hand (to prevent it from sliding up towards the patient's neck) as you and your partner pull the shoulder straps tight and fasten them.

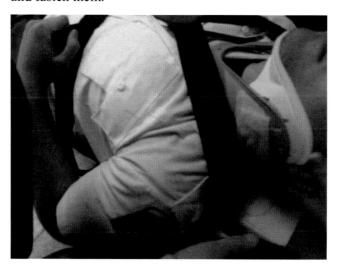

Next, secure the lower leg straps. Pass them through the holes as far down towardsthe foot of the board as possible, so that as you tighten them they will pull the central strap taut. Again, ask the patient to take a deep breath.

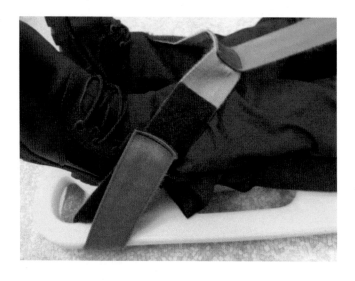

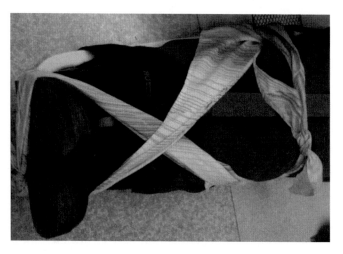

Next secure the chest straps, which go as high on the chest as possible (so as not to interfere with breathing), and through the same holes as the shoulder straps.

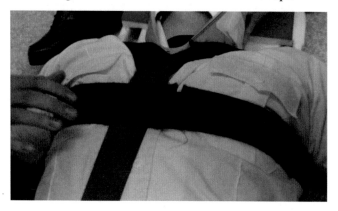

Make sure that the pelvic straps go over the bone of the pelvis, and not the soft part of the abdomen between the pelvis and the rib cage. The thigh straps go between the pelvis and the knees, not on the joints.

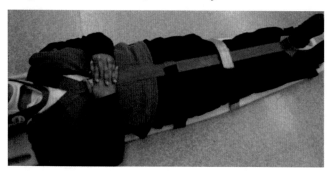

If you will be carrying the patient up or down stairs or a steep slope, add a foot stirrup of webbing or cravats, so as to prevent the patient from sliding down towards the feet during transport. Secure the head last, with a rolled blanket, foam blocks, or a commercial device.

Conclusion

Spinal injury management is a high priority in an accident scene, but not as high as life-threatening hazards or ABCs. If it is necessary to move an unstabilized accident victim away from a hazard, you should keep the spine as straight as possible. If the patient is not breathing, you can use the jaw thrust to open the airway without flexing the neck. But if that does not work, the airway must be opened. After checking for hazards and doing ABCs, do a patient assessment, including head-to-toe exam, medical history, and vital signs, with special attention to neurological signs.

In spinal management, the goal is to get the patient into a neutral position: body and legs straight, arms at sides, neck slightly extended with face forward. Minimize the chance of further spinal injury by moving parts of the body slowly and carefully towards the neutral position, in one plane of motion at a time. Flexing, extending, or especially rotating the spine away from the neutral position is dangerous, because it can damage the spinal cord.

One rescuer needs to stabilize the neck manually and keep it in line with the body until the patient is completely secured to the backboard or other device. This rescuer also should talk to the patient, explaining what the team is doing and monitoring the patient's responsiveness. When directing the tie-down, the team leader needs to make sure that the ties and padding will prevent the patient from sliding, bending, or twisting on the board. By planning each move, you can minimize the chance of further injury and maximize the chance of recovery.

Chapter 12. Chest and abdominal injuries

Most chest and abdominal injuries in wilderness activities are caused by impact from falls or collisions. In these cases, you need to reconstruct the mechanism of injury and ask yourself what damage it could have caused. For example, a rock climber who did a long pendulum and smashed against the rock sideways may have cracked ribs or fractured the pelvis, and the impact (or the broken bone ends) may have ruptured blood vessels or vital organs.

You also need to check and continue to monitor the effects of the accident on the patient's vital systems very carefully, especially if they suggest shock. Vital signs may change because of direct damage to the vital organ in question. For example, breathing may change, because a lung has been torn open by a cracked rib. They may also change from the indirect effects of damage elsewhere. For example, internal loss of blood, which reduces circulation, can change skin signs and level of responsiveness as well as pulse and breathing.

Signs and symptoms in a patient with a chest injury that impairs breathing may include:
- guarding or self-splinting position;
- asymmetrical chest movement;
- rapid breathing;
- labored breathing with use of accessory muscles (tensed neck muscles, flared nostrils);
- voluntary restriction of breathing;
- air under the skin of the chest (crackly to the touch);
- cyanosis (blue lips, gums, skin);
- coughing up blood;
- distended veins in neck;
- and rapid pulse (especially over 130 per minute).

Rib fractures and separations
Any fall or collision with an impact to the rib cage can damage it. A hard impact to the center of the chest can fracture the sternum. In automobile accidents, it can happen to a driver thrown forward onto the steering wheel post, though it is rare in wilderness accidents. The main symptom is sharp chest pain, aggravated by finger pressure on the sternum, especially over the injury site.

Rib injuries are much more common. A cracked rib, like any fracture, usually causes a sharp, local pain, and point tenderness when touched. Moving, straining, twisting, or coughing can cause severe pain. Usually you can locate rib fractures during your patient assessment by putting gentle hand pressure on the sides of the rib cage, then asking the patient to take a deep breath and point to any place that hurts. The fifth through tenth ribs are most often fractured, since the first four are somewhat protected by the shoulder girdle. The eleventh and twelfth ribs are more likely to flex rather than crack, since they are not attached to the sternum.

An impact or a twisting stress on the rib cage can tear the cartilage that connects the ribs (separation). An extensive tear is very painful and slow to heal. It can cause severe pain whenever the patient makes a move that pulls on the torn cartilage, e.g., lying down or getting up, coughing, or sometimes just taking a deep breath.

Emergency care for either injury is to keep the patient comfortable, check for effects on respiration and circulation, and try to prevent further damage, especially to the lungs. It is generally not helpful to tape or splint the ribs. In fact, it may be harmful by restricting breathing even more than the patient will be doing voluntarily. While the patient may be able to walk out on relatively easy terrain, the injuries may prevent safe negotiation of steep or difficult terrain and require evacuation.

Chest injuries and vital functions
Chest injuries account for about 25% of all trauma deaths in the United States. They can interfere with breathing and circulation in several ways: by impairing chest movement, collapsing a lung, bruising the heart, or compressing the heart inside its protective sack with accumulating blood.

If you visualize the mechanism of breathing, then the possible effects of a chest injury on respiration will be easier to assess. The lungs are enclosed in a slippery membrane that is normally pressed against a membrane lining the inside of the chest cavity by air pressure inside the lung. This air pressure varies as you inhale and exhale, but as long as no air or blood gets between the lungs and the chest wall, the lungs should remain inflated.

When the rib cage expands and the diaphragm flattens, the lungs expand with the chest cavity. Since the volume of the lungs has increased, air pressure inside drops below atmospheric pressure, and new air flows in through the airways. When the chest contracts and the relaxed diaphragm domes up, they compress the air inside the lungs and force some of it out. The lungs also contract like balloons because of their elasticity.

What can interfere with this mechanism for moving air in and out of the lungs? If a lung is punctured by a cracked rib, even if the chest wall remains intact, then the lung will begin to collapse like a balloon with a slow leak. This is called a **pneumothorax** (Greek *pneuma* "air" *thorax* "chest"). Blood leaking between the lung and the chest wall can have a similar effect, called **hemothorax** ("blood in the chest").

If the chest wall is pierced, and the hole is too big to be self-sealing, then air will be sucked in through the hole when you expand the chest, collapsing the lung. This is called a **sucking chest wound**. Another injury that will impair breathing is an impact that fractures many ribs and breaks loose a whole section of the rib cage – at least three ribs broken in at least two places (**flail chest**). The broken section will be pushed out when the chest contracts by the increasing air pressure inside the lungs and pushed in when the chest expands (**paradoxical motion**). By reducing the effective volume of the expanded chest cavity, this injury reduces the amount of air moved in and out with each breath. It is called flail chest because of the flail-like motion of the broken section. Similarly, an injury to the heart that causes bleeding inside its protective sack will gradually compress the heart and reduce the amount of blood that it can receive from the veins and pump out

When assessing a patient with a possible chest injury, always go to skin and check for bruising, crackling or an open wound.

Usually a patient with breathing problems will be more comfortable, and able to breathe better, in a sitting position. But a patient with an injury to one side of the chest who cannot or does not want to sit up

should be placed on the injured side to protect the good lung. You should give oxygen (if you have it) to any patient in respiratory distress and protect the airway.

Children and chest injuries

Since children's bones have less mineral content than adult bones, they are more flexible. As a result, their rib cages flex more with the impact of a fall or collision, and transmit more of the impact to internal organs. So even if a child seems all right after blunt chest trauma, it is important to watch vital signs over the next day or two, because a slow air leak or bleed may happen inside the chest. If the child's vital signs do start to change (e.g., more rapid breathing and pulse), then you should assume that a chest injury has occurred and evacuate.

Pneumothorax and hemothorax

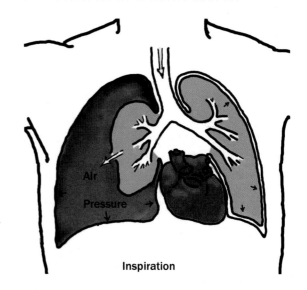

Inspiration

Tension pneumothorax & open wound in the chest

Young people, especially tall thin men who smoke, as well as people with emphysema can get blebs (blisters) or cysts on the lungs that can cause air leaks when they rupture (**spontaneous pneumothorax**). An impact to the chest, or the jagged ends of broken ribs, can also cause an air leak by tearing the lung, even if there is no open wound in the chest. Usually the patient will feel a sharp, constant pain in the chest that gets worse with inhaling. As the lung shrinks, the patient will feel short of breath and breathe faster. A patient who cannot sit up should be placed on the injured side to protect the lung that is still functioning.

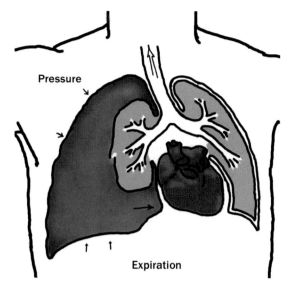

Pressure

Expiration

If the tear in the lung acts like a one-way flap valve, leaking air into the chest cavity on inspiration, which is trapped on expiration, then the increasing air pressure in the injured side of the chest will collapse the lung. This is called a **tension pneumothorax**. The trachea may eventually be twisted to the side by the unequal pressure; and pressure on the heart reduces the amount of blood that can return to the upper chambers to be pumped out again, so the jugular veins in the neck will become distended. The injured side will have no breath sounds and be hyper-resonant when you tap on it (like a drum).

Bleeding into the chest cavity (**hemothorax**) has similar effects. A patient may have both a blood and an air leak. In both cases, you need to evacuate as rapidly as possible and give oxygen if you have it.

Sucking chest wound

If an open wound penetrates the chest and is too wide to self-seal, you will see air bubbling through the blood, and you may hear a sucking sound as the patient inhales. You need to seal the hole immediately with a gloved hand as another rescuer prepares an air-proof patch. If you are alone, have the patient hold a hand over the wound if possible while you prepare the patch.

Your patch should be at least three or four times as big as the hole - otherwise it might be sucked in. A plastic baggie or a piece of aluminum foil over a layer of sterile gauze makes a good patch. Blood and hair on the chest may make it difficult for tape to stick, so reach for the roll of wide duct tape and use a lot of it. If possible, leave one side of the patch un-taped so that it

will act as a one-way flutter valve. When the patient inhales, the patch will be pulled in and sealed by the difference in air pressure. When the patient exhales, some air may be forced out on the untapped side, slightly reducing the pressure inside the chest.

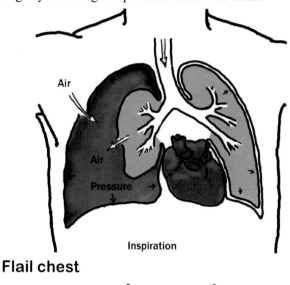

Air

Air

Pressure

Inspiration

Flail chest

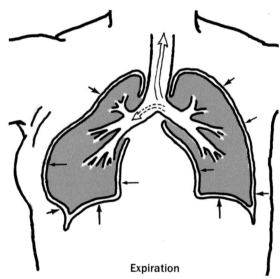

Expiration

If multiple fractures have broken loose a segment of the rib cage, the muscles may self-splint the injury until they tire. Then you will see the paradoxical motion of a flail chest - a section bulging out when the patient exhales, and pulled inward as the patient inhales and expands the chest.

You will also see developing signs and symptoms of respiratory distress. While the patient may feel more comfortable holding or lying on a cushion over the injury, trying to splint it will probably do more harm than good by further restricting breathing that is already impaired. Aside from oxygen, the only treatment is rapid evacuation.

Cardiac tamponade

Since the heart is enclosed in a tough sack called the pericardium (Greek *peri* "around" *kardia* "heart"), any bleeding inside the sack will compress the heart and reduce the amount of blood it can take in and pump out with each stroke. Cardiac tamponade (French *tampon* "to plug up") is usually caused by a penetrating injury such as a stab or gunshot wound that seals up, or a medical problem such as cancer. But it also may occur in a patient who has had a hard impact to the center of the chest that bruises the heart.

The pulse will become rapid and weak as the heart speeds up to compensate for reduced stroke volume. **Pulse pressure** (the difference between systolic and diastolic pressure) will **narrow** as systolic pressure decreases. Heart sounds will become **muffled**. Jugular veins will become **distended** from back pressure in blood returning to the compressed heart. This set of signs (narrowing pulse pressure, muffled heart sounds, and jugular vein distension) is called **Beck's triad**.

The most common cause of narrowing pulse pressure is loss of blood volume from severe bleeding or (indirectly) from severe dehydration. And jugular vein distension can also be caused by right heart failure. So muffled heart sounds is the distinguishing sign of cardiac tamponade.

The only specific treatment for cardiac tamponade is a paramedic level technique - draining the blood from the pericardium with a hollow needle. Aside from that, you should give oxygen if you have it and evacuate as rapidly as possible.

Abdominal injuries

Falls and impacts as well as penetrating wounds can also injure abdominal organs, some of which are unprotected by the ribs. **Solid, blood-filled organs**, especially the liver and spleen, can bleed enough when they are ruptured to send the patient quickly into shock. A blow to the upper abdomen, just below the rib notch, or a blow that fractures ribs on the lower right side of the chest, can rupture the liver. About 20% of patients with multiple rib fractures on the lower left side of the chest have ruptured spleens. The patient may feel referred pain in the left shoulder (Kerr's sign) because it irritates the diaphragm, whose phrenic nerve shares its origin with the supraclavicular nerve. If the kidneys are ruptured, the patient will probably feel lower back pain and may have blood in the urine.

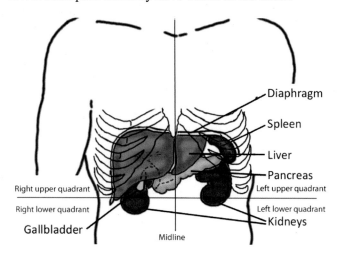

Hollow organs, such as the stomach, intestines, and bladder, may be full or empty. The stomach secretes digestive juices which are very irritating to the peritoneum, a membrane that surrounds the abdominal organs(Greek *tonos* "stretching" *peri* "around"); so rupture of the stomach causes severe pain.

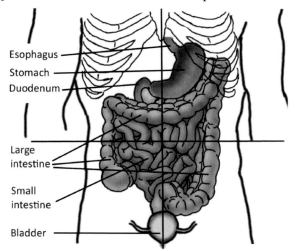

Ruptured intestines can release a semi-liquid mixture of food, enzymes, and bacteria that will cause inflammation. Usually the patient will feel a spreading pain and tenderness from the site of the injury, though at first the pain will not be as great as from a ruptured stomach. As the damaged intestines fill with gas and fluid, the whole abdomen may distend, and you may feel a guarding reaction - rigid abdominal muscles that the patient cannot relax. Blood may appear in the feces. If it is bright red, it is probably from hemorrhoids, but dark tarry blood that is partially digested suggests bleeding in the intestines or stomach.

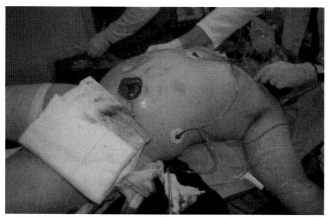

Abdominal injury with protruding intestine.
Photo courtesy of Ben Schifrin, MD

If the urinary bladder is full, it is much more likely to be ruptured by an impact, and it can also be detached from the urethra. This will prevent the patient from urinating. So empty the bladder before doing an activity in which a fall or collision is possible. The urinary bladder and the bowel can also be damaged in a pelvis fracture, either directly by the same impact or by broken bone ends in the pelvic girdle.

If you suspect abdominal injury, go to skin and check the sides and back as well as the abdomen for any bruising or abrasions. Also check carefully for lower rib or pelvis fractures. As with chest injuries, assess for spinal injuries and rule them out if possible.

Impaled objects

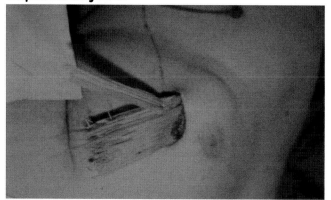

A piece of wood has penetrated the chest wall.
Photo courtesy of Ben Schifrin, MD

In medicine, an impaled object refers to something that penetrates into deeper tissues of the body or limbs, not just skin. Generally you need to immobilize an impaled object with bulky dressings, because trying to pull it out could cause more damage to internal organs as well as more serious bleeding. The only exception would be something going through the cheeks, which you should

pull out because it could compromise the airway, and protecting the airway is the highest priority.

Pelvic fracture

An impact to the pelvis from a fall or collision can fracture pelvic bones, which can then lacerate abdominal organs or blood vessels. The patient can lose several liters of blood internally, and show signs of hypovolemic shock. To control this blood loss, apply a pelvic sling, which goes around the pelvis between the iliac crests and the hip joints. The SAM Pelvic Sling shown in the photo below has a buckle that clicks when adequate force is applied, and prevents over-tightening (www.sammedical.com). Pull the orange and black webbing apart until you hear the click, then secure the webbing to the velcro.

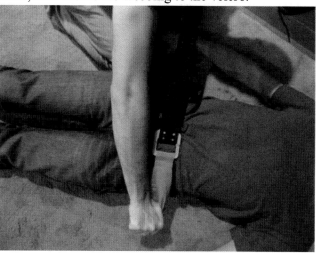

You can improvise a pelvic sling from a jacket or sheet. Wrap it around the pelvis (you may have to logroll the patient to get it underneath) and tie the ends together with a sturdy stick or pole in the knot, like an improvised tourniquet. Twist and secure the stick to apply pressure to the pelvis.

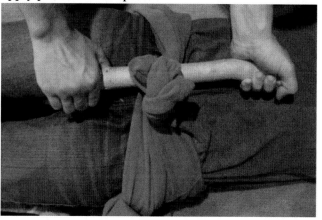

Chapter 13. Hyperthermia
How to beat the heat

Our cells process glucose for energy, but 75% of that energy is turned into heat. If we do not get rid of the excess heat fast enough, it cooks the brain and other vital organs. How does the body dump excess heat? First, the blood must carry heat from the vital organs and muscles to the skin. Fluid flowing from a heat source to cooler surroundings is a very efficient heat transfer mechanism. But blood is also needed in the organs and muscles to deliver oxygen and nutrients. Hot weather requires the circulatory system to do two conflicting jobs, especially if physical activity is increasing the demand for the blood to deliver oxygen and nutrients to working muscles.

Once blood moves heat to the skin, the heat can be lost in four ways: radiation, convection, conduction, and evaporation. But the first three mechanisms only work if the skin is warmer than its surroundings. On a hot, sunny day, the body will actually gain heat by radiation. Only a cool wind will carry heat away by convection, and conduction removes heat only if the body is in contact with something cooler. When air temperature is as high as skin temperature (normally no more than 93° F), evaporation of sweat is the main way that the body can lose heat. You can also lose heat by breathing, which is a combination of convection and evaporation with the breath moving like a wind in and out of the lungs, and water vapor evaporating as you exhale it. Furry animals like dogs, (with no sweat glands under the fur) cool themselves by panting with their moist tongues hanging out.

Water and salt

An **acclimatized** person who is working hard in warm surroundings can sweat up to 3 liters per hour. At that rate, it doesn't take long to get dehydrated. About 60% of the body is water – say 40 liters in a 150-pound (66.6 kilogram) male. But fluid for the sweat glands is supplied by the circulatory system, and only about 3 liters of this water is normally in the blood - the rest of the blood is made up of solids such as red and white blood cells. After losing 3% to 5% of the body's water (1 or 2 liters), which depletes blood volume, the circulatory system stops shunting extra blood to the skin because circulation to vital organs is more critical. When this happens, sweating does little good, because most excess heat is no longer getting to the surface.

Even if you are not acclimatized, you can sweat a liter or more per hour in hot weather, and up to 3 liters when you are acclimatized. You will also be losing water through your breath in dry air and from urination. So if you drink only when you are thirsty while exercising in hot weather, you are liable to get dehydrated. In one experiment with volunteers in the military, they did strenuous exercise in hot weather. Water was available but on average they did not drink until they had lost 2 liters, and when they drank they replaced only two-thirds of the water they had lost (voluntary dehydration).

In the Six Day War of 1967, over 20,000 Egyptian soldiers with no visible wounds died, many of them probably from heat illness and dehydration. But the Israeli army forced solders to drink water and lost almost none to heat illness. In the Gulf War, the American armed forces emulated the Israelis: medics and sergeants regularly ordered soldiers to drink water (11 to 19 liters per day). This regimen seems to have worked, because while there were cases of heat illness, no one died from it.

Conditions in the Arabian desert are extreme (summer temperatures over 120° F), but heat illness is possible at temperatures down to 70° F in people who are exercising or working hard. Also, people working inside industrial structures, or wearing heavy protective clothing (as fire fighters do), may be in a microclimate even hotter and more dehydrating than the Arabian desert. For such conditions, you should drink one cup (one-fourth liter) of water every 20 minutes if possible.

Another extreme condition is exposure to hot weather in an open boat or life raft. When the crew of HMS Bounty mutinied in 1789, they put Captain Bligh and the loyal members of his crew in an open boat. Bligh navigated his overcrowded boat nearly 4,000 miles in hot, tropical weather with almost no water except what they could capture from rainfall. His crew survived, because he had them soak their clothing in seawater. Evaporation of water from their clothes cooled them and conserved sweat. In 1951, the Royal Navy tested this procedure in life rafts. They found that it increased expected survival time in the tropics, with no fresh water, from a few days to several weeks.

Usually, about half a liter is as much as you can comfortably drink at once. Also, it takes time for water to pass out of the stomach (gastric emptying) and be absorbed by the intestine. In an average adult, about 1.2 liters of water per hour can be absorbed, and 3 liters per hour is as much as the stomach can tolerate (the gastric nausea threshold). This makes it hard to catch up with water loss after becoming dehydrated. So you should begin drinking water before you start exercising in the heat.

A little flavoring may make the water more palatable, especially if it is heavily chlorinated or treated with iodine. Also, cool water (50° F) is absorbed faster than warm water. Coffee and regular tea should be avoided because the caffeine in them is a diuretic. It increases water loss through urination. Alcohol also dehydrates by increasing urination.

Sweat and urine contain sodium and potassium. These are electrolytes that control the movement of water in and out of the body's cells. Most American diets, however, include up to 10 times as much sodium, from salt, as the body needs; and acclimatizing to heat reduces sodium loss tenfold. Therefore, sodium loss is seldom a problem, unless you are sweating copiously or not acclimatized to the heat.

But acclimatizing to heat does not conserve potassium, which is found in many foods that were part of the diet throughout human evolution (nuts and many fruits), whereas salt was often scarce. When you're both losing and drinking a lot of water, however, you need to maintain your electrolyte balance with electrolyte drink or salty snacks (such as trail mix) Otherwise, you can suffer water intoxication, also called **hyponatremia** ("too little salt"), in which water cannot cross cell membranes. An electrolyte imbalance can also cause **heat cramps**.

You can make your own electrolyte mixture to add to your water. For each liter, mix 1/2 teaspoon salt (sodium chloride), 1/2 teaspoon baking soda (sodium bicarbonate), 1/4 teaspoon salt substitute (potassium chloride), and sugar or honey to taste. Alternate this drink with equal amounts of plain water.

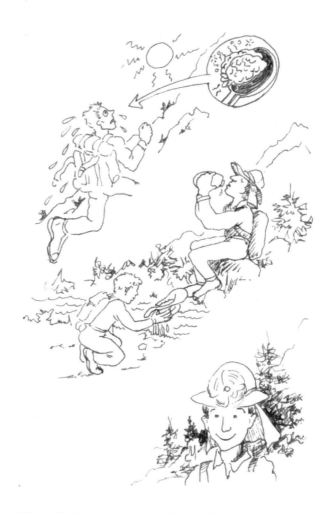

The climber at the top is overheating and getting dehydrated. At the stream, one hiker is hydrating and the other is wetting his hat to cool his head by evaporation. The bottom hiker has a solar-powered fan in his hat.

Cool heads: Dressing for the heat

The brain has its own cooling system using blood vessels that pass through the skull to connect with circulation in the face. Blood picks up heat from the brain and carries it to the skin where it can be dissipated. Wearing a hat with a brim helps this cooling system by shading the face, and a bandanna hanging from the back of the hat can shade the neck. Keeping the hat wet also cools the head by evaporation. A more high-tech solution is a fan built into the hat in front, powered by a solar battery on top. This style of hat is sold by some outdoor and industrial clothing companies.

Loose clothing with an open weave lets air circulate around the skin, cooling by convection. The

Bedouin and other dwellers in the world's hottest deserts wear seemingly heavy robes with cowls. But the layers are loose, so that they allow airflow around the skin. Cotton is comfortable against the skin when it is dry, but it absorbs up to 100% of its weight in water, and then becomes a vapor barrier, preventing your sweat from evaporating through the fabric. So it is not a good choice for vigorous activity in hot (or cold) weather. Also, when cotton is soaking wet from your sweat, it becomes transparent to ultraviolet radiation, so it provides no protection against sunburn. Most sports clothing for vigorous activity is made of synthetic fabrics such as polyester knit, which absorbs only 1% to 2% of its weight in water and dries quickly. So sweat evaporates through the pores (along with your excess heat) instead of saturating the fabric.

Exposing as much skin area as possible maximizes cooling by evaporation, but increases the risk of sunburn, which can shut down the sweat glands. A good sunscreen should prevent sunburn by absorbing the energy of ultraviolet radiation that penetrates the skin. Sunscreen should be applied liberally an hour or so before exposure, so that it can bond to the outer layer of the skin. Also it must be renewed frequently. For sensitive areas, such as the face, you may need a sun block that reflects ultraviolet radiation. Heavily pigmented skin gives more protection from ultraviolet radiation, which causes sunburn, but absorbs up to 20% more heat than light skin.

Heat production and heat loss

How much heat does your body produce, and how much can your sweat dissipate? At rest, a man of average size might produce about 60 kilocalories (kcal) of heat per hour. On a hot day, a seminude person at rest could gain up to 250 more kcal per hour from exposure to the sun, and a clothed person up to 100 kcal per hour (solar load). One kcal will heat one liter of water 1° C (2.2° F). During vigorous and sustained exercise, heat production can be multiplied up to 6 times in a fit person, and up to 10 times in an athlete. If heat production is multiplied 6 times, then an average sized man will be producing 360 kcal of heat per hour. If we assume that the man has 40 liters of water in his body, disregarding the solids, the heat will raise the temperature of the water by 9° C (16.2° F). That would be more than enough heat to broil the victim slowly in

his own fluids, though he would have collapsed long before driving his body temperature so high.

Evaporating one liter of sweat from the skin will take away about 580 Kilocalories of heat. But first the circulatory system needs to carry the heat from the organs and working muscles that produce it to the skin, as well as supplying the sweat glands with water. Blood vessels under the skin can increase their blood flow 10 times. If you are dehydrated, however, your blood volume will be reduced. The circulatory system may not be able to spare enough blood from the vital organs to move heat to the skin or to deliver enough water to replenish the sweat glands.

Sweat can only take heat away from the skin if it evaporates. In very dry air, sweat evaporates insensibly. If water vapor is already in the air, however, it exerts vapor pressure, which resists the evaporation of sweat. Rate of evaporation is proportional to the difference between the vapor pressure of the liquid sweat and the vapor pressure of the surrounding air. If the air is already saturated with all the water vapor it can hold at its present temperature, no sweat can evaporate. It just pools and drips off the skin, not cooling the body. Even at 70% relative humidity (70% of maximum water vapor saturation in the air), sweating is ineffective. So the more humid the air, the lower the temperature at which heat risk begins, especially if you are generating heat with vigorous activity.

Clothing that absorbs sweat also prevents it from dissipating heat by evaporating. Finally, you have only so much skin surface, and even if it is all bared (risking sunburn) you could evaporate about 1.2 liters per hour of sweat at most, no matter how much was pouring off you. That would get rid of about 700 Kilocalories of heat. But heat loss by evaporation of sweat seldom reaches its optimum level because of all the limiting factors. So you should reduce heat risk whenever you can by getting out of the heat when you are resting, sitting, or lying down comfortably to ease the stress on the circulatory system.

Heat risk factors

Some people have risk factors for heat intolerance, or conditions that predispose them to heat illness. Risk factors include being over 50, obese, fatigued, out of condition, or un-acclimatized to heat. Prior heat illness or recent fever may also handicap response to heat. Many medical conditions can predispose to heat illness. For example, cardiovascular illness and diabetes weaken the circulatory system, and thus reduce its ability to cope with heat. Malaria (prickly heat) or healed burns impair sweating. Some drugs also increase the risk of heat illness. Diuretics ("flowing through") including alcohol and caffeine increase fluid loss through urination, and blood volume is reduced with dehydration. Thyroid hormone, amphetamines, cocaine, and trycliclic antidepressants increase heat production. Antihistamines and some medications prescribed for psychiatric problems reduce sweating.

Heat syncope

Even standing in the heat can cause fainting (heat syncope), because blood is drawn to the skin and pools in the legs, reducing blood pressure and cardiac output. Heat syncope is usually relieved by getting in the shade and lying down.

Heat cramps

A sodium deficiency in exercising muscles can cause heat cramps. This means a few muscle fibers at a time will spasm one to three minutes so that the cramp seems to move over the muscle. Heat cramps are usually relieved by an electrolyte drink. It also helps to stretch out the cramping muscle.

Heat exhaustion

Exercising in the heat can cause dehydration and collapse (heat exhaustion) if it overloads the circulatory system. In heat exhaustion, the body core temperature may be normal or a few degrees high. The patient will usually be sweating profusely. Severe dehydration can reduce blood volume, which will make the pulse rapid and weak. Symptoms of heat exhaustion may include headache, faintness, confusion, and nausea, all related to poor blood supply in vital organs from a stressed circulatory system. Treatment is to move the patient out of the heat and gradually rehydrate, adding electrolytes if plain water doesn't improve the patient's condition. If there is no shade, placing wet cloths on the head and neck can help prevent the patient from overheating.

Hyponatremia ("too little salt")

Patients who have been sweating copiously and drinking water regularly to replace it, but not taking in any electrolytes, may have water intoxication, called hyoponatremia. The symptoms are confusingly similar to those of heat exhaustion. Cases of hyponatremia have been reported in endurance athletes, such as Grand Canyon hikers and marathon runners, who were drinking plenty of water but either not eating anything or just eating candy. So if you find someone with these symptoms in hot weather, ask what the patient has been drinking and eating. Also, victims of hyponatremia will urinating regularly, and the urine will be clear; whereas if victims of heat exhaustion are urinating at all, it will be dark yellow or orange.

Heat stroke

If the body core temperature goes up past about 106° F (41° C), the temperature control system fails (heat stroke). Cell membranes leak and sodium ions accumulate inside, stimulating an increase in heat production. Since chemical reactions speed up when temperature increases, heat production in the cells increases, which creates a vicious circle of further heat stress. As fluid leaks into the tissues, less blood goes back to the heart, and the shortage of blood to the intestines and other organs causes damage.

Classic heat stroke (CHS), the slow cooker, may take days to develop. It usually afflicts the elderly unable to get out of the heat. However, even healthy athletes can generate enough heat from exercise to go into exertional heat stroke or EHS (the fast cooker) in as little as 15 minutes. More often than not, EHS victims will still be sweating profusely, with a rapid and bounding pulse. So the appearance of the skin is not a reliable way to distinguish heat stroke from heat exhaustion.

Behavior changes drastically in EHS, and is a more reliable way to distinguish it from heat exhaustion. Patients often become irrational, and sometimes aggressive. They may also have seizures, and if not cooled, go into a coma. The longer coma lasts, the less chance of survival.

Besides watching for behavior changes, the only other reliable way to distinguish heat stroke from heat exhaustion is by the temperature of vital organs. But even a rectal temperature may not be the same as the temperature in the liver, and the brain may be several degrees cooler than the liver. Also, a conscious heat stroke patient is unlikely to cooperate. So in most situations, you will probably have to rely on behavior changes to warn you of heat stroke. When in doubt, cool the patient.

As behavior changes signal possible damage to the brain, tissues in other vital organs also begin to bleed and swell, including the bowels, and eventually the kidneys and liver. The number of platelets in the blood (the circulatory system's materials for stopping leaks) goes down. As temperature in the body continues to increase, cells are destroyed. Fats liquefy and proteins coagulate. Fluid often accumulates in the lungs (pulmonary edema). In pilgrimages to Mecca, 23% of those treated for heat illness, and 58% of those who died from it, had pulmonary edema. So it is important to cool a heat stroke patient quickly.

Cooling

Ice baths cool a patient about 0.3° F (0.17° C) per minute, but take a lot of ice, usually over 80 pounds. Cool water baths at 59° F (15° C) are just as effective if the water is stirred to prevent a warm layer from forming around the body. Monitor vital signs, including level of responsiveness (by talking to the patient), and be careful not to over-cool. Misting (aerosols driven by fans) is used on pilgrims to Mecca. The water droplets act as artificial sweat, cooling the patient by evaporating from the skin. However, this method may not be so effective in a climate where humidity is high. Ice bags in towels against the big veins in the groin, armpit, and the sides of the neck, plus fanning and sponging, will also cool though not nearly as fast as immersion. Do not, however, use alcohol for cooling the skin. It can be absorbed into the blood causing alcohol intoxication.

Acclimatizing

Endurance training helps prepare you for heat stress, because even in cool weather, sustained aerobic exercise can generate enough heat to raise the body core temperature and stimulate some acclimatization. However, full acclimatization requires exercise in a hot environment. The body adapts to repeated heat stress in two ways. First, it becomes more efficient so that the metabolic cost of work and the heat produced by it are lower. Second, it improves heat loss mechanisms.

With aerobic conditioning, the heart pumps more blood with each stroke, so that it needs fewer contractions to move the same amount of blood. Sweating starts earlier when you are aerobically conditioned or acclimatized; and the maximum amount of sweat per hour increases to 3 liters or more. Also, the sweat glands and kidneys conserve sodium, losing only a tenth as much in sweat and urine. If your sweat no longer stings your eyes and tastes bland, you are probably either in good aerobic condition or at least partly acclimatized.

Also, veterans of the heat are usually more aware of how much water they need to drink, as well as more adept at getting out of the heat and minimizing its stress whenever they can.

Reducing the body temperature before heat exposure also enables you to tolerate the same level of heat stress for a longer time, because it will take longer for the body to overheat. Veghte and Webb demonstrated this in 1960 by pre-cooling subjects with cold air or cold water immersion. This experiment was suggested by the way that camels survive heat exposure without water. Their body temperature drops as much as 11° F (over 6° C) during the cold desert night, and it takes a long time for their chilled body mass to reheat during the day. While humans cannot function at such a low body temperature, cooling the body a few degrees Fahrenheit with a cold shower or immersion when you are in danger of over-heating does seem to extend heat tolerance.

Conclusion

Even if you are acclimatized to heat, you need to know how much fluid you are losing to the heat and you must replace it. You should be able to assess heat hazard, and protect yourself against it. You should also know the risk factors and predisposing conditions for heat illness, recognize the early signs and symptoms, and know what to do about them. With knowledge, preparation, fluid replacement, and prompt emergency care, heat casualties in warm weather activities can be avoided.

Chapter 14. Hypothermia
Exposure, immersion, and drowning

If you are losing heat faster than you can produce it, then your body temperature will start to drop. This is called hypothermia (Greek *hypo* "under" *thermia* "heat"). Animals such as snakes and lizards are called poikilotherms (Greek *poikilos* "varied") because their body temperatures vary with the temperature of their surroundings. They can tolerate considerable heat loss and change in their body temperature. When they get too hot, they look for shade or go below ground. When they get chilled, they seek a heat source or a sheltered place where they can survive until their surroundings warm up enough to revive them. Their blood chemistry adjusts with temperature change to keep their metabolism in balance.

Humans are homeotherms (Greek *homoios* "like or similar") meaning that they have evolved to keep their body temperatures within a narrow range where their vital processes work most efficiently: between about 96° and 102° F. The disadvantage is that if a homeotherm's body core temperature drops below the optimum range, vital functions are impaired. Below about 86°F core temperature, humans become poikilothermic, which means that their temperature is no longer regulated from within. Unlike lizards, we are not evolved to survive this experience without help.

Internal climate

Within the human body, the temperature normally varies by several degrees F depending on the time of day. For most people, metabolism and body core temperature peak in mid or late afternoon, and are at their lowest a few hours after midnight.

Temperature inside the body also varies from the core of vital organs to the shell of fat and muscle. While the liver may be 101° F, resting muscles will usually be several degrees cooler, and the skin temperature in cold surroundings may be 70° F. As a result, you would get different readings on a thermometer depending on where you took the temperature. A rectal temperature would be several degrees higher than an oral temperature. In cold weather, the temperature of the body core is most critical, because vital organs, especially the brain,

rapidly get less efficient when they are chilled. For this reason, hypothermia has probably caused many more accidents and deaths in the wilderness than accident statistics suggest.

The range of air temperatures in which the body's heat loss balances resting heat production is called the thermoneutral zone (TNZ). In air, it is 82°-93° F; in water about 91.4° F. When you start exercising, your heat production increases, so the range of comfortable air temperatures drops. In the TNZ, it is easy for the body to maintain its core temperature. Human bodies can function unprotected in somewhat colder surroundings by generating more heat and withdrawing warm blood from the skin, but to survive very long at air temperatures below 70° F (or in water below 77° F), most humans need to create a microclimate with clothing and to keep that microclimate in the TNZ.

As heat production increases with muscular activity, clothing must be opened up or layers removed. This will dissipate heat by convection and allow sweat both to evaporate and escape. Even in the TNZ, humans can sweat insensibly. If clothing absorbs sweat or blocks its escape as water vapor, humidity in the microclimate increases, which inhibits evaporation of sweat. Overheating triggers more sweating, increasing dehydration. Severe dehydration reduces the volume of circulating blood, and good circulation is essential for resisting the cold.

Size and shape

Body size, shape, and composition also affect cold resistance and survival, as do health and fitness. Heat loss depends on the surface area of the skin, which increases roughly as the square of the height. Heat production depends on the volume of lean body tissue, which increases as the cube of height. Big people, therefore, have an advantage over small people in cold weather, because their ratio of heat-producing tissue to skin area is higher.

For example, a 3-foot child will generally lose heat at least twice as fast as a 6-foot adult; a 1-foot tall infant at least 4 times as fast. Smaller people also transfer heat faster by conduction from the core to the

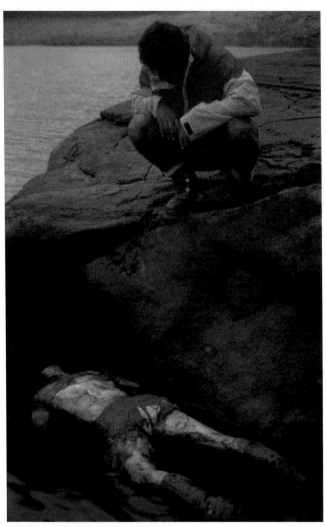

Victim who died of hypothermia
Photo courtesy of Ben Schifrin, MD

skin, because their organs and muscles are closer to the surface. A rounded shape with small hands and feet (typical of Eskimos) helps conserve heat. However, a lean, fit person may compensate for the lack of insulating fat by greater heat-producing activity, so long as the muscles have enough fuel.

Elderly people tend to have less lean muscle mass to produce heat and weak circulatory systems. As a result, their body temperatures may be below average even before exposure. They are more likely to have chronic diseases, or to be taking medications that can interfere with heat production or with temperature regulation. They also may not sense the cold as well as younger people and often fail to shiver.

All of these factors should be at the back of your mind when assessing a possible hypothermia patient. You should know the effects of cold on each vital system, not only to help detect hypothermia, but also to recognize when other things may be going on, such as illness, injury, or drug overdose.

Hypothermia and the brain

Chilling progressively affects all brain functions, including temperature regulation. For every degree Fahrenheit that brain temperature drops, cerebral metabolism decreases 3.3-3.9%. This can increase brain survival time without oxygen up to 1 hour, but it soon makes a patient incapable of self-care. Down to about 90° F, neurons become hyper-excitable, and reflexes are more easily triggered than normally. This does not mean, however, that cooling makes brain and spinal cord functions more efficient. Below 95° F brain temperature, memory and concentration are impaired, thinking slows down, and auditory or visual hallucinations are possible. Speech becomes slurred and increasingly difficult. Fine coordination (especially of the fingers) deteriorates.

Hypothermics often lose emotional expression (flat affect). Even mild hypothermia can bring out and exaggerate pre-existing behavioral problems, such as anxiety, poor judgment, or psychosis (living in a separate reality). This situation is especially alarming in someone with leadership responsibility.

As the core temperature falls below 90° F, neurons become less and less excitable, and reflexes get more and more sluggish. Muscle strength also declines. Usually the knee jerk reflex is the last to go and the first to come back with rewarming. Voluntary movements are slowed, and the patient has serious problems with coordination and balance. A patient who is still conscious at an 86° F core temperature may take 15-30 seconds to touch the nose. Pupils become dilated and eye movement may be uncoordinated (i.e., the patient becomes cross-eyed). In an unresponsive hypothermic, pupil response to light will be so slow that you may miss it.

Breathing and circulation

In the early stages of hypothermia when the body core temperature is 95°-90° F, breathing speeds up. Pugh's experiments on humans in an environmental chamber showed that a 1.1° F drop in body core temperature increases oxygen consumption, even while resting, by 360%. Also, subjects chilled by about that amount used half again as much oxygen to do the same amount of

114

work as those who were not chilled. Metabolism in cold tissues, including muscles, is less efficient.

Because blood vessels in the limbs constrict to conserve heat (peripheral vasoconstriction), muscles and nerves in the limbs get less circulation and chill even more rapidly than the body core. At high altitude, where one begins with less oxygen per lung-full, hypothermia can come on much more quickly and be harder to treat. Because of changes in blood chemistry as body temperature drops, hemoglobin does not release oxygen as easily to the tissues.

As body temperature drops below 90° F, however, the hypothalamus no longer responds to carbon dioxide (CO_2) as a trigger for breathing, so breathing slows, and CO_2 accumulates in the blood. If breathing paradoxically speeds up in deep hypothermia, the patient may be a diabetic, have high blood alcohol from drinking, or have a brain injury. Often the breath of a hypothermic has a fruity (acetone) odor, like that of a diabetic who forgot to take insulin, because of incomplete metabolism of fats. Mucus secretion increases and may clog air passages. The patient may become nauseated, so you need to be alert to prevent the aspiration of vomit.

Although the pulse usually speeds up slightly as body temperature begins to drop, it soon slows down, sometimes to one-half of its normal rate, because the chilled heart pumps more slowly. It also pumps less with each stroke, so a hypothermic patient's pulse is hard to find, especially in the limbs, where circulation is reduced by peripheral vasoconstriction. If the pulse remains rapid, then something else is going on (e.g., drug overdose, hypoglycemia, or hypovolemic shock).

Another problem that can occur in deep hypothermia is embolism or blood clots because cold and thickened blood clots more easily. Water moves from blood to the tissues and can reduce blood volume as much as 25%. Cold suppresses the thirst sensation, so dehydration from increased urination and the failure to drink water can further reduce blood volume.

Digestion and metabolism

Even when a person is at rest, heat production is increased by cold stress, so long as the cells have enough fuel, water, and oxygen and body temperature remains normal. At lower blood temperatures, however, it is harder for glucose to cross cell membranes, less insulin is released by the pancreas (which is slowed down by cold like other vital organs), and cells become insulin resistant. Glucose may then accumulate in the blood (hyperglycemia) or be excreted in urine. Also, chilled kidneys cannot concentrate urine, so increased urination dehydrates the body. This is called cold weather diuresis ("flowing through"). Urine-soaked clothing is common in cases of profound hypothermia.

Metabolism slows down, so the body produces less heat. At 82.4° F, heat production will be only one-half of normal. Below about 90° F, the gastrointestinal system stops functioning, which means that no new fuel goes into the blood from food. There will be no bowel sounds, and the abdominal muscles may be rigid. You should still, however, try to rule out injuries or illnesses that also cause guarding or rigidity of the abdomen, in case their signs are masked by hypothermia.

It is dangerous to give drugs to hypothermics, because the chilled liver metabolizes them more slowly, so the drugs stay in the system longer. Their effects are also exaggerated as the metabolism slows. What would be a normal dose at normal body temperature becomes an overdose to a hypothermic.

Alcohol, which increases the risk of hypothermia, reduces the chances of survival in several ways. First, it impairs judgment and concentration. Second, it gives an illusory sense of warmth by dilating blood vessels near the skin, which suppresses shivering and may increase heat loss. Third, it seems to act directly on the temperature regulation center and turn the body's thermostat down, reducing heat production. Fourth, alcohol can double urinary output, which is already increased by exposure to cold, thus dehydrating the patient much more rapidly.

Other drugs that increase the risk of hypothermia are barbiturates (sedatives), which slow down metabolism and reduce core temperature; narcotics, which reduce body temperature; and phenothiazines (used to treat psychiatric problems), which suppress the heat regulation center. Carbon monoxide (from driving a vehicle with an exhaust leak or cooking in a tent) increases hypothermia risk, because it reduces the oxygen-carrying capacity of the blood.

Diabetes or hypothyroidism can also reduce heat production. A stroke can affect the temperature regulation center in the hypothalamus. Some signs of stroke (e.g., slurred speech) may mimic those of hypothermia.

All of these possibilities suggest questions to ask a responsive patient after doing urgent first aid and evacuating to a warm environment. If hypothermia is secondary to an illness, medication side effects, or injury, then the cause must be treated.

Treatment

Patients who are still alert, shivering, and coordinated should be able to restore their own body temperatures to normal if their heat loss is reduced by shelter and warm, dry clothing. Also, their heat production can be increased by re-hydration and energy food. Even patients who are confused and uncoordinated may respond to passive rewarming, if they are in a warm environment. In the field, however, when rapid evacuation is not possible, you may need to add heat.

Warmed, humidified oxygen delivered by mask will rewarm a shivering patient slowly, but probably be ineffective on a patient who is too cold and unresponsive to shiver. Dry and unwarmed oxygen will cool the patient even more.

Heat packs (carefully wrapped to prevent burning) can warm blood going to the brain and other vital organs, if placed against the sides of the neck and in the armpits. Skin to skin warming should only be to the upper body, and the sleeping bag should be pre-warmed before putting the patient in it. Never massage a hypothermic. Warming the skin can suppress shivering, and stimulating circulation in the limbs would return cold, acidotic blood to the heart.

In the hospital, rewarming techniques may include procedures such as forced heated air under an insulated blanket (shown in the photo) and immersing the body in warm water. Since 1970, the Danish Navy has rewarmed hypothermic sailors by immersing their arms and legs in warm water, which warms the blood in the limbs before it returns to the heart. These techniques usually rewarm the patient fast enough to avoid afterdrop, which is a sudden drop in the temperature of the heart when chilled blood from the arms and legs returns. With slower and less effective rewarming methods, afterdrops of up to 9° F (5° C) have been measured.

Hypothermics must be handled gently, especially if they are cold enough to be stiff and unresponsive. Heart tissue becomes very irritable when chilled, so jarring or rough handling, as well as exertion, can trigger ventricular fibrillation. This is a condition in which the heart muscle fibers twitch irregularly so that the heart does not pump blood.

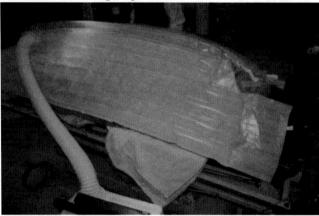

Rewarming in the hospital
Photo courtesy of Ben Schifrin, MD

A patient in profound hypothermia (stiff and unresponsive) cannot be rewarmed with the resources you will have in the wilderness. The most you can achieve is to reduce or prevent further heat loss with a hypothermia wrap and arrange for an evacuation:

- Carefully strip off wet clothes (or cut them off if necessary to avoid jostling the patient).
- Dress the patient in dry clothes.
- Lay several foam pads and a pre-warmed sleeping bag on a tarp.
- Gently slide the patient into a sleeping bag and cover the head.
- Wrap the tarp around the bag.

CPR on hypothermic patients is rarely successful without rapid transport to an emergency department, and at a core temperature of 86° F or less, the heart is unlikely to respond to electrical defibrillation. Patients in profound hypothermia should be evacuated immediately to a hospital equipped for rewarming as well as advanced life support. In addition to ventricular fibrillation and embolisms, rewarming complications may include pneumonia from aspiration of mucus or vomit, and damage to the pancreas.

A Night in the snow

On Friday, December 29, 1978, two sisters in their 20's went cross-country skiing on the Forest Service trails at Pinecrest, California. They started at 2 p.m., leaving their parkas and survival gear in their jeep.

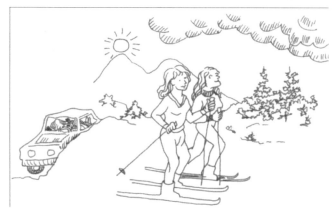

On the way back, they got lost. Windy blowing snow made it hard to see, and the deep snow pack covered many landmarks, including the STOP sign at the turnoff to the trailhead. As it began to get dark, they dug holes in a snow bank with their bare hands and tried to keep each other awake. The temperature dropped to 13° F that night. Ironically, they were only a mile from Dodge Ridge ski resort and less than a mile from their car.

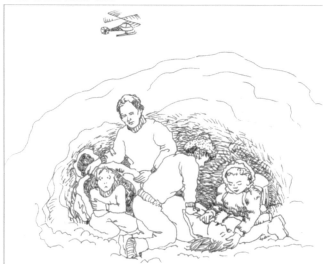

At 10:30 Saturday morning, three skiers (who were patrolling the trails for the Forest Service) found one of the sisters awake and the other stiff and unresponsive with no perceptible vital signs. One of them was a member of the National Ski Patrol. They performed CPR on the unresponsive one for 3 hours, until she and her sister were loaded onto a Medi Flight helicopter and taken to Doctor's Hospital in Modesto, California.

On arrival, the unresponsive sister had a core temperature of 68° F, and her blood was crystalline. She remained comatose for five days but recovered with no neurological damage. According to Dr. McMillan (who treated the sisters), this was the only known case of a non-immersion patient in deep hypothermia surviving after 3 hours of CPR. The other sister was treated for frostbite.

Ben Schifrin (then a paramedic on the Tuolumne County Search and Rescue Team that evacuated the sisters) said, "They did absolutely everything wrong. They were wearing the wrong type of clothing, and they had no hats on when found. They didn't know the area and didn't have a map or trail guide. They should have been on their way back at the time they were leaving. They didn't notify anyone that they had gone on a cross-country tour."

Yet they did survive, thanks to a strenuous rescue and intensive medical care for the comatose sister. So what did the rescuers do right? According to Dr. Schifrin (who now practices emergency medicine at the Valley Medical Center in California), the hypothermic sister may have had a pulse that was too faint to palpate. But once the rescuers started CPR, they continued without interruption until she was loaded onto the helicopter with life support equipment. They were able to do sustained CPR because they were fresh, properly clothed for the weather, and close to the trailhead. Also, there were three of them, so they could relieve each other before they became exhausted.

Members of the National Ski Patrol are all trained in CPR as well as Outdoor Emergency Care. While they may not do CPR in the snow very often, they probably prevent many emergencies by finding and helping skiers who are getting cold, dehydrated or lost.

Immersion hypothermia

In cold water, we lose heat much faster than in air, because water conducts heat 25 times as fast as air and has a huge heat capacity. The top three meters of the oceans can hold as much heat as the entire atmosphere of the earth. Body shape and composition, however, make much more difference in water than in cold air. Seals, walruses, and whales are insulated with a thick layer of blubber. At 48° F water temperature, an unprotected lean survivor will lose heat about 100 times as fast as in equally cold air, and up to 9 times as fast as a fat survivor in water. A wet suit or dry suit will reduce heat loss considerably by reducing heat loss from convection – cold water pushing away warmed water or air around the skin. Personal flotation devices (PFD) also help keep you warmer in water, because they have a layer of insulating foam and keep your head out of the water. But without a flotation device, you will lose the ability to keep your head above water and drown long before you could die of hypothermia.

If you are wearing a PFD, you can conserve heat by doubling up and grasping your knees, or huddling with other survivors; but getting even part of your body out of the cold water by climbing onto floating wreckage is much more efficient.

Immersion in water colder than about 60° F causes changes in breathing and circulation, as the body reacts to the sudden loss of heat (**cold shock response**). First, there is usually a reflex gasp, which may cause you to aspirate water. Then for several minutes, hyperventilation (up to five times normal) flushes out CO_2. Hyperventilation can cause confusion and muscle rigidity, and it decreases underwater breath-holding time (from 60 to 20 seconds in one experiment). This means less chance of survival in rough water or of escape from a submerged vehicle.

However, after the first few minutes of immersion, breathing slows to a rate and volume just sufficient to maintain metabolism. Systolic blood pressure rises: in one experiment from 130 to 180-190 for most of a two-hour immersion in 50° F water. Pulse rate will increase for the first few minutes, then slow down. Blood vessels near the surface dilate, probably because their muscular sheaths are paralyzed by cold, which may increase the rate of heat loss.

All of your muscles will get weaker and less efficient as they are chilled, so you may not be able to swim more than 15 minutes without protection in cold water. Even wearing a PFD, the average person can swim only about half a mile in 50°F water. Soon you may not have enough strength left to grip anything or climb out of the water (**cold incapacitation**).

Victims of immersion hypothermia should be pulled out of the water horizontally if possible and never be allowed to get up and walk. Blood pressure usually drops when someone emerges from cold water, and the effect is aggravated by standing and walking.

Some reports tell of shipwreck survivors who were able to climb out of the water, then collapsed and died.

Submersion and drowning

Reactions to immersion in cold water increase the risk of drowning: loss of decision making ability as the brain is chilled; weakening of chilled muscles; and aspiration of water from the reflex gasp. Aspirating even a small amount of water can cause a laryngospasm – a reflexive constriction of the larynx – that normally keeps water out of the lungs, but also prevents breathing. If the laryngospasm does not release until the victim becomes unconscious, then (without a PFD) that victim will usually aspirate water and sink, because buoyancy depends on the amount of air in the lungs, as well as body fat and clothing.

Salt water is hypertonic (more saline than the body's fluids), so aspirated sea water draws fluid into the lungs by osmosis; and aspirated fresh water will be absorbed into the blood stream by osmosis, because it is hypotonic (less saline). But any aspirated liquid disrupts the surfactants that help keep the alveoli in the lungs open; and the more alveoli collapse, the less oxygen exchange surface remains in the lungs. Aspirated water can also have delayed effects on a drowning victim who has been revived, especially if the water was polluted – acute respiratory distress syndrome (ARDS), or secondary drowning. So after a wilderness water rescue, any drowning victim who survived the experience should be evacuated - even one who seems fully recovered.

While it is possible to attempt rescue breathing on a drowning victim in the water, it is better to remove the victim from the water before starting any resuscitation attempts. The classic mantra for water rescue is: reach; throw; row; go. Reach from land with something the victim can grab if possible. Throw a rope or floatation device to a victim too far to reach. If that is not possible, approach the victim in a boat. Swimming to the victim with a floatation device or rope is the last resort, and should only be attempted by those trained in water rescue, especially in swift water and other dangerous conditions. If you are caught in swift water, try to turn on your back with your feet downstream so that your legs (and not your head) can absorb the impact of any collisions.

Once the victim is out of the water, check the airway, give oxygen if available, and do CPR if necessary (following the ABC sequence, not CAB since a drowning patient will almost certainly be hypoxic). While techniques for draining water out of the lungs (including the Heimlich maneuver) are no longer recommended, about 86% of drowning victims vomit during CPR (usually from swallowed water); so you must be prepared to turn the victim quickly onto the side (preferably the left side) and clear vomitus from the mouth and nose. Victims of warm water submersion who do not revive after 30 minutes of resuscitation are usually considered dead; but victims of cold water drowning have been revived after 60 minutes of submersion, so the same principle applies to them as to victims of hypothermia by exposure: not dead until warmed and dead.

CPR and hypothermia

Hamilton and Paton surveyed 37 mountain rescue teams, asking whether they would start CPR on hypothermics in the field. Interestingly, 28 teams (76%) said yes, but only if rapid evacuation was possible. But 5 teams (13%) said no, and 4 teams (11%) said probably not. Reasons given by all the teams for not doing CPR included:

* Death obvious   22
* Long downtime   9
* Risk to rescuers   6
* Long evacuation   6
* Too cold   4
* Leader says no   3
* Patient has pulse   6

In the example above [A night in the snow], the patient was not obviously dead. There was no lividity, there were no injuries, and the chest was compressible. There was no apparent risk to the rescuers. They were near the trailhead, so they anticipated a short evacuation. The morning temperatures were moderate, and there was no palpable pulse. Any of the mountain rescue teams that said, "Yes" to the survey would presumably have done CPR.

Would it have made any difference if they had not done CPR until the victim was in the hospital? A survey of hypothermia cases by Danzl, et.al., showed no significant difference in outcome (see the bibliography). Of 27 patients who were given CPR in the field, 9 survived (33%). Of 14 patients who were not given CPR until they arrived in the hospital, 6 survived (43%). Admittedly, the samples are small, but they suggest that a decision not to begin CPR on a hypothermic in the field is not a death sentence. Either way, the chance of survival is not good; but it is much better than the chance of someone in cardiac arrest on a city street, with a normal body temperature, who isn't defibrillated until an ambulance arrives.

Practical guidelines

What should you do if you find a hypothermic victim in the wilderness with no detectable vital signs? The above study supports a decision not to begin CPR on a hypothermic patient in the wilderness when it would be impractical to perform, or impossible to continue until the patient was in the hospital. Whether or not you begin CPR in the field, however, you should:

* Handle hypothermics gently, since a chilled heart is very irritable. If it is still beating, perhaps too faintly to produce a palpable pulse, rough handling (including chest compressions) can trigger ventricular fibrillation.
* Prevent further heat loss with a hypothermia wrap: dry clothes, head covering, sleeping bag, thick foam pad, and a tarp around it all. But do not try to re-warm an unresponsive hypothermic in the field.
* Intubate if you are trained and equipped to do so. It does not increase the risk of cardiac arrest in a hypothermic.
* Give oxygen if it is available.

Conclusion

Chilled patients who are still alert and coordinated (especially if they are shivering) can usually rewarm themselves by getting out of the wind, adding dry clothing, rehydrating, and munching energy food. Patients having problems with speech and coordination usually need to be protected from further heat loss in a sleeping bag, and (if they do not improve) rewarmed with well wrapped hot water bottles or body heat. Stiff and unresponsive patients, however, cannot usually be rewarmed in the field, so they need to be evacuated (and handled gently) while preventing further heat loss.

Chapter 15. Frostbite and Raynaud's disease

Photos courtesy of Ben Schifrin, MD

Napoleon's surgeon-in-chief, Larrey, recommended rubbing frostbitten flesh with snow or ice. His disastrous treatment was generally used for frostbite until 1956, when laboratory tests and clinical tests in Alaska showed that rapid rewarming in hot water was best. However, even if frostbite is properly thawed out, it can cause devastating damage and excruciating pain. You therefore need to know how frostbite occurs, and what factors increase the risk, so that you can protect yourself and others from it.

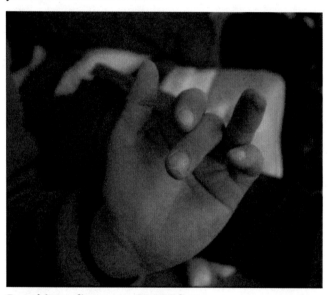

Frostbitten fingers at 21,000 feet

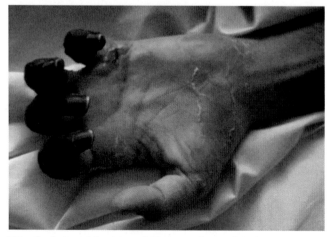

Weeks later, blackened tissues show the damage.

Reactions to cold

In cold surroundings, heat from underlying tissues warms the skin, so skin must be super-cooled below 25° F in order to freeze. As the skin cools, blood flow to it decreases, dropping to a tenth of normal in the hands and feet at 59° F. But skin temperatures below 59° F trigger a protective reaction called cold-induced vasodilation (CIVD), also called hunter's response. Blood vessels dilate at short intervals to bring surges of warm blood to the skin. People who grow up and work in cold climates, such as Inuit, Lapps, and Nordic fishermen, tend to have strong CIVDs.

If the body core temperature is dropping, however, or temperature in the exposed tissues drops to the 37°-50° F range, circulation withdraws from the surface and the extremities, because the vital organs have higher priority. Then temperature in the extremities can drop as rapidly as 1° F per minute.

Raynaud's disease

Some people have a negative circulatory response to cold – Raynaud's disease. Their circulatory systems withdraw blood from the extremities in cold weather even when the air temperature is well above freezing, which means that their hands and feet can easily go numb. In sub-freezing weather, they have no natural defenses against frostbite.

Any sudden drop in skin temperature can trigger Raynaud's disease in a susceptible person. Hands or feet turn pale as blood withdraws, and the victim may also feel tingling and numbness. It can happen in mild as well as cold weather. Circulatory problems and some drugs can bring it on, but the mechanism of primary Raynaud's disease, caused by cold or stress, is unknown.

Murray P. Hamlet, who ran the U.S. Army's Cold Research Division, developed and tested a simple procedure for treating primary Raynaud's disease, which reconditions the circulatory system to increase blood flow in the hands and feet when the body is exposed to cold. He claims to have a high success rate. You need a warm place and a cold place, with a tub of water, kept at 110° F, in each place. Dress lightly.

In the warm room, immerse your hands in the hot water for two to five minutes. Then wrap your hands in a towel, go to the cold area, and immerse your hands for ten minutes. Repeat the cycle three to six times on alternate days, for a total of about 50 trials. The reconditioning usually lasts for years and can be quickly restored if it lapses. Some mountaineers with normal circulatory response to cold try to improve it with this treatment before doing cold weather expeditions.

Freezing

We lose sensation at a skin temperature of about 50° F, so numb skin is not necessarily frozen. To test for actual freezing, dent the skin with your fingernail. If the skin remains dented like wax, it is frozen, but the frostbite is superficial. If the skin cannot be dented, then underlying tissues are also frozen. Some authorities recommend rewarming superficial frostbite in the field with body heat if you can't get indoors, but deep frostbite should never be deliberately thawed until the patient is in an environment that can be kept warm. Victims can walk on frozen feet, if necessary, but thawed frostbite is crippling as well as being very painful. Moreover, the damaged tissues quickly refreeze in sub-freezing weather.

When tissues begin to freeze, ice crystals form between the cells because the fluid there has a lower concentration of electrolytes than fluid inside the cells. The crystallizing ice draws water out of the cells, dehydrating and shrinking them. Electrolyte concentration inside the cells becomes toxic. Sudden temperature change (thermal shock) also does damage, and the cell membranes may break down. If the tissues are frozen rapidly, which can happen by contact with cold metal or liquid, ice crystals also form inside the cells, which do even more damage. Prospects of recovery are therefore poorer with contact frostbite than with the slower chilling of frostbite from cold air.

Our extremities are most vulnerable to frostbite, because they are furthest from the heart, their tissues are close to the surface, and they have a high surface-to-volume ratio. This makes them efficient at radiating heat. Feet are frozen more often than hands, because feet also lose heat by conduction to cold ground, rock, or snow. Tight boots greatly increase the risk of frostbite because they impair circulation to the feet, which have little heat-producing tissue of their own and depend on a constant supply of warm blood to keep from freezing in very cold weather. Ears and noses are also vulnerable, and some winter joggers have suffered frostbitten scrotums and penises. Also, keeping unprotected eyes open against a cold wind can freeze the corneas, for example when snowmobiling or cross-country skiing,.

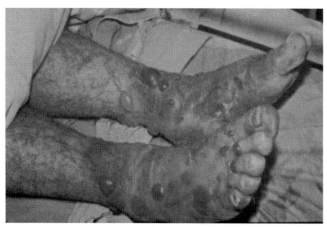

Effect of tight boots, showing blistering after the feet were thawed, and progressive necrosis.

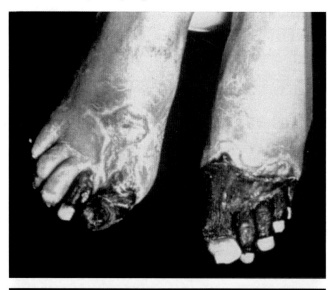

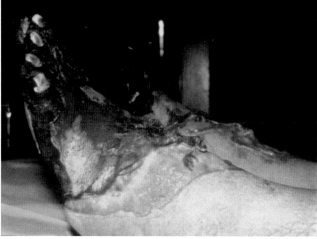

About a month after thawing, necrosis has spread.

Risk factors

Wind chill greatly increases the risk of frostbite. Also, wet skin cools faster than dry skin and can trigger ice crystallization in the tissues. Other risk factors are:

- hypothermia (circulation withdraws to vital organs);
- alcohol consumption (increases heat loss and lowers heat production);
- smoking (causes blood vessels to constrict);
- impaired circulation to hands or feet, e.g. from tight boots;
- immobility (e.g., when trapped by a storm);
- accident (physical and psychological effects);
- fatigue or apathy (slows heat production);
- previous frostbite injury (causes lasting damage to blood vessels).

Contact with very cold metal can freeze skin instantly, especially a full metal fuel container. To prevent contact, wear glove liners, and cover metal (such as fuel bottles for backpacking stoves) with duct tape. Petroleum fuels can chill far below the freezing point of water and remain liquid, so they can also freeze skin on contact. Liquified petroleum fuels such as butane, which are pressurized natural gas, are even more dangerous. They can freeze skin on contact in any weather, as they suddenly expand from liquid to gas.

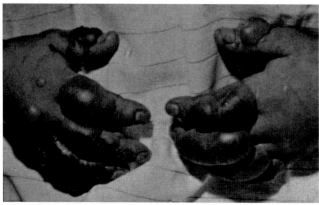

Swelling and blistering in frostbitten hands hours after rewarming

Treatment

If the skin is getting numb, it is close to the temperature at which circulation will withdraw, leaving the tissues defenseless against freezing. Outdoors, body heat may be the only way to rewarm the skin (putting your fingers into your armpits or inside the clothing, for example). Another technique is to force circulation back into the hands by shaking them vigorously or windmilling the arms. It is more difficult to rewarm your own feet, unless you are an advanced yogi. Sometimes the only alternative is to find a friend with a warm belly, as Thomas Hornbein did on his ascent of the west ridge of Mt. Everest. He came back with all his toes, but his companion (who did not rewarm his feet) lost all his toes to frostbite.

Portable handwarmers, which weigh only a few ounces, can deliver heat to a small area for hours. They may be the only way to prevent frostbite in a fractured limb, if evacuation is delayed. Even superficial frostbite is better rewarmed indoors, because if it refreezes after thawing, the damage will be worse and probably go deeper. Napoleon's army was crippled on the retreat from Moscow by partially thawing frostbitten limbs in front of roaring fires every night, and then refreezing them.

For deep frostbite, prevent further heat loss during evacuation with dry, loose wraps or clothing, and pad or splint for protection if the injury is to an extremity.

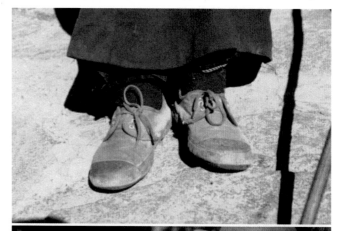

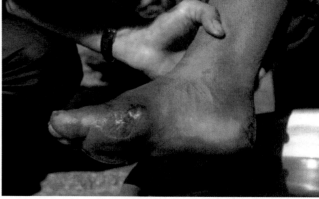

This Tibetan nun walked over the Himalayas in tennis shoes that were too tight.

Transport to a hospital or, if that is not possible, to another place where the patient can be kept warm. Thaw an extremity by immersing it in water at 104° to 108° F. Stir when adding new hot water. Have the patient move the thawing digits, if possible, but do not massage. Continue warming until the skin is red and pliable (up to 30 minutes). The patient will know that the tissues are thawing because they will hurt. After removing the thawed digits from the water, gently separate fingers or toes with loose, sterile dressings, elevate, and handle as little as possible.

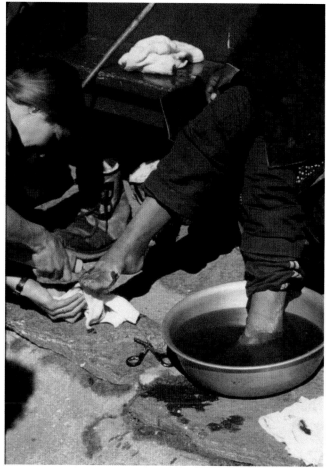

Rewarming the nun's feet

The goal of rewarming is to restore circulation as fast as possible, without damaging the tissues. As the tissues rewarm, their oxygen demand increases, so they will die unless circulation is restored quickly enough to meet this demand. Radiant heat (e.g., standing in front of a heater or fire) is too slow and inefficient. Water transfers heat about 100 times as fast as air and quickly brings the chilled flesh up to a temperature at which blood will return.

After rewarming, the goal of treatment is to maintain circulation in the thawed tissue while preventing infection. Swelling and blisters develop within hours.

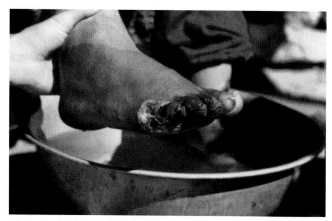

The nun's feet had partially thawed and re-frozen several times, so they already show necrosis.

Damage to blood vessels in the thawed tissues continues, probably caused by clots (embolisms). Physicians no longer amputate, unless the limb dies from impaired circulation, or infection gets out of control. Nature does a slower but better job of separating the living tissue from the dead.

Dead tissues blacken and wither over a period of weeks or months. If the damage is bone-deep, the dead part of the limb eventually self-amputates. If enough tissue survives to keep the limb viable, the blackened tissue will peel off, revealing new skin underneath.

Wind chill chart

A National Weather Service chart shows the relation of wind velocity to air temperature, hypothermia, and frostbite: http://www.nws.noaa.gov/os/windchill/wind-chill-brochure.pdf.

Conclusion

Recovering from deep frostbite is very painful and usually takes months even if you do not lose digits or limbs. Moreover, even healed frostbite leaves the patient more vulnerable to cold injury in the future, probably because of lasting damage to blood vessels. But by knowing how the body reacts to sub-freezing weather and recognizing the risk factors, you can usually avoid frostbite and help to prevent it in others.

Chapter 16. Dressing for survival

Genetic engineers may someday enable us to grow winter coats of fur. Until then, however, we will need an artificial substitute – clothing – to survive in cold weather. Clothing, like fur, controls heat transfer by controlling the layer of air around the body. Air is an excellent insulator, so trapping it against the skin keeps heat in. Conversely, venting and circulating warmed air away from the skin carries heat away. And since our body's heat production can increase up to ten-fold when we are exercising hard, we often have to get rid of excess heat even in cool weather.

Water is an excellent conductor, and it can also absorb far more heat than air. If water displaces the trapped air around the skin, it will turn clothing into a refrigerator. Clothing therefore needs to control the movement of water as well as air. Keeping rainwater and snow out would be a simple function to design into clothing, if it did not also have to allow our sweat to evaporate into the air. Performing both these functions during active use requires clothing to have good design and the right materials.

The right stuff
Wool keeps sheep warm and dry, but the sheep have oil glands that keep the fibers water-repellent. We have only the oil that is left in the wool after manufacture. "Virgin" wool is best, especially if it comes from sheep that grew up in cold and wet surroundings. "Oiled wool" has some of the oil lost in processing restored to the fibers. Wool that is not virgin is recycled from old fabric, so it is unlikely to have much water-repelling oil left. It will also be weaker than virgin wool, because the fibers are chopped up during recycling.

Wool garments can absorb up to half their weight in water, although they may not feel wet until they are 35% to 50% saturated. Also, wool dries very slowly. These limitations make wool best for clothing in which its toughness and resilience count: long-wearing socks, durable mittens, and tightly woven pants or shirts.

Cotton can quickly soak up 100% of its weight in water, and it loses 90% of its insulating value when wet, so it makes good bath towels but terrible cold-weather clothing. Down-filled garments are tempting because down's springy plumules expand more and trap more insulating air than any other material of the same weight. But down, like cotton, has high affinity for moisture and loses almost all of its insulating power when wet. Down clothing is, therefore, most useful in arctic conditions where it is unlikely to get wet, and where its warmth-to-weight ratio significantly lightens the burden of clothing.

Silk absorbs about 20% of its weight in water, so it makes a better inner layer than other natural fibers, and some people like the feel of it next to their skin. But it usually requires careful hand washing, and does not perform as well as synthetics.

Synthetic fibers have much more survival value than natural fibers in cold and wet weather, because they absorb very little water. Nylon can absorb only 4% of its weight in water, while polyester and polypropylene absorb 1% to 2%. If these fabrics get soaked, they feel clammy, but do not lose much insulating value. They dry out very fast, because the water does not wet the fibers in the fabric. In natural fabrics, by contrast, water bonds to the fibers, displacing trapped air bubbles. It requires a great deal of energy in the form of body heat to displace it.

Layering
Clothing for the body and limbs should be layered, so that it can easily be added or taken off to fit conditions and activity level. The inner layer should be stretchy, so that it hugs the body without binding, and should allow sweat to move freely between its fibers ("wicking off"). The middle layers are insulation, stabilizing the layer of air warmed by body heat next to the skin. They should also allow sweat to pass through. The outer layer, or shell, should keep wind and water out of the insulating warmed air. But like the other layers, it must allow evaporated sweat to escape. These conflicting functions make the shell the most difficult layer to design and sew, and often the most expensive.

The inner layer
Specially knit polyester has largely replaced polypropylene for winter underwear, because polyester

does not pick up body odor so easily, and it is less likely to shrink or pill in the wash. It comes in several thicknesses, from lightweight (for active use in moderate temperatures) to expedition weight (for severe cold). Polypropylene fishnet, however, is an excellent inner layer because it gives a lot of warmth for its weight. The open mesh allows sweat to escape, which makes it comfortable over a large range of temperatures and activity levels. It is made by Brynjie (www.brynjie-shop.com), a Norwegian company. Some people still prefer a wool inner layer because it doesn't feel wet until it has absorbed quite a bit of water, but it has less survival value than synthetic because it is harder to dry. Silk is also harder to dry than synthetic, but it absorbs less water than wool.

Insulating layers

For active use, these should usually be of polyester pile or fleece. Fleece is synthetic fur with a short nap, inside and out. Its most common brand name is Polartec®, which all comes from the same mills. Microfleece or regular fleece with a wind-proof layer is more expensive, but useful in cold and windy conditions where it may be enough protection by itself when you are moving. Wind-Pro® is more tightly knit Polartec®, which has about four times the wind resistance, but is more breathable than Windbloc® which has a wind-proof layer sandwiched inside. Pile is thick synthetic fur. Polyester is also used as fill, like down, for jackets that are sewn into compartments. These are good for staying warm when you're not moving, but not so good for active use because they do not vent sweat or excess heat. Also, they do not dry as easily as fleece or pile, because the compartments trap water.

Outer layer: Wind and rain shell

Shells (parkas or anoraks, and rain pants) are of nylon or polyester, with a water-repellent layer laminated inside. To protect the water-repellent layer, they have either another layer of fabric laminated to the inside or a liner. They may also have a waxy coating sprayed or washed onto the outer layer that resists wetting.

Water repellency is tested by hosing the fabric with water at a measured pressure. The water repellency rating depends on how much pressure the fabric can withstand without leakage. These tests do not tell you about the ability of water to leak through defective seams, or to wet the outside fabric and wick around the edges to the inside. They do not tell you how durable the water-repellent layer is. They also do not tell you how well the garment conforms to your body when you move, or pulls away to expose you to the elements.

Evaluating wind and rain shells

Since a good wind and rain shell is expensive, you should check its design and construction carefully before buying.

*   How many layers are there? The minimum is two: a water-repellent film laminated inside the fabric. An exposed film can easily be worn away as your body rubs against it. Three layers are best -- stretchy nylon tricot laminated inside, over the water-repellent film. Many parkas have a liner instead of the inner layer, stitched only at the seams and hanging loose.

*   Look at the seams, inside. They should all be sealed with waterproof tape. Look closely at tape intersections, because that is where tape most often delaminates. Seam tape is laminated by heating it to a temperature very close to the melting point of nylon, so the temperature of the heating element needs to be controlled precisely. If the garment has a liner covering the seams, you might still be able to see and feel them through the outer fabric.

*   How thick and tough is the outer layer? A thin fabric will save weight, but then the water-repellent layer inside can more easily be shredded by abrasion, e.g. by sliding down a snow slope, even if the outer layer isn't cut. You've had a similar experience if you've ever scratched or scraped your skin through a layer of clothing. The fabric was undamaged, but your skin was raw or bleeding underneath.

*   What happens when you move? When you turn your head, does the hood turn with you or does it blind you? When you raise both arms, does the parka continue to cover your body or does it hike up halfway to your armpits?

*   Is there a wind skirt, which you can cinch around your waist, to prevent wind and rain from blowing in from below?

- Check the zippers: the front zipper should be 2-way, and the armpit zippers (essential) should be long enough so that you can slip your arms through them and tuck the sleeves inside the parka. Most water-repellent layers on garments, like Gore-Tex®, are more or less breathable, because they have microscopic pores to let out the water vapor of evaporated sweat. However, if you are sweating heavily, you will quickly saturate the pores. Then you need the pit zips to vent steam.
- Heavy rain or wet snow will also prevent evaporation by saturating the outer layer of the garment with water, though this layer can be made more water repellent by treating it with a spray such as Nik-Wax®.

For many years, some Gore-Tex® shell garments carried a lifetime guarantee, and some manufacturers would replace them if they began to leak no matter how old they were. So it paid to buy the best. But Gore Associates now claims a lifetime of only about eight years for its product with normal use, or ten years with little or no use. Other manufacturers of water resistant layers claim similar lifetimes for their products.

If you do serious outdoor activities in extreme conditions, where your survival may depend on your clothing, then you need high quality outerwear. And if you spend much of the year outdoors, the comfort and safety margin of the best outerwear is still a good investment. But for occasional trips in moderate conditions, where you have an easy escape route, cheaper outerwear may be adequate. If you're huddling in the rain, or hiking on an easy trail, advanced design features aren't going to make much difference.

Head, hands and feet

Head protection: The hood of your parka should fit comfortably over your head insulation. A warm cap of synthetic or wool that pulls down over the ears, and a lightweight balaclava that can cover the whole head and neck, are a good combination. For very cold, windy conditions a neoprene facemask may be needed.

For the hands: Synthetic glove liners, gloves or mitts (wool or synthetic), and water-repellent overmitts are the three layers. The middle and outer layers may be combined into insulated gloves, but on a back-country trip, these are hard to dry out when they get

wet. Glove liners are essential so that you don't expose bare skin when you need full use of your fingers.

For the feet: Leather boots require preparation to make them waterproof. First, seal all seams, especially in the welt (connecting the uppers and the soles) with a liquid such as Stitch-Lock. This saturates the threads and makes them swell, sealing the stitch holes. Then seal the leather uppers by rubbing in a waterproofing compound for leather. Plastic ski and mountaineering boots are waterproof and insulated with foam. If they don't fit well, however, they can pinch and impair circulation. This problem in rented boots has caused more than one case of frostbite.

For cold winter skiing or mountaineering, gaiters should completely cover the boots and have pockets inside to insert insulating foam. Inside the boots, you need thin, synthetic inner socks that cling to the foot and protect the skin from abrasion. Thick wool or synthetic socks provide insulation, but be careful not to cram so many socks into the boots that you cut off circulation. To reduce heat loss by conduction through the bottom of the boot, add an insole of foam neoprene.

Vapor barrier liners

Since we lose heat by insensible sweating, even in cold weather, some people use waterproof liners between layers. For example, one plastic produce bag between the inner and outer sock, and another between the outer sock and the boot, seals in sweat and keeps the insulating sock dry. Similarly, a plastic liner can go between glove liners and mitts. For the body, a thin waterproof shirt or jacket goes just over the synthetic underwear. Some people have more tolerance than others for the clammy feeling of vapor barrier liners, but they are seldom used during vigorous activity unless the temperature is well below freezing.

Putting it all together

When selecting cold weather clothing, bring along the other layers that you will be wearing with it, to make sure that they will fit together comfortably, and not bind or bunch when you move. If you will be snow camping, try lying down and turning over a few times, because you will probably be wearing at least some layers in the sleeping bag. Do the clothes stretch and move with you, or do they bind and shift?

Cold weather clothing has not quite caught up with the natural insulation that caribou and wolves have evolved. But by knowing how clothing works, and selecting clothes that fit our activities as well as our bodies, we can survive and even enjoy winter weather.

Sleeping warm

Getting chilled at night can lower your resistance to hypothermia, altitude illness, and respiratory infections, as well as making you more susceptible to accidents the next day by reducing your physical and mental efficiency. So making sure that you sleep warmly and comfortably is good preventive medicine. Your choice of sleeping bag and insulating pads can make a big difference, but certain tricks can help you make the most of equipment.

Preparing the ground

Before laying down your tent or ground cloth, remove any pebbles, twigs, or pine cones that could dig into you through your pad and bag. Remember the story of the princess and the pea. Avoid tall grass, because on a cool night it will collect a lot of dew, and so will your sleeping bag or shelter. Also avoid the bases of big gullies or descending valleys that can turn into wind tunnels as cold air flows down them at night.

If you can't find level ground, sleep with your head uphill. In a snow shelter, sleep on a shelf with a deeper trench beside it to collect and carry out the cold air. When digging a snow shelter in moderate temperatures, wear only your underwear under your waterproof outer layer. In colder temperatures, add only the minimum of synthetic layers to keep you warm while digging. Then put on more layers when you finish digging. If you tend to sleep on your back, a little padding under the sleeping pad at knee level will prevent hyper-extension of the knees.

Down sleeping bags

High quality goose down has the most loft of any sleeping bag fill, and so gives the most warmth for the weight. But it has two limitations: it collapses when wet; and because it is so compressible, it provides very little ground insulation under the body. As a result, you may need more thickness of foam pad underneath you than with a synthetic bag. Some down bags have shells of water-resistant but breathable fabric, which gives

them considerable protection from both water and wind, but you still must be careful not to saturate them from within. As a result, down bags work well in dry climates, including arctic conditions, but have little survival value in climates where they can get wet.

The best down comes from mature geese - long, springy, branching plumules that provided insulation for the geese's bodies. If you take good care of a down bag, it will last for many years. Don't keep it stuffed any longer than necessary. Never dry-clean it, because the chemicals strip the natural oils from the down plumules and make them less springy, reducing the down's loft. Some laundries specialize in washing and drying down bags in large drum-type machines.

Synthetic sleeping bags

Synthetic bags are filled with fibers, usually polyester, that are crimped at a temperature of about 160° F to give them loft. They are heavier and bulkier than good down for the warmth they give. Also, they can lose loft if they are kept stuffed, especially in a hot car. The temperature inside a parked car or the trunk of a car driving on a hot summer day can be high enough to re-crimp synthetic fibers in the compressed position. And even if the fibers are not forcibly re-crimped, they lose their loft with use much faster than high-quality down. Transporting them in loose storage sacks, however, will extend their life.

The advantage of synthetic bags is that the fibers do not absorb moisture, so they keep most of their loft and warmth even when the bag gets wet. Also, since they are less compressible than down, they provide more ground insulation. The first synthetic fill, kapok, consisted of loose fibers with a solid cross section. The loose fibers now used for fill are hollow, which gives them more trapped, insulating air at a lighter weight. In the 1970s, a company called Snow Lion began sewing mats of continuous fibers used for furniture stuffing into sleeping bags and jackets. They called it Polarguard®. It is now a common synthetic fill for sleeping bags. Unlike loose fills, it doesn't spill out if the fabric of the shell is torn.

Shape and construction

Sleeping bags come in a variety of shapes, from the rectangular bags that give you space to move around inside, to the mummy bags that are designed to be worn like a garment – when you turn, the bag turns with you. The advantage of mummy bags is that they keep the insulation right next to your body, thus providing maximum warmth for their weight.

Bags with loose fill also have baffles to keep the insulation from shifting. Polarguard® is usually cut into strips that are stitched in an overlapping shingle design, to provide flexibility without cold spots. When you're checking a bag for size, wear the clothes that you would on a very cold night, zip it up, and snug up the hood around your head so that only your eyes, nose, and mouth are exposed. Then stretch out completely. You should have just a little room beyond your feet so that you can extend them freely. But if stretching out pulls the bag taut, it is too short for you.

Dressing for sleep

You can sleep warmer and get by with a lighter sleeping bag by wearing clothes inside it, but they need to be the right kind of clothes – stretchy synthetics. These clothes will not wrinkle or bind, and will also not absorb water from your sweat. An inner layer of synthetic underwear and a pullover or jacket of fleece or pile work well. Dry socks will keep your feet warm - it is impossible to feel warm if your feet are cold. A fleece cap or balaclava will prevent heat loss through your head. As you warm up inside the bag, you can remove layers of clothes.

In very cold weather, some people use vapor barrier liners (VBLs) inside their sleeping bags - bags of waterproof nylon that prevent evaporative heat loss by sweating and keep the moisture out of the insulation. The disadvantage is that VBLs may make you feel damp and clammy, even if you wear your synthetic underwear underneath.

Breath, fuel and water

When you breathe dry air, your circulatory system humidifies it with water from a network of blood vessels in the air passages, and you lose most that moisture when you exhale. If you breathe inside your bag, that water will soak into the bag's insulation. So you should keep your mouth and nose out of the bag, even when you cinch up the hood around your head.

Inside a tent, you should always have some back-to-front ventilation that will carry your warm, moist breath outside. Ideally, cold air comes in through the low vent at your feet and warmed moistened air rises to pass out the higher front vent. Otherwise moisture will condense on the tent fabric and rain down on your bag.

Digestion generates heat, so eating a good dinner will help keep you warm at night. You also need to be well hydrated, because dehydration can reduce blood volume. This in turn can slow down heat-generating metabolism and impair circulation to the hands and feet, making them feel cold. But if you let yourself get dehydrated all day then tank up before crawling into the sleeping bag, that guarantees some late night excursions to empty your bladder, which on a cold night can chill you down fast. Caffeine and alcohol before sleeping can also send you out with a full bladder, because they are diuretics. Keeping a plastic pee bottle (and a pee funnel for ladies) in reach just outside the tent can save you from a cold trip. The half-gallon size with a handle and a screw top works best.

Insulating pads

Closed cell foam pads are the most reliable ground insulation. Traditionally, they were just flat sections of foam, but now several models are available with patterns of ridges or nubbins that increase the effective insulation for the weight and bulk. The old pads stiffened in very cold weather, but the newer pads of EVA (ethylene vinyl acetate) and improved Ensolite® remain flexible.

Thermarest® pads are inflatable, which adds insulating air to the foam inside. Their drawbacks are that they can be punctured and start leaking (so it is important to carry a patch) and the valve can fail. Also, the nylon shell is slippery, even if you spray it with an aerosol that makes it a bit tacky, so you can slide off it at night, especially if the ground under you is not quite level. The advantage is that it gives you much more insulation than a closed cell pad for its weight, and that it conforms more to your body, like a mattress. So it is less likely to impair circulation. For a very cold winter trip, a three-quarter length Thermarest® and a full-length closed cell foam pad is a good combination.

A small pillowcase of soft-textured nylon can be stuffed with any soft surplus clothing. Or you can make a pillow by zipping up a fleece or pile jacket, turning it inside out so that the sleeves are inside, then folding it with the zipper on the bottom.

Chapter 17. Effects of high altitude

Photos courtesy of Ben Schifrin, MD

Before birth, we all live at high altitude for nine months. Fetal blood has about the same oxygen concentration as the blood of a mountaineer breathing the air on top of Mt. Everest. But the fetus has a special kind of hemoglobin, with more affinity for oxygen than adult hemoglobin. Some adult animals, such as the llama of the Andes, have hemoglobin that also works better at high altitude, but not humans. We must adjust to low atmospheric oxygen pressure in other ways.

In this chapter, we will review the oxygen transport system, see how it responds to the challenge of high altitude, and how an ineffective response can cause illness. We will also see how to help the body respond well to altitude, and how to treat patients with various forms of altitude illness.

Air and oxygen pressure at altitude

Atmospheric air is 20.94% oxygen, a percentage that remains constant at terrestrial altitudes. At sea level, atmospheric pressure is about 760 millimeters of mercury (760 mmHg) measured with a barometer, though it varies with the temperature of the air. Part of atmospheric pressure, however, comes from water vapor pressure. This varies with humidity, but averages about 47 mmHg. So to calculate the partial pressure of oxygen, subtract 47 from the barometric pressure, and take 20.94% of the result. At sea level, 760-47=713. 20.94% of that is 149.3 mmHg. At 18,000 feet, barometric pressure is about one-half what it is at sea level, and at the top of Mt. Everest (29,029 feet), about one-third of sea level pressure; but partial pressure of oxygen is only about one-fourth what it is at sea level, because the lower the barometric pressure, the more significant water vapor pressure becomes.

Oxygen transport

Inhaling mixes fresh air with the oxygen-depleted residual air still in the lungs, which lowers the percentage of oxygen to as little as 13% in the alveoli. So partial pressure of oxygen decreases when it is inhaled from the atmosphere into the alveoli (air sacs) of the lungs. Inhaling and exhaling more deeply makes the mixture richer, reducing the drop in oxygen pressure from atmosphere to alveoli (below).

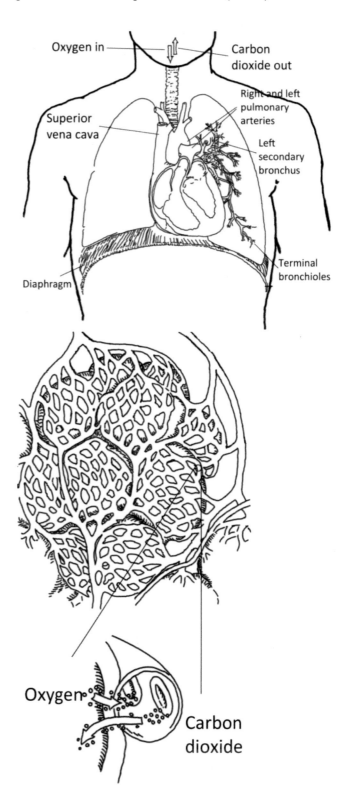

Oxygen is driven through the body by pressure differences, from higher to lower concentrations. From the alveoli, it moves across the membranes and thin capillary walls into the blood, which carries oxygen through the pulmonary veins to the left side of the heart. The left ventricle then pumps the oxygenated blood through the aorta to the whole body. However, the body's blood supply (about a quart for every 25 lbs. of body weight) could not hold nearly enough oxygen in solution to supply the cells. Oxygen is therefore carried by hemoglobin in the red blood cells. Hemoglobin binds to oxygen where oxygen pressure is high (in capillaries around the alveoli) and releases oxygen from capillaries to the working cells, where oxygen pressure is low. Iron in hemoglobin gives blood cells their color: bright red when it binds to oxygen, and darker red when the oxygen is released.

Oxygen depleted blood, returning to the right side of the heart, is pumped to the lungs by the right ventricle through the pulmonary arteries. This blood also carries dissolved carbon dioxide (CO_2), a waste product of metabolism, and some of it is expelled as you exhale. Carbon dioxide is about 50 times more soluble than oxygen in water. Concentration of CO_2 in the blood helps control breathing.

Breathing and altitude

Carbon dioxide, dissolved in blood, forms a weak acid. As it accumulates, it makes the blood more acidotic, which stimulates the respiratory center in the medulla of the brain to increase breathing. As we flush carbon dioxide out of the lungs by breathing more rapidly or deeply, however, the blood becomes more alkaline, which decreases breathing. Two small sensors, the carotid bodies, detect oxygen concentration in the blood flowing through the two big arteries of the neck. As oxygen concentration decreases, they also signal the respiratory center to increase breathing.

Up to about 5,000 feet, oxygen saturation in hemoglobin remains about as high as at sea level - at least 96%. As we go higher, the body struggles to get enough oxygen from the thinner air. In order for the body to acclimatize, breathing must become both deeper and more regular. The body dumps bicarbonates from the blood through the urine, which allows a lower concentration of carbon dioxide to make the blood acidotic, and to stimulate the breathing center of the brain. This is the most important way that the body acclimatizes to high altitude.

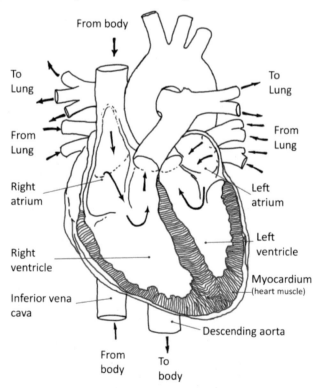

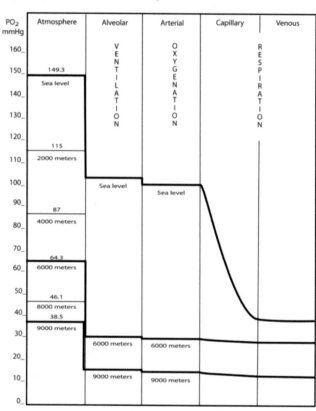

Oxygen cascade and altitude

The graph shows the drop in partial pressure of oxygen that moves it through the body. As inhaled air mixes with residual, oxygen-depleted air still in the lungs, the partial pressure of oxygen drops. As you become acclimatized, you breathe more deeply and regularly, which makes the mix in the alveoli richer in oxygen. So there is less of a drop in partial pressure of oxygen with **ventilation** (Latin *ventilare* "to air"), the movement of air in and out of the lungs. But deeper breathing cannot completely compensate for the lower oxygen pressure in the atmosphere at higher altitudes, as shown in the graph, so the amount of oxygen that reaches the cells is less than at sea level. On the highest mountain peaks (over 8,000 meters), air and oxygen pressure are less than a third of air and oxygen pressure at sea level.

As oxygen moves from the alveoli into the blood and bonds to the hemoglobin in the red blood cells (**oxygenation**), there is a slight drop in partial pressure. Oxygenated blood flows back to the heart in the pulmonary veins, and is pumped out by the left ventricle. As blood saturated with oxygen reaches capillaries around the body's cells, oxygen is driven into the cells by the difference in partial oxygen pressure and carbon dioxide moves from the cells into the blood. This gas exchange by cells and blood is called **respiration**, though the word comes from Latin *respirare* ("to breathe"), so it is also used (confusingly) as a synonym for breathing.

At high altitude, the heart has less blood to pump, because of dehydration and a shift of fluid out of the circulatory system. To compensate and meet oxygen demand, the heart rate initially increases (up to 50% at 19,000 to 25,000 feet). Blood pressure also increases slightly, but usually returns to normal in a few days (except in the pulmonary arteries) as climbers acclimatize to altitude. Heart rate decreases with acclimatization, but remains above sea-level values.

One factor in acclimatizing to altitude is the hypoxic ventilatory response (HVR). It means the increase of ventilation when there is less oxygen getting into the body. According to Houston in *Going Higher* (see the bibliography) there is considerable variation in people's HVR, and it tends to decrease with age. To quote Houston, "A low HVR has been implicated in acute mountain sickness and high altitude pulmonary edema." Aerobic fitness at sea level, however, does not seem to guarantee a strong HVR, or to make climbers less vulnerable to altitude illness. Even elite climbers are generally not exceptional athletes at sea level. They owe much of their performance at high altitude to good acclimatization. Hundreds of climbers who were well acclimatized have gone to the top of Mt. Everest without oxygen, but this seems to be very close to the limit of what is possible. Above 5,000 feet, even acclimatized people lose about 3% of their work capacity for every 1,000 feet of further elevation gain. At the top of Mt. Everest (29,029 feet or 8,848 meters) an acclimatized climber's work capacity (without supplemental oxygen) would be only one-quarter what it was at sea level.

Helping the body to acclimatize

Although the physiology of the body at high altitude is complex, the ways in which we can help our bodies to acclimatize are simple:

- Give the body time by gaining altitude gradually.
- Drive to the high trailhead the night before starting the climb and sleep there to start acclimatizing.
- Climb high, and sleep lower.
- Drink water regularly to maintain blood volume and prevent clots from increased red blood cell production. Dehydration also dries up the urine supply and prevents the body from dumping bicarbonates.
- Eat a high-carbohydrate diet, starting days before the ascent. Carbohydrate loading maximizes the supply of fuel (glycogen) in the muscle cells and liver, and carbohydrates require less oxygen to digest and metabolize than fats or proteins.
- Stay warm. Muscles become much less efficient as they chill. A drop of 0.9° - 1.8° F. in body core temperature can increase the oxygen requirement (for the same amount of work) by up to 50%.
- Avoid respiratory depressants such as alcohol and sleeping pills.
- Don't climb high with a respiratory infection. Colds and flu set you up for altitude illness.
- Grow older. Susceptibility to altitude illness seems to decrease with age, and children are at greater risk than adults. However, that may be because younger climbers tend to go faster and push themselves harder.

Other responses to altitude

Hemoglobin production starts within two hours of ascent, and new red blood cells are in circulation within four to five days. Total body water decreases at high altitude because of losses through urination, sweating, and breathing. Loss of the thirst sensation and the difficulty of melting snow reduce the chances that lost water will be replaced. Blood volume is reduced because water that the circulatory system delivers to the sweat glands and various parts of the body is not fully replaced. More red blood cells make the blood even thicker, which slows circulation and increases the risk of blood clots. Severe dehydration can also pack red blood cells tightly in the capillaries, so that less surface of the cells is exposed for picking up and releasing oxygen.

Because altitude exposure reduces mental and physical efficiency, it increases the risk of accidents. Another problem is that wounds heal more slowly with altitude gain, especially in the extremities, because too little oxygen is reaching the tissues. On the American Medical Research Expedition to Everest in 1981, there were 4 expedition members (including 2 Sherpas) with minor wounds on their hands and feet. These wounds would not heal at Base Camp (17,700 feet), but healed when they descended to 14,000 feet.

About 18,000 feet is the highest altitude at which people can live for more than a short time, and without proper acclimatization it can be fatal. During the border conflict between China and India, there was fighting at that altitude. The Chinese were well acclimatized from living for months at 15,000 feet in Tibet. But many Indian soldiers, who were rapidly transported to the mountains from sea level, died of altitude illness. Thousands of Indian and Pakistani soldiers in the Kashmir Border War have also died of altitude illness. When they move up to a pass that is over 20,000 feet, they usually last about a week.

Even if climbers are well acclimatized staying at very high altitude usually causes weight loss, including fat and some lean body mass as well as fluid. As oxygen pressure in the blood goes down, cerebral blood flow increases so as to maintain the brain's oxygen supply. Pulmonary arterial pressure (PAP) also goes up as blood flow to the lungs increases in response to lower oxygen pressure. But at about 14,000 feet, there is a measurable decrease of higher brain functions, such as the ability to calculate. Climbing to extreme altitude (over 24,000 feet) without oxygen may also cause some permanent brain damage.

The effects of altitude form a spectrum or continuum. Patients often progress from a mild to a more serious condition. But for convenience, altitude illness is classified into several clinical types.

Acute Mountain Sickness (AMS)

Acute Mountain Sickness may begin with ascent above 6,000 feet, but is more common 6 to 48 hours later. About 20% of those who go to 7,000 feet get AMS, and about 50% of those who go to 15,000 feet. In the United States, 95% of all altitude illness is AMS. Symptoms vary, but headache (often intense) is the most common. It is usually not relieved by aspirin, though ibuprofen may help. Other symptoms may include weakness, lassitude, shortness of breath, nausea, loss of appetite, and insomnia. AMS often interferes with sleep, and sleep loss can aggravate the effects of altitude.

Even though most AMS victims are probably dehydrated as well as being short of oxygen, fluid leaking out of the blood vessels water-logs the tissues in the brain, lungs, and digestive system. Diuresis (increased urination, encouraged by drinking plenty of water) makes climbers less susceptible to altitude illness. In the face and limbs, edema can be uncomfortable, but it is not dangerous unless it affects the lungs or the brain.

Treatment of AMS is to stop ascending until the body catches up with the altitude, rehydrate, and watch for improvement or worsening of the condition. If the symptoms persist, go down. Often just going down 1,000 feet or so will enable you to sleep, recover, and then continue the ascent.

Medications

Acetazolamide (Diamox) may relieve or prevent AMS. Acetazolamide speeds up the process of dumping bicarbonates from the blood. This increases the effective level of carbon dioxide in the blood and thus tends to make breathing deeper and more regular, especially while sleeping. Since it does this by increasing urination, it is especially important to stay hydrated when taking acetazolamide. But people who are allergic to sulfa drugs cannot take acetazolamide.

And there are other possible side effects. Another prescription drug, dexamethasone, may relieve the symptoms of AMS. The effects of dexamethasone are not so well understood, but it probably reduces leakage from capillaries in the brain, and thus reduces fluid accumulation.

An herbal remedy, Ginkgo biloba (which dilates blood vessels and increases arterial oxygen saturation) has also been shown to help prevent AMS and reduce its severity. It is also used to treat several other conditions, including dementia. A study published in *Wilderness & Environmental Medicine* recommends taking an 80 mg tablet twice a day, starting at least a day before the ascent.

High Altitude Pulmonary Edema (HAPE)

If parts of the lung are poorly ventilated (hypoxic), the pulmonary arteries supplying them constrict, directing more circulation to the rest of the lung. This hypoxic pulmonary vasoconstrictor response (HPVR), is advantageous at sea level, because it sends the blood to where the oxygen is. But at high altitude, the whole lung is hypoxic, so the response increases pulmonary arterial pressure (PAP). Some animals that live at high altitude, such as the Tibetan snow pig, have thin-walled pulmonary arteries that lack muscle to constrict, so there is no danger of increased PAP.

Herbert Hultgren has proposed a very plausible explanation of HAPE in *High Altitude Medicine* [see bibliography]. He points out that if the HPVR is uneven, because of differences in anatomy or function within the lung, some arteries may develop so much pressure that they leak. Laboratory experiments on sections of blood vessels have shown that pressures measured in climbers are enough to open spaces between arterial wall cells, and to let not only fluid but also large protein molecules and blood cells leak through. All of these have been recovered from the lungs of live climbers. First the leakage accumulates in the tissue around the air pockets (alveoli), slowing the transfer of oxygen. Then it starts to fill the alveoli. In x-rays, the accumulations of fluid (edema) look like fluffy snowballs scattered through the lung.

A climber getting High Altitude Pulmonary Edema (HAPE) will be short of breath and tired, even after resting, because the edema is reducing oxygen transfer in the lungs. Resting pulse rate will probably be over 100 per minute (or at least 30 more than what is normal for that patient), in response to low oxygen delivery. This speeding up of the resting pulse is perhaps the most reliable way to distinguish HAPE in its early stages from AMS. A climber who has these symptoms after resting needs to go down immediately.

As HAPE progresses, the patient will be coughing, dryly at first, and the congestion will produce a breath sound, called crackles, like the sound of hairs being rubbed between your fingers. Crackles can be heard with a stethoscope, or by putting your ear against the patient's rib cage under the armpit. As more fluid accumulates, the sound may turn into gurgling, and coughing may bring up sputum that is tinged pink with red blood cells. Lying down may make it worse because then fluid in the lungs will cover more surface and reduce oxygen exchange; and sleep depresses respiration.

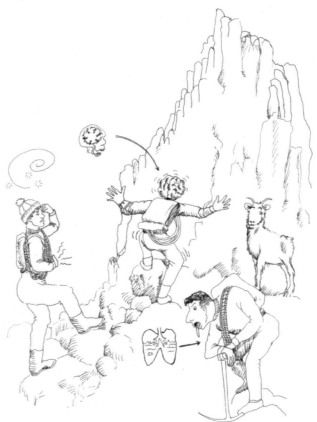

The climber on the left is feeling the typical headache and malaise of AMS. The climber in the center is losing his sense of balance because of HACE. The lungs of the climber on the right are filling with fluid (HAPE). The mountain goat, however, is having no problems with the altitude.

Oxygen will help, especially if given through a positive pressure mask, but it will not reverse the course of HAPE, which is 50% fatal if not treated. Immediate treatment is descent to lower altitude. Nifedipine, which lowers pulmonary arterial pressure, has been successfully used to treat HAPE. Nitric oxide, which has similar effects, has also been used to treat or prevent HAPE.

The Gamow bag, a portable nylon tube pressurized by a foot pump, can simulate lower altitude. Putting the patient inside may relieve the symptoms of altitude illness until the patient can be evacuated. After recovery, the patient should be monitored for respiratory infection.

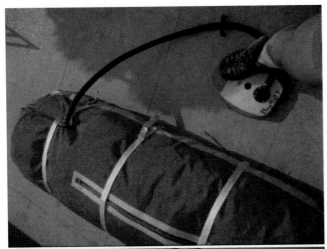

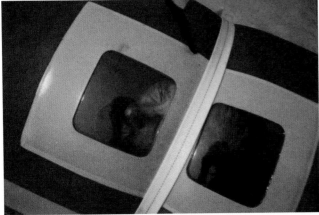

Gamow bag in use: The foot pump increases air pressure inside the bag.

High Altitude Cerebral Edema(HACE)

When the brain does not get enough oxygen, it swells. Shortage of oxygen stimulates increased cerebral blood flow, which stretches blood vessels. Then fluid accumulates in and around the cells, further increasing brain volume. Since the brain is enclosed in the skull, it cannot expand, and pressure increases.

This oxygen shortage and swelling may have many effects on brain function, ranging from confusion and irritability in a mild case to amnesia, hallucinations, or irrational behavior in an advanced case. But the effect on the balance center of the brain, called ataxia, is the most important warning sign of HACE (high altitude cerebral edema), and the easiest to test. The Greek word "ataxia" means "without order," but what the ataxic patient lacks is a normal sense of balance.

To test for ataxia, have the patient walk a straight line, heel against toe. Doing it easily rules out HACE. Swaying indicates a mild case, going off-line a moderate case, and falling a severe case. Another ataxia test is to have the patient stand within (but not touching) your circled arms for 30 seconds, with feet together, hands on shoulders, and eyes closed. A stable posture rules out HACE. Swaying indicates a mild to moderate case, and a patient who falls against your arms has a severe case.

Treatment is to descend immediately, because otherwise the patient will probably be in a coma within 12 hours, and die. Most patients with HACE also have HAPE. Pumping up pressure in a Gamow bag can simulate lower altitude during (or while waiting for) evacuation, and oxygen will help. However, a patient with HACE must always be evacuated. Fortunately, HACE is the least common form of altitude illness, and almost unknown below 11,000 feet.

Vision and altitude

Since the retina is very sensitive to oxygen level in the blood, altitude affects vision. Night vision starts getting dim at 4,000 feet, and at higher altitudes you may suffer night blindness. Much less common are temporary visual changes, such as blurred or double vision. flashing lights, or blindness. These problems usually stop after descent.

Climbers who have had an eye operation to correct their vision called radial keratotomy (RK) have reported changes in their vision at high altitude. After a day or more at high altitude, their cornea flattens, making them more far-sighted and blurring their vision. In a keratotomy, the eye surgeon makes deep radial incisions in the cornea to change its shape. These incisions apparently weaken the cornea enough so that it moves in two dimensions when it swells in response to the shortage of oxygen in the cells.

Since the closed eyelids during sleep further reduce the supply of oxygen to the cornea, a climber with a radial keratotomy may wake up at a high base camp with drastically blurred vision, and have trouble climbing or descending safely; and vision would continue to change with changes in altitude.

Studies by Mader and White on Pike's Peak in 1995 (cited by Butler – see bibliography) measured the hyperoptic shift over 72 hours in subjects who had had RK. But subjects who had had another corrective operation called laser refractive surgery showed no change in vision. In this operation, the eye surgeon peels back a flap of the cornea surface and uses a laser to correct the curvature of the underlying tissue, then replaces the flap. On the Mt. Everest climb organized by two ophthalmologists, Geoff Tabin and Jason Dimming, they reported minor blurring of vision in a few climbers whose corneas had been reshaped with laser refractive surgery. However, they point out that even people who have not had eye surgery can sometimes experience similar vision problems at high altitude.

Using contact lenses at high altitude is problematic. They reduce the oxygen supply to the cornea if left in overnight, but can be hard to keep clean in a wilderness environment if they are frequently removed and replaced. Also, they may freeze in their containers at night. But climbers on the British Everest Expedition used them successfully up to 24,000 feet. Guidelines for military personnel include some sensible suggestions: use disposable lenses for up to 1 week; carry eye drops and contact lens re-wetting solution; and always carry back-up glasses, including prescription sunglasses or goggles that will fit over regular glasses.

Another problem, which over half the people going to 17,000 feet or higher experience, is high-altitude retinal hemorrhage (HARH). Blood flow in the vessels of the retina, and the diameter of these vessels, can double. This can force blood through the stretched vessel walls or even rupture them. But these small leaks seldom cause any symptoms, and usually clear up on return to sea level.

Other altitude problems

Altitude can cause other problems as well, some of them serious. Dehydration plus increased red blood cell production from altitude exposure thickens the blood. Mountaineers who are immobilized by a storm, or in an evacuation litter, are susceptible to embolisms (clots in the thickened blood). These embolisms can break loose and be carried through the heart to block arteries carrying oxygen-depleted blood to the lungs (pulmonary embolism). Climbers have also died of ischemic strokes (blood clots in the brain), probably also brought on by dehydration and thickened blood.

Perhaps the most notorious altitude problem is HAFE (high-altitude flatus expulsion). Because atmospheric pressure is lower, gasses inside the gut expand. HAFE is only dangerous, however, to the noses of other people in the tent.

Conclusion

Even at moderate altitudes, AMS is common. More serious forms of altitude illness (HAPE and HACE) are rarer. But they can occur, especially in those who drive up to a high trailhead and immediately start ascending. Knowing how the oxygen transport system works, and how the body is affected by altitude, will help you to make sense of signs and symptoms otherwise hard to interpret. Knowing how the body acclimatizes will help you to stay healthy at high altitude.

Chapter 18. Lightning strike

On August 29, 1991, a marathon runner and his wife hiked up to the peak of Mt. Lassen. When they saw storm clouds approaching, they began to descend. Lightning struck the ground near the husband. His wife heard the strike and saw pieces of his hat fly by. She ran back and found him motionless, not breathing. When she could not find a pulse, she started CPR. When she re-checked his vital signs after a cycle of CPR, pulse and breathing had returned.

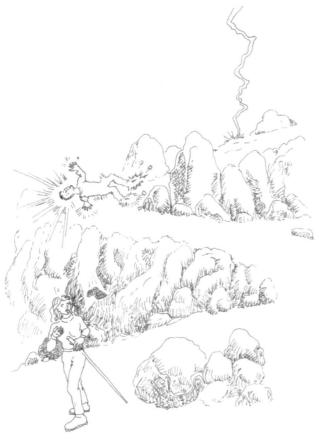

He was carried down, evacuated by helicopter, and treated for superficial burns, two broken ribs and ruptured eardrums. He still remembers nothing of the accident, but as he reconstructed it later from the evidence, "It [ground current from the strike] jumped the rubber sole of my boot and went through the nylon upper and into my ankle. From there it traveled up my left leg to the pelvic region, back down my front leg, and exited through the other ankle. Along the way it melted my nylon running shorts and both boots." His doctors attributed his quick recovery to his excellent aerobic condition, but his wife's prompt CPR almost certainly saved his life.

Immediate effects of lightning strike

Lightning can:

- strike directly if the victim is a prominent object in the area (about 5% of strikes);
- splashover from another prominent object such as an isolated tree (about 1/3 of strikes);
- flow through the ground from a nearby strike to shock the victim (about half of strikes);
- flow through a conductor such as water or a wire fence.

Current through the brainstem can damage the cardiorespiratory control centers, which would make resuscitation more difficult. This happens to about 75% of the victims in a direct strike, and about 67% in a splashover; but to only about 8% of victims injured by ground current, because typically most of the current goes up one leg and down the other. Victims of direct strike or splashover are also more likely to suffer temporary paralysis (two-thirds of them in the upper limbs only) or temporary blindness. Sometimes loss of vision can be permanent.

In about one-half of lightning strike victims, the concussion ruptures the eardrums. Lightning can also cause trauma from muscle spasms, or from throwing the victim some distance. Burns are usually superficial, in a streaking pattern if the current flashing over the skin vaporizes sweat. Punctate burns may be caused by vaporized sweat droplets, or be exit wounds from current passing through deep tissues. Full thickness burns can be caused to skin in contact with synthetic clothing that the current melts.

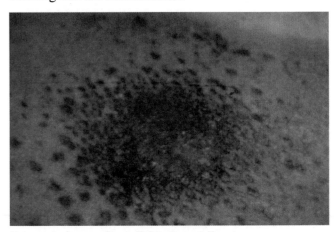

Punctate burns from lightning strike
Photo courtesy of Ben Schifrin, MD

Many lightning strike victims survive, because most of the current flashes over the surface of the body.

Flashover of current can also blast clothes off the body.

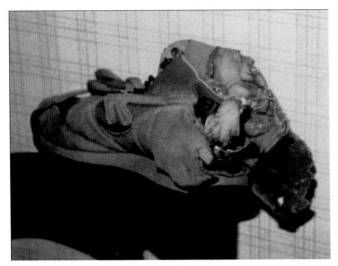

Shoe blown off lightning strike victim
Photo courtesy of Jim McBride

Treating the victims

What can we learn from the example of the marathon runner?

- There is a good chance of saving a lightning strike victim with no vital signs by doing prompt CPR.
- Since the heart has its own electrical backup system, there is a good chance that the pulse will come back spontaneously if rescue breathing begins before the heart runs out of oxygen.
- If several people are down after a lightning strike, the quiet ones need to be checked first because they might not be breathing.
- Since the concussion of a strike can rupture eardrums, even a responsive victim may not be able to hear questions.
- A lightning strike with multiple victims is an exception to the START (Simple Triage and Rapid Treatment) system for sorting mass casualties.

According to START, an unresponsive victim who does not start breathing spontaneously when the rescuer opens the airway is considered dead. The START system, however, is designed to deal with trauma in mass casualty situations, and a victim with injuries severe enough to prevent breathing usually has a poor chance of survival.

A lightning strike victim may have secondary injuries from being hurled to the ground (like the man in the example above) or thrown through the air by the blast wave. But unless these injuries are severe enough to compromise the vital systems, there is a good chance of reviving the victim with prompt CPR. Even if the cardiorespiratory centers in the brain are damaged, and the victim does not resume breathing spontaneously, there is a good chance that the pulse will come back. In this case, continuing rescue breathing until the helicopter arrives can save a life. Rescue breathing is much easier to do than full CPR.

Historical note

Attempts to revive lightning strike victims have a long history, which Cooper et al relate in their chapter on lightning strike in *Wilderness Medicine* (see the bibliography). In the 1750s, Ben Franklin supposedly electrocuted a chicken in a lightning experiment and revived it with mouth-to-beak breathing. In 1807, a human lightning strike victim was revived by mouth-to-mouth breathing.

Other historical techniques for reviving lightning victims included dousing the chest with cold water and gentle electric shocks from Galvanic batteries. In 1859, Alfred West described how his rescuer revived him after a lightning strike, by putting his feet in warm water and "[drawing] out the electricity" by pulling on his toes with one hand and milking a cow with the other. Concepts of how electricity works have changed since the days of Franklin and West, however, so treatment of lightning strike survivors no longer includes cows.

Long-term effects

Fatality from lightning strike is about 30%. Only 100 to 300 deaths are reported each year in the United States. But survivors can suffer long-term neurological effects that are still poorly understood. One survivor, Gretel Ehrlich, has written a vivid account of her experience (see the bibliography). She was struck twice, first by ground current flowing up the legs of her horse and bouncing a spark off her head, then years later by a direct hit. When she woke up after the direct hit, her eye crusted with blood, she thought she was dead. Her heart was beating erratically, and she was partially paralyzed. Her dogs did not recognize her and ran away whining. When some feeling returned to her limbs, she dragged herself to her ranch house and managed to call for help before she passed out again.

Although her wounds healed, she continued to have headaches, chest pains, and trouble staying conscious. Doctors denied her problems or were unable to help. Finally a cardiologist referred her to Joseph Ilvento, who specializes in the effects of electrical impulses (including lightning) on the heart. He found that damage to her brain stem prevented it from sending speedup signals to the heart in response to oxygen demand. Instead her heart slowed down, so she would often pass out when she stood up. Now she takes medications that maintain her heart rate and blood pressure.

At a conference on lightning strike and electric shock, she met other survivors. Harold Deal, for example, was thrown 50 feet by the blast. Since then he cannot feel cold or pain, or taste food. Other survivors suffer amnesia, erratic brain functions (such as the loss of the ability to read and write), or lasting paralysis and muscle weakness in parts of their bodies.

Avoiding lightning strike

In a process that is not completely understood, the collision of rising and condensing moisture with falling ice particles in a cloud strips electrons that accumulate at the bottom, turning the cloud into a giant capacitor, with visible discharges within the cloud. When the potential difference between the bottom of the cloud and the surface of the earth is high enough, it equalizes in a sudden discharge between the cloud and the earth, usually lasting less than 1/1000 of a second. One discharge can dissipate more power than all the industrial electricity generated in the United States for that instant. Since electricity follows the path of least resistance (POLR), high points in the landscape are likely targets. So the best way to avoid lightning strike is not to be a POLR and not to be on or near a POLR during thunderstorms. Clouds do not even have to be overhead for lightning to strike - many survivors report "blue sky" strikes.

In an open field or near a solitary tree, you are very exposed. Staying inside a forest is much safer. Failing that, huddling in a depression may reduce your exposure. Peaks and ridges are doubly dangerous, because lightning can blast you off them. Mountaineers have often reported tingling, humming through metal objects, and even St. Elmo's fire (a bluish glow or corona as the air is ionized). Sometimes they feel these sensations through their own bodies as static electricity builds up during a thunderstorm. These are urgent signals to get down to a less exposed place. If a group is caught in an exposed place, they should stay at least 20 feet apart because lightning can jump at least 15 feet (splashover) if it strikes one person.

Caves or overhangs are tempting, but unless a cave is deeper than it is wide, ground current from a nearby strike can flow over the surface. A group of hikers once learned this the hard way, when they continued their trip up Half Dome in Yosemite National Park in spite of storm warnings. When a thunderstorm caught them on top, they took shelter in a shallow cave near the edge. Ground current from a nearby lightning strike blew them out, and they fell to their deaths.

Conclusion

While the number of people struck by lightning is small, those who do outdoor activities are at the greatest risk, especially in the mountains, in open places, and on water. Survivors often say that they knew they shouldn't have been outside in the storm. If you are caught in an exposed position, try to get to shelter or a place less exposed, and don't be a POLR. If lightning does strike, and one or more people in your group are down, check the ones who are still and quiet first. If someone is not breathing, you have a good chance of saving a life by promptly doing rescue breathing or CPR if necessary.

Chapter 19. Solar radiation and eye protection

By Stephen R. Chun, OD, FAAO

Solar radiation ranges from very high energy X-rays and gamma rays, with wavelengths shorter than 10 nanometers (nm), to low energy radio waves. In between are ultraviolet radiation, visible light, and infrared (which we perceive as heat). These are the wavelengths that we call sunlight. Most very high-energy radiation is absorbed by the atmosphere before it can reach the ground, which is fortunate because it can cause serious damage to living tissues. When high-energy radiation (also called ionizing radiation) penetrates tissues, it strips electrons from atoms, producing charged particles or ions.

Ultraviolet and infrared radiation

Even though the wavelengths we call sunlight are not ionizing, they can also cause damage to living tissues, including the eyes. Ultraviolet (UVR) is the most dangerous, because it has the shortest wavelength, and therefore the highest energy. It is divided (by wavelength) into three parts for convenience.

UVA: 380 nm to 320 nm

UVB: 320 nm to 290 nm

UVC: 290 nm to 200 nm

Ultraviolet C is almost completely filtered out by the ozone layer of the atmosphere. Ultraviolet B is only partially filtered, so it causes most of the damage to skin and eyes. Little ultraviolet A is filtered out by the ozone layer, but it carries less energy. It does, however, contribute to the forming of cataracts, along with UVB.

Unlike UVR, infrared radiation (IR) is readily absorbed by atmospheric moisture, carbon dioxide, and dust, which reduces its total energy; so on overcast days the sun will not feel hot, but 60% to 80% of UVR passes through clouds and moisture (even rain). Without the warning sensation of heat, it is possible to suffer severe damage from UVR to skin or eyes before realizing it. Moreover the eyes, unlike the skin, have no way of adapting to UVR exposure.

Ultraviolet exposure

About 13% of the sunlight reaching the ground is UVR, 43% is IR, and the remaining 44% is visible light. As the position of the sun in the sky changes, both with the season and with the time of day, the amount of atmosphere through which UVR is filtered varies. Over 60% of the day's UVR reaches the ground between 10 a.m. and 2 p.m. Only about 25% as much UVR reaches the ground at 4 p.m. as at noon, and less gets through in winter than in summer because of the lower angle of the sun in the sky. The ozone layer also varies with latitude and season. It is thinnest at the equator and in late summer and fall; and thickest at the poles and in winter. Because of ozone depletion from fluorocarbons, however, UVB reaching the ground in the Antarctic has doubled, and increased significantly in the rest of the world.

The higher you climb, the greater the UVR exposure, with an increase of about 5% for every 1000 ft. of altitude gained. UVR exposure is also increased if you are on a reflecting surface. Grass reflects only about 3%, sand 10% to 15%, and fresh snow 85% to 90%. How much reflected UVR reaches your eyes also depends on the angles: water absorbs more UVR striking it vertically than at a glancing angle. At noon, still water may reflect only about 5% of incident UVR, but earlier or later in the day, it will reflect 20% to 25%. Choppy water provides reflecting surfaces at a variety of angles, no matter where the sun is in the sky, and can reflect up to 100% of incident UVR.

Probably the greatest UVR exposure, however, comes when you ski at high altitude in snow bowls. All of the variables are maximized: more UVR reaching the ground; highly reflective surface; and landscape that focuses much of the reflected radiation on you. UVR is also scattered by clouds, moisture or dust, and this diffuse radiation or skylight can still reach you even if you are not exposed to direct sunlight. There is a higher percentage of skylight in areas more open to the sky: mountains, deserts, beaches and water.

Climate can also increase the risk of damage to the eyes from UV, which is more dangerous when the air is dry and hot. Holidays in the tropics during midwinter can be particularly harmful because the sudden change in luminosity and climate (from winter to tropical) are both a shock to the eyes.

Damage to the eyelids

Eyelids can be sunburned like other skin, especially if a sunbather is lying face up with unprotected eyes. Any ultraviolet B radiation that is not reflected by the skin penetrates until its energy is dissipated. Special light-absorbing molecules called chromophores are located in the skin. Absorbing energy causes chromophores to release free radicals and other products that trigger some reactions. Capillaries become congested, reddening the skin (erythema).

If cells are damaged by UVR, they accumulate fluid, causing swelling (edema). These changes may be seen within three to four hours after exposure. Since they are caused directly by UVR, not indirectly by heat, the victim may not feel the effects before the damage is done.

The sensitive skin of the eyelids can become acutely inflamed and swollen, causing great pain and discomfort. The conjunctiva (mucus membranes lining the insides of the lids) can also become swollen and bloodshot from UV exposure. Repeated exposure may even cause them to thicken and spread to the point where they need medical treatment. Watering, pain and irritation are the usual signs and symptoms.

Since sunscreen on the lids invariably gets in the eyes, causing stinging, burning and redness, the best protection is to wear a brimmed hat and UV absorbing glasses with side shields or wraparound lenses. First aid for UV damage to eyelids or conjunctiva is to apply cool compresses wet with isotonic saline solution (used to rinse contact lenses) or water if saline is not available. In the wilderness, be sure that the water is disinfected, preferably with a method leaving no chemical residue that might irritate the eye. Applying an over-the-counter topical decongestant to the lid may reduce redness and swelling. Medical treatment may include oral antibiotics to reduce infection and dermatological cream to assist healing.

Damage to the cornea

Damage to the epithelium (outer layers) of the cornea from UVB can cause these layers to begin sloughing off. Since the loss of epithelium can expose the corneal nerve endings, victims feel intense pain and photophobia (inability to tolerate light). This is often called snow blindness, because activities on snow expose unprotected eyes to so much reflected UV, especially at high altitudes. Brief but intense UVR exposure from a welder's arc (welder's flashburn) and commercial tanning booths can also burn the cornea.

First aid is to apply cool compresses (moistened with sterile saline if possible), as for sunburned eyelids, and give an over-the-counter pain killer. Apply loose patches to reduce eye sensitivity to light, but do not leave the patches on overnight because they might promote secondary infection. Medical treatment may include oral antibiotics and systemic steroids.

Damage to the retina

While long-term UV exposure can cause cataracts in the lens, these can usually be treated surgically. However, gazing at the sun even for a minute or two will burn the retina. Sun gazers may experience persistent afterimages and visual distortion. Eventually they will lose some visual acuity and possibly lose the central visual field.

Sunglasses that do not absorb 100% of UV may actually increase the amount of UV going into the eye by dilating the pupil. The more visible light the lenses block, the more the pupil will dilate. At 10,000 feet, lenses of crown glass (poorest in UV protection) can increase the amount of UVA going into the eye by 100%. Pupil diameter changes from about 2 mm on a bright day with a high reflective environment to about 8 mm on a dark night. Average pupil diameter in ambient light conditions (indoor room lighting) is about 4.5 mm. The older the person, usually the smaller the pupil is under ambient light conditions. Also, the pupil reacts more sluggishly to changes in light level, because the dilator muscle of the iris atrophies with age.

Sun glasses: Lens tinting

Ultraviolet filtering or absorption depends on the lens material, thickness and the way it is processed. High-index plastic, polycarbonate, and CR-39 (hard resin ophthalmic plastic) absorb more UV than crown glass, but unless they are treated with UV additive, they will still transmit considerable UVB. UV additive is a clear coating on the surface that absorbs much of the UV striking the lens. An absorptive tint may be processed into the lens either while it is being made or in the final stages while it is being ground to prescription. Most glass lenses are tinted during the early stages of production. Glass solid tints are metallic oxides melted into the glass. This kind of tint is permanent, and its light transmission does not change over time. It also reduces internal reflection, because the tint is distributed throughout the lens. Most plastic lenses are tinted toward the end of production. Lenses may also have absorptive surface coatings.

Plastic lenses are tinted by surface absorption, in which the tint solution penetrates uniformly 3-4 microns into the resin surface. In darker lenses, the solution does not penetrate any deeper, but more pigment ions attach to the molecules of the lens polymer. This type of tint fades with time. Also, high index plastic lenses, unlike CR-39 and polycarbonate, have a clear, abrasion-resistant coating on the front surface that is non-porous and cannot usually be penetrated by the tint. In this case, only the back surface is tinted.

Either glass or plastic lenses can be surface coated. In a high temperature vacuum chamber, metallic oxides are vaporized onto the concave (inside) surface of the lens, producing a thin film. Different oxides yield different colors. Coatings adhere best to glass surfaces. Plastic may deform with changes in temperature. The main advantage of coatings is that they are independent of prescriptions. However, because coatings are on the surface, they can easily be damaged by scratches.

Cosmetic tints (light pink, rose, rose brown, flesh, pale brown and similar hues) on glass or plastic have UV transmission similar to clear lenses. With CR-39 hard resin lenses, UV absorbers added to the lens resin during fabrication, and organic tints, absorb all UVB and the shorter UVA wavelengths.

Photochromic lenses

Glass lenses that darken when exposed to light were introduced by Corning Glass Works in 1964. Silver and chloride ions are included in the glass melt, where they form silver halide microcrystals. When exposed to ultraviolet or blue light, these crystals dissociate into silver ions, which cluster into specks, absorbing all UVB, most UVA, and some visible light. In darker conditions, the specks split into atoms which form crystals again, transmitting more light. This process is reversible indefinitely and will work without deterioration as long as the lenses last.

Photochromatic or variable tint lenses called Transitions are available in plastic and polycarbonate. They are 50% lighter than glass and block 100% of the UV rays. Transitions quantum (also known as velocity lenses) get 22% darker than other Transitions. They darken and fade in just 30 seconds, which is 28% faster than other transitions lenses.

Photochromatic lenses are temperature dependent: they darken as it gets cooler, and lighten as it gets warmer. A cooling of 15°C (27°F) will darken the lenses 50%. Blocking of UV, however, is not affected by temperature. These lenses can protect the eyes from all harmful light, both visible and invisible in both dark and light conditions.

Polarizing lenses reduce the intensity of reflected glare from horizontal surfaces. This glare is not only bothersome but reduces visual performance. Yellow and brown lenses are best for reducing scattered blue light. Gray lenses reduce overall brightness with the least change in color perception. Mirror-coated lenses are good at blocking glare from reflected light.

UV absorption and optical clarity tests

Image distortion in sunglasses can cause eyestrain and headaches. It is also dangerous in activities that require accurate vision. A good test for distortion (in a non-prescription lens) is to hold the lens in front of a movie or slide projector. If the image is unchanged, then the lens has good optical clarity. Alternatively, hold the lens at arm's length and look for any bending of a straight line, such as a doorway or window frame. Another test is to hold the lens up to a fluorescent light and rotate it. If the fluorescent tubes appear to change shape, the lenses do not have consistent optical clarity.

Sunglass design and shape

Larger lenses give more protection, but they should not be so large as to rest on the cheeks. Lenses should be as close to the eyes as possible without touching the eyelashes or causing the back surface of the lenses to fog up. Prescription lenses should be mounted in their frames so that the center of the lens is about 1 cm. from the surface of the eye.

Light, including UV, can strike the eye from around the sides of the lenses, especially when there is much reflected or diffuse radiation. Wraparound lenses block more sidelight, but it is important to check them for peripheral distortion, which can cause eye fatigue, headache, and even double vision. Use the same distortion tests as for a regular lens, but be sure to sight through the whole width of the lens. Avoid wraparound designs for high power prescription lenses, especially if they have a lot of correction for astigmatism. Side shields block side light, but the opaque ones may block enough peripheral vision to be a safety hazard for outdoor activities, and are illegal to wear while driving.

Standards

The Standards for maximum transmission of UVB and UVA are recommended by the American National Standards Institute (ANSI), which puts sunglasses and fashion eyeglasses in three categories based on their main intended use. Special purpose sunglasses, for skiing, mountain climbing, beach or boating should have a UVA level no greater than half the visible range, and a UVB level no greater than 1%.

Impact and scratch resistance

Prescription glass lenses must pass an impact resistance test. A 5/8" steel ball (weighing 0.56 oz.) is dropped 50" onto the center of the lens, which must not fracture under the impact. Raised edge multifocal lenses and laminated lenses, however, are not tested.

Plastic and especially polycarbonate lenses are safer and more impact-resistant than glass. They are now made of high-grade optical polymers which are lightweight and resistant to shock and scratches. CR-39 is the hardest plastic, though it is not as hard as glass. High index plastic comes next, and polycarbonate is the softest. A prescription lens should be tested and UV treated before applying a scratch-resistant coating.

Does age make a difference?

Our age affects how we react to UV rays. Children and older adults are more vulnerable and should be protected in order to maintain good eyesight. Long-term, chronic exposure to UV can cause eyesight to deteriorate. Small children are especially sensitive to light. Their pupils are wider than those of adults, and the tissues of their eyes have less pigment, which makes their eyes particularly susceptible to UV. In infants without eye protection, 90% of UVA and 50% of UVB reaches the retina.

In children under twelve, 60% of UVA and 25% of UVB reach the retina if they do not have eye protection. Children with lower levels of pigment (blond with blue eyes) are even more likely to suffer damaging effects from UV exposure. In adults over 25, less UV reaches the retina because more of it is absorbed by the lens of the eye.

To protect children from UV exposure, dress them in wide-brimmed hats and make sure that they have effective sunglasses, preferably made of optical plastic or polycarbonate. Avoid toy sunglasses, as tinted glass or plastic lenses cause the child's pupils to dilate, allowing more harmful UV rays to reach the retina.

Older people should also take precautions for UV protection, especially two groups: those who suffer a loss of pigment in the retina called macular ["spot or dye"] degeneration; and those with cataracts. Macular degeneration affects 25% of older people, especially those with light-colored eyes and those who live in areas of high UV exposure. People with cataracts should wear sunglasses with extra-powerful filters, tinted brown or orange. Smoking is a risk factor for both macular degeneration and cataracts.

Emergency eye protection

For every serious wilderness trip, the group should have at least one pair of extra sunglasses. Plastic lenses and nylon frames are the toughest and most likely to survive accidents. A hat with a visor shades the eyes. If you don't have a visor, use a small branch with foliage. Sun shades can be cut out of cardboard or heavy paper in the shape of glasses, with a pinhole in the center of each cardboard lens. These will protect your eyes from UV and enable you to see short distances, but they will restrict your peripheral vision.

Conclusion

Sunglasses for wilderness activities should protect your eyes from UVR, including reflected light. They should also have uniform optical clarity, so as not to distort your vision. Their effectiveness has little relation to price or brand, so you should check the specifications carefully, and test them in the store before buying.

Chapter 20. Sunburn and skin protection

Photos courtesy of Ben Schifrin, MD

Exposure to sunlight stimulates the production of vitamin D in the body. Pale skin (the result of a mutation 50,000 years ago) synthesizes vitamin D six times faster than dark skin, and enabled humans to thrive in northern climates with less sunshine. After the industrial revolution, many city-dwelling children (who were deprived of sunlight) developed rickets, a softening and bending of the bones. But vitamin D, the only vitamin that is a hormone, controls the expression of over 200 genes, and vitamin D deficiency can increase the risk of many other medical problems. Too much exposure to strong sunlight, however, can cause skin damage and increase the risk of skin cancer.

Before the industrial revolution in Europe and England, most poor people worked outdoors, tending crops or herding animals. So they were exposed to the sun all day, and their skin showed it (though most of them did not live long enough to develop skin cancer). Pale skin, especially in women, was therefore a sign of high social status, and "fair lady" a common phrase in lauding a woman's beauty. But as more and more men and women spent their long working days in factories and offices, sun tans became a sign of high social status as well as beauty, with sun lamps and tanning salons eventually augmenting natural sunlight; and the increase in average life span allowed time to develop skin cancer.

In the next 50 years, an estimated 12,000,000 new cases of skin cancer will occur in the United States, many of them caused by sun damage. As the ozone layer erodes, this number will probably increase. According to the Environmental Protection Agency, ozone depletion is already causing 4,000 more deaths per year in the United States from skin cancer. In the United States, one person in five born today will get skin cancer; in Australia and New Zealand (because of the hole in the ozone layer), one in three. Sun damage also ages skin prematurely, causing it to wrinkle and lose its elasticity. So if you do outdoor activities, you need to know how to protect your skin.

Sunscreens help to prevent skin damage by absorbing the energy of ultraviolet radiation. Sun blocks (also called physical sunscreens) form a layer over the skin that reflects ultraviolet.

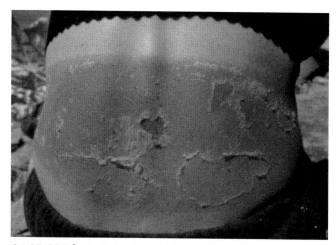

At 15,000 feet, it took only 15 minutes of exposure to cause this sunburn.

Sunscreen ingredients

For many years, the most popular sunscreen agent was PABA (paraminobenzoic acid). About 4% of the people exposed to PABA have a reaction to it, either on contact or on exposure to light. The reaction may include itching, redness, or scaling of the skin. PABA also can stain clothing yellow. So PABA is seldom used in sunscreens any more. PABA esters (padimate A and padimate O), formed by a chemical reaction with alcohol, are much less allergenic. Cinnamates absorb much less UVB than padimate O and can cause allergic reactions. They also do not bond as well to the skin. Other ingredients may be included because they are insoluble in water, or absorb UVA. Although UVA has less energy than UVB, it can cause skin damage.

Sun blocks

Sun blocks (physical sunscreens) contain either zinc oxide or titanium dioxide particles that reflect UV, but to do this they need to stay on the skin. The ones with greasy bases are messy, but more tenacious. If the particles are ground very fine (micronized) the sun block is transparent to visible light, and does not have the classic clown-white effect.

Sunscreen hazards

A percentage of sunscreen ingredients absorbed through the skin enters the bloodstream, and can be detected in blood, urine, and breast milk up to two days after application. Of the 15 chemicals approved by the FDA for use in sunscreens, 9 are endocrine disruptors, which could interfere with the normal functions of hormones and possibly increase the risk of some cancers. The non-profit Environmental Working Group has a useful guide to sunscreens, with lists of brands whose ingredients (based on the latest research) appear to be safe: www.ewg.org/sunscreen/.

Sunscreens and sun protection

Sunscreen labels have numbers that supposedly tell you how effective a sunscreen is – SPF (sun protection factor). If you multiply this SPF number by the time your unprotected skin could be exposed to sunlight without burning, you get the length of time that the manufacturer claims the sunscreen will protect you. Let's look at that claim and see what it actually means.

Your skin has some natural protection against the sun. It secretes a sunscreen called urocanic acid, and in response to UV exposure produces melanin, which absorbs, reflects, and scatters UV. As melanin oxidizes, it darkens the skin (tanning), though the skin may already be sunburned by the time that the new melanin gets to it. People with more melanin-producing cells have darker skin and more natural sun protection. For example, a dark-skinned person may have enough natural protection to survive two hours of sun exposure without burning. One application of a sunscreen with an SPF of 6 would theoretically protect that person for the whole day. But a light-skinned person, who would burn in the same conditions after 20 minutes, would need an SPF of 36. Sunscreens with SPF numbers over 30, however, provide no significant additional protection.

In practice, several factors affect how much protection a sunscreen actually gives:

- Apply sunscreen an hour before sun exposure, so that the active ingredient can bond to the outer layer of skin. Until that happens, the sunscreen may not be giving you full protection.
- You are exposed to 8%-10% more UV for every 1,000 feet that you climb, so at 10,000 feet, your exposure can be double what it is at sea level.
- Choppy water could double UV exposure by reflection from the waves at a shallow angle; and other reflecting surfaces such as snow or polished granite can greatly increase UV exposure.
- Clouds do not block UV, so it is easy to burn on an overcast day because you don't feel the need of sun protection.
- Insect repellent applied over sunscreen will reduce its effectiveness by at least one third, because the repellent is in a solvent that will also dissolve part of the sunscreen. So apply sunscreen well before exposure, and insect repellent after the sunscreen has had time to bond to the skin.
- Some sunscreen bases are more tenacious than others - the oily or waxy types adhere better than the creamy or alcohol bases.
- The active ingredients of a sunscreen can lose up to 90% of their effectiveness in an hour of exposure.
- The layer of sunscreen that has not actually bonded to the skin can be sweated or rubbed off.
- Wet skin burns faster than dry skin, and salt water makes skin even more susceptible to burning.

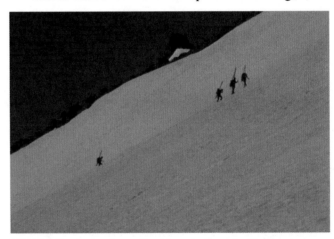

High altitude and a reflective surface both increase UV exposure.

Sunscreens advertised as "very water resistant" are supposed to stay on for 80 minutes of immersion or heavy sweating; "water resistant" for 40 minutes; and "sweat resistant" for no more than 30 minutes. So unless you have strong natural protection, you will have to reapply sunscreen frequently to exposed skin when you are sweating in hot weather. No sunscreens could accurately be called waterproof.

Clothing

An alternative to sunscreens is protective clothing. A hat with a wide brim will help to protect the face, especially from the mid-day sun. Pinning a bandana to the back of the hat, Legionnaire style, will protect the back of the neck. For extreme conditions (e.g., spring skiing at high altitude) consider wearing a hood of lightweight cloth with eye, nostril and mouth holes that hang over a hat. Mold the eyeholes around your sunglasses to maintain your field of vision.

Some clothing fabrics are tested for UV protection and given a UV protection factor (UPF) similar to the SPF for sunscreens. The UPF number means how many units of UV are blocked or absorbed by the fabric for each unit that goes through. So a UPF of 30 means that if 30 units of UV fall on the fabric, it blocks or absorbs 29 units, and only 1 unit passes through. Tightness of weave and the material of the fabric are the most important factors. Some materials (like 100% polyester) absorb as well as block UV radiation, and others may have UV absorbers added to the fabric. Also, most wet fabrics transmit more UV than dry. For example, a dry white cotton T-shirt has a UPF of 5 or more, but it loses most of its protection when it is drenched with sweat.

Photosensitivity and allergic reactions

Many medications can cause photosensitivity in some people. This results in exaggerated sunburn, out of proportion to exposure. The medications include some antidepressants, antipsychotics, antihistamines, antimicrobials, diuretics, hypoglycemics, nonsteroidal anti-inflammatory drugs, and (ironically) sunscreens containing benzophenones or cinnamates. Those with very fair skin who burn easily are most susceptible. At least 10% of Caucasians can get another reaction if exposed to more sunlight than usual - sun poisoning or polymorphous light eruption. This is especially likely at the first exposure of the season. As the name suggests, the reaction can take many forms, including swelling, blistering, and scabbing. A much rarer problem is photoallergy, in which the victim becomes sensitized to a chemical added to soap, cosmetics, or perfume, and then has a reaction triggered by sunlight, usually a rash.

Vitamin C and morning after lotion

Dr. Sheldon Pinnell, Chief of Dermatology at Duke University School of Medicine, showed in 1991 that vitamin C could reduce skin damage from UV if applied directly to the skin. It is not a sunscreen and does not replace sunscreen, but it will reduce the amount of damage done by the UV that penetrates the screen. Just dissolve vitamin C crystals (available in any health food store) in water and rub the solution on your skin before going out into the sun. The solution will be absorbed by the skin in concentrations 20 times as great as you can achieve by eating the vitamin. The body retains no more than 1.2 g per day of ingested vitamin C and dumps the rest through the urine. When rubbed on and absorbed by the skin, however, vitamin C has a half-life of 10-20 days, which means that at the end of that time half of what you originally applied will be left.

Traditional sunburn remedies such as over the counter anti-inflammatory drugs (ibuprofen) and aloe vera lotion may help alleviate some of the symptoms. Some sunscreens and skin care products include an enzyme called plankton photolyase, found in marine algae. When exposed to light, it reverses DNA damage to the cells and also blocks the inflammation called sunburn. Since sunburn occurs two to six hours after exposure, and peaks 15-24 hours later, the enzyme could prevent much of the pain and discomfort of sun exposure, as well as reversing permanent skin damage. The study was described in the *Proceedings of the National Academy of Sciences* for February 15, 2000 [See the bibliography].

Conclusion

We need sunlight to stimulate the production of vitamin D. But too much exposure can cause painful sunburn as well as long-term skin damage, and increase the risk of skin cancer. Many factors can increase exposure to UVB (which causes the most damage); and some medications and chemicals (including ingredients of some sunscreens) can aggravate the body's responses to sunlight exposure. So understanding and using clothing and sun screens to control exposure to UVB is essential for avoiding painful sunburn and long-term skin damage as well as skin cancer.

Chapter 21. Contaminated water and disinfection

Organisms that cause intestinal disease (enteric pathogens) can be transmitted by contaminated hands, food or water. They include parasites, bacteria and viruses. Parasites may pass out of the intestine as cysts, which have tough, protective outer layers. Cysts, as well as some bacteria and viruses, can survive in water for weeks or months, even in winter. Water may also contain parasite eggs.

While the risk of infection is greatest in water that has been obviously polluted by campers, cattle or pack animals, even lakes and streams that appear pristine may be contaminated. Since the incubation period of some disease organisms may be a week or more, wilderness travelers may not always realize where they picked up an infection. However, an infection may have come from contaminated food or poor group hygiene, rather than from water.

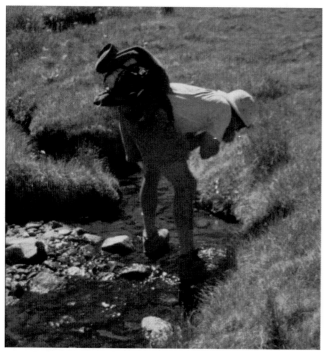

Trusting the water.

Waterborne diseases

Giardiasis is caused by a protozoan parasite that lives in the upper intestine, *Giardia lamblia*. In the U.S., about 7.4% of the population is infected. In some countries with poor sanitation, the infection rate is 20% to 30%. Only about one-fourth of those infected show

any symptoms of the disease, but they can still transmit it to others. Some of the organisms encyst and pass out with the feces. The feces can then contaminate hands, utensils, diapers, or drinking water.

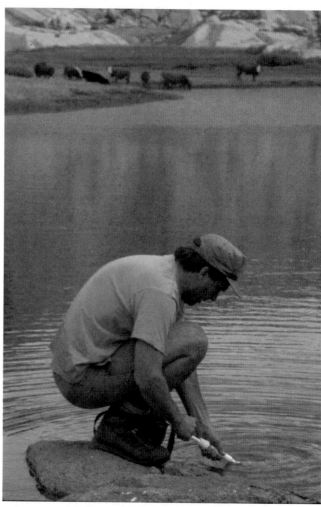

Hiker using a filter on suspect water. Note the cows across the lake. *Photos courtesy of Ben Schifrin, MD*

As few as 10 cysts can cause infection, and 25 or more cysts guarantee it. Once cysts get into the system, it takes one to three weeks for them to become active (incubation period). In heavily used wilderness areas, as much as half of the surface water may be contaminated with *Giardia*; and even some towns with chlorinated water supplies have had giardiasis epidemics. At high altitudes in the mountains, however, there may be little contamination if the water is above any cow pastures or camp grounds.

In a severe infection, the organism can cover much of the mucous membrane in the upper intestine, interfering with digestion, especially of fats. Signs and symptoms may include nausea, abdominal cramping, diarrhea, and weight loss. Mucus and blood may appear in the stools. The disease may fluctuate and go on for months. It may even become chronic. The cure usually takes 10 days or more, and the drugs used for treatment can have unpleasant side effects.

Diagnosing giardiasis by looking for cysts in the stools with a microscope is difficult. Even if the sample was taken when the patient was shedding cysts, they might be missed. Immunoassay tests of stool samples, or testing for antibodies in the blood, are more reliable.

Cryptosporidium is another protozoan whose cysts are found even in chlorinated water supplies. Some recent studies have shown that it is very resistant to chemical disinfection. Iodine and chlorine treatments used in the wilderness do not work. It is, however, very sensitive to heat and can be removed by filters with pores that are 1μ (micron) or smaller. Water polluted by sewage or agricultural runoff is very likely to be contaminated with cyyptosporidium. Pristine water, however (not polluted by animals or backpackers), is unlikely to contain enough concentration of cryptosporidium to cause illness.

Many bacteria can cause gastrointestinal disease. *Escherichia coli* is a common intestinal parasite, which is usually kept under control by the body's immune system. But infection with an alien strain, or by a large dose, can cause disease within two days and sometimes within a few hours. Usually it causes diarrhea and nausea for just a few days, but it can go on for weeks.

Salmonella is often transmitted by meat and dairy products (food poisoning), but it can also be picked up in contaminated water. Incubation takes 8 to 48 hours, and the disease usually runs its course in a few days, though the feces will be contagious for a month or two.

Some other enteric bacteria that may contaminate water are *Shigella*, *Campylobacter*, and *V. cholerae*. *Shigella* can cause bloody stools (disentery). Cholera kills by dehydrating the patient, and has caused epidemics for thousands of years. Cholera is now rare in the U.S., but still common in developing countries with poor sanitation.

Several **viruses** also cause gastrointestinal disease. They spread from person to person, by direct and indirect contact, as well as through contaminated drinking water. Norwalk-like viruses, rotaviruses, and hepatitis A are the most common. Over 90% of adults in developing countries, and 50% of adults in the U.S., have antibodies to hepatitis A, which means that they have been exposed to the disease even if they are not currently infected.

The Norwalk-like viruses usually cause only mild disease, lasting a day or two. Rotaviruses are more serious. They are the most common cause of diarrhea in young children, and often require hospitalization for dehydration. After incubating for one to three days, they usually cause several days of vomiting, followed by three to eight days of diarrhea.

Hepatitis A can last one to two weeks in children and four to six weeks or longer in adults. Immunization for hepatitis A may be worthwhile for people who are likely to be exposed to it (e.g., those who work with children). No cure is available for any of these viral infections, though Human Immune Globulin (HIG) can reduce the severity of hepatitis A. Treatment is mainly fluid replacement.

Prevention

Before defecating, dig a hole (4 to 6 inches deep) well away from water (100 feet if possible) and campsites and NOT in a gully that may become a runoff stream during rainfall or snow melt. Wash your hands with soap and water after defecating and before handling food. If water is scarce, use a benzalkonium chloride towelette. People who show signs of intestinal disease should not handle food for the group. Filter or disinfect all ground water.

Water disinfection techniques

Cloudy water can be clarified by letting it stand overnight in above-freezing weather, then dipping clarified water after sediment has precipitated out. This will speed chemical disinfection and help avoid clogging of filters. A pinch of **alum** in the water will speed the settling out of sediment. Shake or stir it in for a minute, agitate the water frequently for about 5 minutes, then let it settle for at least 30 minutes. Dip clarified water from the top. If you use chemical disinfection, warm the water by carrying it in a translucent dark plastic Nalgene® bottle, exposed to the sun, because warming speeds up chemical reactions. Carry two water bottles, so that you'll have one to drink from while the other disinfects

Heating

Bringing water to a vigorous, roiling boil (at any altitude to which you can climb) kills all organisms that can make you sick and makes the water safe to drink. As altitude increases, the boiling temperature decreases, to 187° F at 14,000 feet and 166° F at 24,000 feet. But as the water heats to the boiling point, it is killing microorganisms, and any temperature over 140° F. should kill them within seconds. Some older sources recommend boiling water for up to 10 minutes, but according to more recent lab tests, cited by Dr. Howard Backer, this is not necessary (see the bibliography). Boiling for one minute should give you an ample margin of safety, by making sure that the water really has come to a full boil.

Chemical disinfection

Chlorine and **iodine** in water can disinfect it, but several factors can interfere with the process.

- Chlorine and iodine molecules kill microorganisms by oxidizing their enzymes and cellular structures. Any particles in the water, however, may react with the chemicals and take them out of action.
- CAUTION: do not add anything (e.g., flavoring) to the water until disinfection is complete.
- Concentration of a saturated solution depends on temperature. In cold water, much less iodine or chlorine will dissolve than in warm water.
- Disinfection, like any chemical reaction, depends on temperature. The colder the water, the slower the reaction.
- In alkaline water (pH over 7.5), higher doses of chemicals are required to disinfect.
- The largest microorganisms (e.g., Giardia and Cryptosporidium cysts) are most resistant to chemicals, because of their tough outer covering. But they are very sensitive to heat, so boiling easily kills them; and they are easy to filter out.

Chlorine

Halazone tablets release chlorine as they dissolve in water. But exposure to air, heat, or moisture rapidly reduces their potency, and even if they are stored in a cool, dry place, shelf life is only about six months.

Bleach is another source of chlorine, but in 1% concentration it takes up to 20 drops per liter and 45 minutes contact time to disinfect cold and cloudy water. Even warm, clear water requires 10 drops per liter and 30 minutes contact time. Water that is so heavily chlorinated will taste unpleasant, and smaller doses are not reliable. Moreover, chlorine is unlikely to be effective against Giardia or Cryptosporidium cysts. Many outbreaks of giardiasis have occurred in small cities with chlorinated water systems.

Miox Purifier (www.miox.com) is based on technology used in large commercial processes, adapted by the military to a portable device. It uses salt, water, and electrical current from camera batteries to produce a disinfecting solution that you add to drinking water. The 8-ounce kit includes the device (Pen), batteries, salt packet, and test strips to check the treated water for adequate concentration of disinfectant. LED lights signal low battery or inadequate salt or water. Retail price is high but test results show that it seems to be slightly more effective than other chemical disinfection systems, killing viruses and bacteria in 15 minutes, Giardia in 30 minutes, and Cryptosporidium in up to 4 hours (or less if the water is clear). However, it only generates enough disinfecting solution in each cycle to treat 1 liter of water.

Iodine

Iodine also comes in tablets (Potable Aqua, Globaline, EDWGT), but these have the same problems as chlorine tablets. While sealed bottles of iodine tablets have a shelf life of four to five years, frequent opening reduces their useful life to about two weeks, so you should get a new bottle for each trip. Iodine crystals are more reliable. Adding water to the crystals makes a saturated iodine solution, which is poured into the drinking water. The Polar Pure® system has iodine crystals in a bottle with a thermometer on the side. This is useful because the concentration of a saturated iodine solution depends on its temperature.

Recommended doses of iodine are calculated for a temperature of 68° to 77° F. In a transparent bottle, you can tell how saturated the solution is by its color. Pale yellow is weak and dark orange is strong. If the solution is weak, you can warm it up next to your body. Let it equilibrate for 30 to 60 minutes before using, or increase the dose by 30%.

Doses from a 2 oz. bottle are usually given in bottle caps. One capful holds 2.5 cc. For clear water, use five caps of the solution. Be careful not to let any crystals into the water bottle. Shake the bottle well. You should allow at least 15 minutes contact time if water is warm or 60 minutes if it is cold. For cloudy water, use ten caps of solution. Allow 30 minutes if the water is warm or 60 minutes if it is cold.

Alcohol solutions of iodine also work. For 2% tincture of iodine, just substitute one drop for each capful of the water solution and allow the same contact times. For 10% Povidone/iodine solution (Betadyne), use eight drops instead of five capfuls, sixteen drops instead of ten capfuls. You can also add 100 cc of 95% ethanol to 8 grams of iodine crystals. Just 1 cc of the ethanol solution equals five capfuls of the water solution. CAUTION: use only U.S.D.A. food-grade resublimated iodine crystals. Other iodine crystals intended for industrial use contain impurities that may be toxic.

About 7% of the population may have a reaction to iodine, usually diarrhea. Iodine is not recommended for pregnant women or people with thyroid problems. Also, the longer you use it the more likely you are to have problems. So on a long trip, iodine is probably best reserved as a backup to other disinfection techniques, such as boiling or filtering.

Making the water palatable
You can remove the taste of iodine by sprinkling vitamin C crystals in the water or using a powdered drink flavoring that includes vitamin C (ascorbic acid). Be careful not to do this until disinfection is complete because it will inactivate the iodine. It will not, however, remove iodine. To do that, you would need to run the water through a block of granular activated carbon, available as an attachment on some filters.

Water filters
Intake hoses attached to water filters usually have screens to keep out large particles, and there may be one or more pre-filters. But the **absolute size** of the pores in the final filter tells you what size organisms the filter can remove. "Absolute" means that all pores are that size or smaller. Nothing that is much larger than the absolute pore size can get through, although microorganisms can deform and squeeze through openings slightly smaller than their diameter. Some manufacturers deceptively use **nominal pore size** in their advertisements, which means that the filter only stops 90% of the organisms that size or larger. For example, a filter advertised as 0.1μ (micron) pore size may be 0.4μ absolute pore size. Nominal pore size is meaningless for water disinfection, because a breakthrough of up to 10% of an organism may be more than enough to make you sick. So be sure that the specifications refer to absolute pore size.

All of the commercial filters with an absolute pore size of 1μ or smaller remove protozoan parasites, such as Giardia lamblia. A giardia cyst is about 5μ across, a Cryptosporidium cyst about 2μ. Some bacteria, however, are as small as 0.3μ. For example, Escherichia coli are from 0.3μ to 0.9μ. So a filter with an absolute pore size of 0.2μ should remove bacteria as well as larger organisms. Viruses are about 0.01μ, much too small for filtration in the field. While many of them will be removed because they tend to clump or attach to larger particles, some will get through.

Some filters use an iodine resin matrix to kill any organisms that pass through the filter. This element may be built into the filter or sold as an optional attachment. Filters with an iodine matrix remove viruses almost completely, though in some tests they do not quite meet the Environmental Protection Agency standard of removing 99.99%.

Some filters include a block of granular activated carbon, which may remove chemicals, such as pesticide, or the residue from chemical disinfection. This is a useful feature for filters that include an iodine resin matrix, and essential for filtering water that may be polluted by agricultural or industrial runoff. While it will not remove all iodine residue, it will greatly reduce the concentration.

Filter types
Filters are of two types: **membrane** and **labyrinth**. Membrane filters are thin and delicate and cannot be cleaned, so you need to carry replacements, especially on a long trip. Labyrinth filters are solid structures that can be cleaned. The pores are twisting paths through the thickness of the filter, so the filter element would have to be seriously damaged to fail. It is also harder

for organisms to get through than a thin membrane with the same pore size.

Ceramic filter elements last at least ten times as long as the others and can be brushed off when they get clogged, so they have an advantage on long trips. Katadyn impregnates its filter element with silver, which it claims inhibits bacterial growth, but independent laboratory tests do not support this claim.

How resistant are the filter elements to damage? Ceramic cylinders, used in some Katadyn and MSR filters, are brittle, so they could be cracked if dropped or if frozen with water inside. The **borosilicate labyrinth filter** used in the Sweetwater Guardian, and the **pleated glass fiber** used in PUR and other filters are rugged, and also cleanable, though they will not last nearly as long as ceramic filters.

Sweetwater filters are now owned by MSR (www.msrcorp.com). PUR (www.purwaterfilter.com) has a range of products for household use that purify water (remove inorganic contaminants), but their portable water filters are now made by Katadyn (www.katadyn.com), the Swiss company that has been providing filters to international relief organizations such as the Red Cross for many decades. Katadyn makes the Pocket Filter (which weighs 23 oz.) and an 11 lb. Expedition Filter, which pumps 4 liters per minute, both with 0.2µ ceramic filter elements. They also make the smaller Hiker with a 0.3µ pleated glass fiber element. PUR makes the Guide and the smaller Hiker, both with 0.3µ filter elements. The trade-off for the smaller sized filters is slower pumping. While the Katadyn Pocket filter is the most expensive in its class, the long service life of its ceramic filter element, and the 20 year warranty (unique in the industry) may justify the cost. The Sweetwater Guardian, on the other hand, has the lowest price of any 0.2µ labyrinth filter. Several manufacturers also make gravity filters, which can be useful in a base camp where you have time to let the water slowly seep through.

UV radiation

One device uses UV radiation to disinfect water – Hydro-Photon Steripen (www.hydrophoton.com). It works by inserting the UV bulb into a container of water and irradiating it with ultraviolet. It weighs 8 oz. with batteries, and costs about $200. The advantages are that it works quickly and leaves no taste or odor.

However, it can be used only on small quantities of water. A liter bottle (the maximum size) requires two doses of UV; a half-liter bottle one dose. Also, the batteries may be affected by cold weather, and any particles in the water will block some of the UV, so cloudy water should be pre-filtered before disinfecting, e.g. by straining through a coffee filter.

Convenience

How easy and convenient are the filters to use? The Katadyn Pocket filter is the hardest and most awkward to pump, because you have to brace it against something solid when you depress the piston. The SweetWater and the MSR filters, with lever handles, are the easiest to pump, requiring only 2 to 3 pounds of force. The MSR has an adapter on the bottom, which screws onto a standard Nalgene® water bottle or an MSR water bag. The SweetWater has an adapter on its output hose, which fits onto several different sizes of water bottle mouths.

How easy are the filters to maintain? The MSR filters are very well designed. The Waterworks II has four filter elements of decreasing size, which greatly reduces clogging. But it must be taken apart regularly to clean and dry out, and includes a number of small parts that can be misplaced. So it tends to be popular with people who are mechanically adept and don't mind doing regular maintenance. Most other filters seem to require little maintenance. Pumps may need occasional lubrication, and the pressure relief valve in the Sweetwater Guardian may need occasional cleaning.

Conclusion

There are many techniques for disinfecting water in the wilderness, but none of them is without disadvantages. Boiling is the most reliable technique, but it requires time and fuel. Chemical systems are very light and compact, but many factors can interfere with their disinfecting action and the chemical residue in the water can cause problems. Filters are expensive, heavy, and bulky, and can be damaged or clogged. Consider the length of your trips, the number of people in the group, and the probable quality of the water where you are going when selecting a system. You should always carry a backup, especially for long trips.

Chapter 22. Mosquitoes, ticks and disease

Blood is about one-half solids, which makes it a rich source of protein for the many arthropods that feed on it. Some, like mosquitoes, use the protein only to make eggs, which means that only the females bite. Others, like ticks, also live on blood. When they feed, these arthropods may transmit disease, so they are called disease vectors. In the United States, ticks currently transmit more than 90% of the disease that arthropods transmit to humans. Fleas carry plague, and in the tropics, other blood-sucking flies carry diseases.

Worldwide, however, mosquitoes transmit the most disease agents to humans. In the United States, mosquito abatement programs in the first quarter of the 20th century reduced disease by reducing mosquito populations, and the North American climate is less hospitable than the tropics to the mosquitoes that carry major human diseases – a condition that global warming may be changing.

However, there are more than enough mosquito vectors to cause epidemics in the United States, and we are protected from some tropical diseases only because there are no reservoirs (animal or human hosts carrying the disease) from which the mosquitoes can pick them up. Large numbers of returning military personnel or immigrants infected with those diseases could change that. For example, cases of malaria in a Girl Scout troop camping near the California coast were traced to an infected Vietnam veteran who was camping nearby.

Mosquitoes & other blood-sucking flies

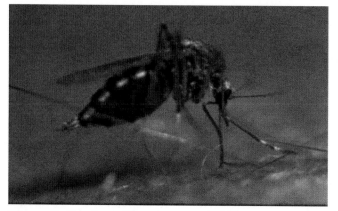

Mosquito feeding *Photo courtesy of Elton J. Hansons*

There are 3,000 species of mosquitoes, and 200 species inhabit the United States. They need still or slow-moving water to breed. The larvae hang just below the surface and feed on detritus and microorganisms in the water. The larvae of Anopheles (Greek "not useful"), which transmits malaria, hang horizontally, supported by air bubbles in their float hairs and body notches. Aedes (Greek "unpleasant") and Culex (Latin "gnat") larvae hang down at an angle, breathing through siphons. When the adult emerges from the pupa, however, it needs to dry its wings and groom its mouthparts while standing on the water's surface before it can fly away. Turbulence or wind can knock it over and drown it.

Mosquitoes, therefore, tend to be thickest in marshy terrain, and most mosquito abatement programs in the past depended on draining marshes, or killing the larvae with pesticides or oil at the cost of polluting the water. Mosquitoes can also breed in snowmelt pools, tree stump holes, ditches, or piles of used tires left outdoors. Most mosquitoes in the United States breed in spring and summer.

They are active at temperatures above 60° F, and some are active down to 50° F in early spring. The higher the altitude, the lower the temperature, and the fewer mosquitoes will be active, especially at night. Some species feed by day, especially in woodlands, and some feed at dusk or at night if it is warm enough; though a strong freeze kills adult mosquitoes. Since anopheles mosquitoes (which transmit malaria) are night feeders, it is important to use bed nets in warm countries where malaria is endemic.

Mosquitoes sense hosts from a distance by odors. Midrange, carbon dioxide triggers a random flying reflex. If the flying brings the mosquitoes in close, heat and moisture attract them to the skin and trigger the blood-sucking reflex. The needle-like proboscis pierces the skin and injects blood-thinner with the saliva. Then if the mosquito is carrying disease, it infects the host.

Some species, such as *Anopheles* spp, also inject an anesthetic, so that the host does not feel the bite. Foreign proteins injected in the saliva can cause an allergic reaction around the bite, with swelling and itching. As the mosquito feeds, it excretes the liquid part of the blood, leaving a little droplet of water on the skin and keeping only the protein-rich solids. A blood meal enables a female mosquito to lay hundreds of eggs, instead of just a few.

Other blood-sucking flies have mouth parts like daggers. They slash the skin and create a pool of blood. Since the larger flies feed mainly on animals with thick hides, such as deer, their bites can be painful. Except for mosquitoes, however, most blood-sucking flies in North America (which feed only during the day) do not transmit blood-borne diseases. Only the deerfly (*Chrsops discalis*) infrequently transmits the tularemia bacterium in the Southwest.

Protection

Repellents are chemicals that seem to interfere with the senses of bloodsuckers, making it hard for them to locate you. For North American mosquitoes and other bloodsuckers, repellents with **DEET** (N-N-diethyl-meta toluamide) have been effective, though some species seem to become resistant to its effects after a few hours of exposure. A 30% solution seems to be optimum. About 3% to 5% of the DEET applied is absorbed through the skin, and some studies suggest toxic effects. So it is probably best to minimize the amount of DEET that you put on your skin. One strategy is to use a mosquito shirt – a shirt made of mosquito netting that is kept in a bag saturated with DEET when you are not wearing it. DEET can also eat holes in plastic and synthetic fabrics, so you should keep it away from clothing, packs, and tents.

Picaridin (brand name Bayrepel) is an alternative to DEET which seems to be at least as effective. It has much less odor than DEET, and does not damage plastic or synthetic clothing. Repellents with 30% oil of lemon eucalyptus (extracted from gum eucalyptus trees) have also scored well in *Consumer Reports* tests. Many other substances have some repellency, but are not very effective and do not last long on the skin.

Spraying clothing and mosquito netting with permethrin also helps. **Permethrin** (which is sold under various brand names) attacks the nervous systems of arthropods, usually causing them to drop off or fly away if it doesn't kill them on contact. Tropical uniforms for the United States military have been treated with permethrin for many years.

Permethrin is recommended only for spraying or soaking clothes and netting, not for use on the skin because it breaks down in contact with skin, and can cause dermatitis. Avoid inhaling it. Spray clothing outdoors while standing upwind. Once sprayed on clothing, it will stay active for weeks, and for months in clothing that was soaked in a permethrin solution. Be careful with permethrin treated clothing around pet cats or dogs, however, because they may rub against it, then ingest the permethrin by grooming themselves with their tongues; and ingested permethrin can cause liver damage.

Malaria

Although about 1,000 cases of malaria are reported per year in the United States, almost all of them are acquired in other countries. But it is a serious threat to travelers in the tropics. Malaria is carried by an estimated 500,000,000 people, including more than half the population of Africa. About 90% of the deaths are in Africa, where many people have little access to medical care and diagnosis; so estimates of malaria deaths vary, up to 1,200,000 per year according to a report published in *The Lancet* in 2012 – twice the number estimated by the World Health Organization, but down from 1,800,000 deaths estimated for 2004. Window screens are almost unknown outside the United States, and programs to control mosquito-borne diseases in Africa have been disrupted by civil wars. But since the *anopheles* mosquitoes that carry malaria are night feeders, **bed nets** treated with permethrin are an effective way to reduce malaria infections – if people actually use them.

The Italian word *malaria* means "bad air," and records a long-standing misconception about its cause, which was supported by the observation that the disease was common in swampy and malodorous areas. But malaria is caused by a **protozoan parasite** that infected mosquitoes transmit when they take blood. Five species infect humans (and some other primates): *Plasmodium vivax* ("long-lived"), *P. falciparum* ("sickle shaped"), *P. malariae*, *P. ovale* ("oval or egg-shaped"), and *P. knowlesi. P. falciparum* and *P. vivax* cause most malaria infections, and *P. falciparum* causes 95% of the deaths, because it has many ways to invade red blood cells, and infects up to 60% of them. Other species of the parasite only infect up to 2% of the host's red blood cells. *P. vivax* has only about 1% fatality, but can be very debilitating. Also, *P. vivax* can remain in the liver for years after the host has apparently recovered, whereas when someone survives an infection by *P. falciparum*, the immune system usually clears out the parasite completely.

In West and Central Africa, where *P. vivax* has been endemic for millennia, 97% of the population has a mutation (Duffy negativity) that makes them immune. It removes the proteins on the surface of red blood cells (Duffy antigens) to which *P. vivax* attaches. Some people whose ancestors lived in parts of Africa where *P. falciparum* was endemic have another mutation that makes their hemoglobin resistant to that species, so that they get only mild symptoms from an infection. But if they inherit the gene from both parents, the abnormal hemoglobin stretches red blood cells into a sickle shape, making them fragile and short-lived, which causes **sickle cell anemia**. Even without this mutation, survivors of *P. falciparum* who are repeatedly infected become somewhat resistant.

Malaria parasites are transmitted by many species of *Anopheles* mosquitoes. From the mosquito's salivary glands, injected sporozoites (Greek *sporos* "seed", *zoon* "animal") move through the blood to the liver. In liver cells they multiply for about two weeks, forming many merozoites (Greek *meros* "part", *zoon* "animal"). Then the merozoites burst out of the liver cells into the blood stream, invade red blood cells and digest the oxygen-carrying hemoglobin. They grow and split into from 8 to 24 merozoites, then burst into the blood again to invade more red blood cells.

This is when the disease can be diagnosed by identifying the parasite in blood samples. This is also when the patient experiences the symptoms of a malarial attack, which can last from one to eight hours and recur every third day (or every fourth day for *P. malariae*). These symptoms include fever, shaking chills, sweats, headache, muscle pain, and malaise. Victims of malaria also develop a palpably enlarged spleen, because one of its functions is to recycle worn out red blood cells.

After several cycles, some of the merozoites develop into male and female gametocytes (Greek *gamein* "to marry", *kytos* "cell"). When gametocytes are taken in by another feeding mosquito, they begin the process of developing into sporozoites.

Unsuccessful efforts to produce a malaria vaccine date back to 1910. In clinical trials of the latest vaccine (for *P. falciparum*) three shots gave only partial protection. *Plasmodium* species have 5,200 genes (compared to several hundred genes in most bacteria) which gives the parasites many resources for eluding the host's immune system. Also, malaria parasites go through several different life stages in the human host, which makes it harder to target them with a vaccine; and there are several species that infect humans. Moreover, surviving malaria does not confer long term immunity, so neither would a vaccine.

In the 17th century, Jesuit missionaries noticed that Peruvian natives drank infusions of powdered bark from the cinchona tree to relieve the shaking chills and fever of malaria – which, ironically, was probably introduced to the Americas by Europeans. So they began exporting "Jesuit bark" to Europe. One active ingredient, an alkaloid called **quinine**, was isolated in the early 20th century. Because of its side effects, which include ringing in the ears and (with repeated use) possibly deafness, quinine was supplanted by synthetic anti-malarial drugs, such as chloroquine and atabrine; but it is still sometimes used for treating *P. falciparum* infections resistant to newer drugs.

The most recent remedy for *P. falciparum* infections, **artemisinin**, made from the leaves of *Artemesia annua* (sweet wormwood) trees, was discovered in an ancient Chinese herbal manual. Artemisinin combination therapy (ACT) combines several artemisinin derivatives with another anti-malarial drug. Some studies by doctors in Africa (reported in www.malariaworld.org) seemed to show better results (without the side effects of ACT) using *Artemesia* leaves in tea or ground up in capsules. These results suggest that the leaves contain more than one antimalarial ingredient.

Since conditions and treatment may change rapidly, travelers should get the latest information about malaria and other diseases in their destination countries from the Centers for Disease Control and Prevention website (www.cdc.gov).Travelers should also bring all the necessary medications with them, because Africa and Asia are flooded with **counterfeit medications**, some of which mimic authentic appearance and packaging so closely that they fool even medical professionals.

Yellow fever

Yellow fever infects monkeys in Africa and South and Central America, but only humans in the United States and Canada. The yellow fever epidemics in the United States from the 17th to the early 20th centuries were in seaports such as New Orleans, where travelers and sailors infected in the tropics provided a reservoir. It is caused by a virus, and transmitted mainly by *Aedes aegypti* and *A. albopictus* (Asian tiger) mosquitoes. Yellow fever infects about 200,000 people a year, with about 30,000 deaths, 90% in Africa and about 10% in South America.

Early signs and symptoms, which can come on very suddenly from three to six days after being infected, may include fever, chills, headache, muscle aches, nausea and vomiting. Jaundice – skin turning yellow – gives the disease its name. In more serious cases, the patient can also bleed from the nose and gums. No treatment is available for yellow fever, but a **vaccine** can provide protection for up to ten years.

Dengue fever

Dengue is caused by a virus related to the yellow fever virus, and seems only to infect humans. The word may come from the Swahili for "sudden cramp or seizure." Dengu is transmitted by several species of *Aedes* mosquitoes. Most cases are mild, but symptoms may include fever, headache and pain behind the eyes, and bone and joint pain (which is why it is also called breakbone fever).

Dengue is a tropical disease, so most cases in the United States are brought back by travelers. Usually it lasts a week or less. But children can get a potentially fatal variation called dengue hemorrhagic ("bleeding") fever, which is an over-reaction of the body's immune system after they have started to recover from the virus. A number of cases have been reported in Texas, which borders Mexico.

Zika virus, which has been spreading through Latin America, is related to Dengue and transmitted by the same species of *Aedes* mosquitoes, so it could easily spread to North America. Its symptoms are similar to those of Dengue, though three out of four victims may not realize they are infected because they have mild or no symptoms. Some researchers suspect, however, that it can cause birth defects if a pregnant mother is infected.

Encephalitis

Encephalitis means "inflammation of the brain," and mosquitoes transmit many viruses that can infect the brain. No specific treatments or vaccines are available for any of them. Most forms of encephalitis rarely infect humans in the U.S. Reported cases per year usually number in the hundreds, at most, though they can be very serious. Eastern equine encephalitis (so called because it infects horses as well as humans) has a mortality rate of 30-60%, and St. Louis encephalitis 3-20%. Other forms of encephalitis, such as Western equine encephalomyletis, LaCrosse, and Venezuelan usually cause mild, flu-like symptoms at worst.

West Nile virus

West Nile virus has spread rapidly over the United States since 1999, when it was first reported, because its animal reservoirs include many species of birds, and it is transmitted by 64 mosquito species. It is now found in all states except Alaska, Maine, and Hawaii. Symptoms may include fever, headache, nausea and vomiting. In fewer than 1% of the victims, the virus invades the brain, and about 10% of these victims die. About 80% of people infected, however, experience no symptoms; and as with other infectious diseases, mild cases are rarely reported, or even diagnosed, so West Nile virus infection is probably much more common than the statistics indicate. In 2015, 2175 cases (serious enough to require treatment) and 146 deaths in the U.S. were reported to the Centers for Disease Control and Prevention (www.cdc.gov). They also estimated that 345 blood donors were infected with the virus.

Plague

Caused by bacteria (*Yersinia pestis*), this disease devastated the Byzantine Empire in the 6th century, killed about one-third of the population in 14th century Europe and 10,000,000 in the late 19th century. Since plague is carried by rodents, especially black rats, shipping routes have traditionally spread it from seaport to seaport. For millennia, when humans shared their homes with unintentionally domesticated rats, they also shared the rats' fleas, which transmit the disease from host to host. Plague was probably introduced to the United States in San Francisco in 1899, and spread through the Western United States (as well as parts of Canada and Mexico) in wild rodent populations that live in burrows, including ground squirrels, deer mice, voles, and prairie dogs.

Yet only about ten human cases are reported per year in the United States. Humans enter the cycle only when they live near rodents and their fleas, like an Asian family in California whose house had a thatched roof inhabited by roof rats. And campgrounds are sometimes closed when infected rodents are found nesting in the grounds.

But infection is possible whenever a die-off of the wild rodent population leaves hungry fleas on their carcasses or their burrow entrances. So it is wise not to walk within flea-jumping distance (three feet or more) of a dead animal or to camp near rodent burrows. And before traveling to countries where human plague is more common, you should get the latest information from the Centers for Disease Control and Prevention web site.

Bubonic plague, so-called because it causes the lymph glands in the neck, armpits, and groin to swell, is the most common form (Greek *boubon* "swelling in the groin"). Other signs and symptoms may include high fever, headache, delirium, nausea, and a rapid, irregular pulse. Early diagnosis and treatment with antibiotics (such as streptomycin and tetracycline) reduces mortality to about 15%. If it is not treated, mortality is about 50%. **Pneumonic plague** (infecting the lungs) is much more contagious, because it can be spread rapidly, like flu, by coughing and sneezing. It is almost always fatal if not treated promptly.

Ticks

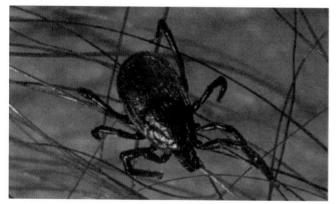

Female western black-legged tick on skin
Photo courtesy of Jack C. Clark

Only seven of the 86 tick species in the United States feed on humans with any regularity and can transmit disease agents to them. Soft ticks, which are found in burrows, caves, nests (and occasionally human homes) seldom contact humans and carry only one human disease – tick-borne relapsing fever. Hard ticks, so called because they have a shield-like cuticle (scutum) over the front half of their bodies, are much more likely to find and feed on humans.

Hard ticks wait for hosts in vegetation, and concentrate along animal trails, especially the uphill side when the trails traverse slopes and vegetation overhangs the trail, and at the boundaries (ecotones) where trails go from one type of vegetation to another (e.g., meadow to forest). In some habitats, 80%-90% of the ticks will be at ecotones. Host animals may brush against them when crossing the boundary and become infested. Larvae and nymphs are usually in leaf litter on the ground, in dense woodlands. Nymphs of some species may also be on logs or the lower parts of tree trunks. Adults wait on the tips of grass blades or other low-lying herbaceous vegetation in a questing posture, holding on with their rear and middle legs while extending their forelegs.

Ticks have carbon dioxide sensors in their forelegs. Exhaled breath can stimulate the tick to climb onto a passing host or crawl up to 15 feet. Entomologists use dry ice (which emits carbon dioxide) to collect ticks and test them for disease agents. At close range, heat and moisture trigger a reflex to grip and crawl upward on the host, against gravity. Then serrated mouthparts open the skin, and the barbed, harpoon-like hypostome (Greek "under the mouth") secures the tick. Once attached, a hard tick will secrete a cement-like substance to hold it in place, and feed for up to a week, or even longer. An adult female can increase its weight a hundred-fold or more during blood feeding while regurgitating the liquid part of the blood back into the host and using the protein to make eggs. Larvae and nymphs also need blood meals to develop to the next stage of their life cycle.

Lyme disease: History and geography

Lyme disease is the best-known tick-borne infection and the most common in temperate regions of the Northern Hemisphere. It was first diagnosed in Europe in 1883, and in the United States (in Lyme, Connecticut) in 1975. About 30,000 cases of Lyme disease are reported in the United States each year, out of 300,000 per year estimated by the Centers for Disease Control and Prevention.

However, Lyme disease has probably been in the United States for millennia. It was often unrecognized or misdiagnosed, because its signs and symptoms can mimic those of several other diseases, including syphilis. Early settlers in New England described ticks boiling out of the ground whenever they sat down in the woods. But as land clearing for cultivation and urbanization reduced or eliminated the habitats of tick hosts, the disease declined. Now it is increasing as more people move into the suburbs or semi-rural areas, or engage in wilderness activities.

In 1982, Dr. Willy Burgdorfer identified the corkscrew-shaped bacterium that causes Lyme disease, so it is named after him – *Borrelia burgdorferi*. It lives in the gut of an infected tick, and is stimulated to reproduce when the tick starts feeding. After a day or two, it begins to cross to the circulatory system and migrate to the salivary glands, where it can be injected into the host. But if the tick is properly removed before that, there is very little chance of infection.

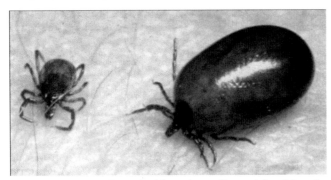

Ticks starting to feed (left) and swollen with a blood meal (right). *Photo courtesy of TickedOff.com*

In the far Western United States, the nymph tick that carries Lyme disease bacteria (*Ixodes pacificus*) can have an infection rate of 10% or higher. But the adult tick has only a 1-2% rate of infection, because the primary hosts of its juvenile stages (larvae and nymphs) are resistant, especially the western fence lizard and the southern alligator lizard. When the host's immune system kills the bacteria, it breaks the cycle of infection. So there is very little chance of catching Lyme disease from a single bite from an adult tick, but more chance of being infected by a nymph tick.

In the Eastern United States, however, the adult tick that carries Lyme disease (*Ixodes scapularis*) has a much higher rate of infection – up to 60% or more in parts of New England – because more of its hosts support the disease. Even the nymphs of *I. Scapularis* usually have infection rates about one-half those of adult ticks, because lizards (which are resistant to the disease) are uncommon.

Lyme disease: Signs and symptoms

Lyme disease can have up to three stages:
- Early flu-like symptoms and (usually) a rash;
- Delayed infection of joints, neurological system, or the heart;
- Chronic, recurring condition.

It begins from 3 to 30 days after infection with flu-like symptoms, which may include chills and fever, fatigue, joint and muscle pain, and loss of appetite as the organism spreads through the blood stream. A rash around the bite, **erythema migrans** (spreading or "migrating redness"), appears in about 60% to 80% of infected adults and 90% of children. As the red spreads slowly over days or weeks, it may fade in the center. After a tick bite, this rash is an almost certain mark of Lyme disease. Without it, diagnosis is tricky, so it is important to find a doctor who is familiar with Lyme disease, and knows which lab tests to order.

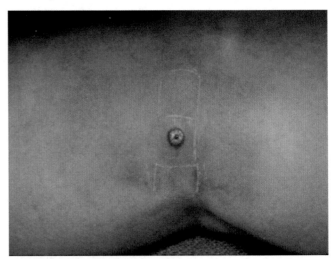

Rash of early stage Lyme disease (erythema migrans) surrounding the tick attachment site
Photo courtesy of Ben Schifrin, MD

In its early stages, Lyme disease is usually easy to cure with antibiotics. In its later stages, it may be more difficult to treat, and there is an ongoing controversy about late stage Lyme disease between researchers and health care providers, who have different criteria for diagnosis and treatment; and several Lyme disease survivor organizations provide patient education and advocacy. If untreated, Lyme disease can persist for months or years. Signs and symptoms vary depending on where the bacteria go, possibly because there are many different strains of *Borrelia burgdorferi*. If they move to the synovial fluid of a joint, they cause arthritic symptoms, usually on just one side of the body. This is the most common form of late stage Lyme disease in the United States. In the cerebrospinal fluid, the bacteria can cause neurological problems, such as Bell's palsy, meningitis, encephalitis, or radiculoneuropathy. In **Bell's palsy**, one or both sides of the face can be paralyzed for weeks to months.

Symptoms of **Meningitis** (inflammation of the membranes around the brain or spinal cord) include headache, a stiff neck, and over-sensitivity to light. In **radiculoneuropathy**, the nerve roots coming out of the spinal cord are infected, which can cause local tingling, numbness, and pain. **Encephalitis** (inflammation of the brain) can cause sleeplessness, memory loss, and mood changes. Infection of the heart can cause **arrhythmia**, which usually clears up within weeks, but may require a pacemaker. If untreated, Lyme disease can become a chronic, recurring infection; but one possibility that may account for some seemingly intractable cases is that the patient had an undiagnosed co-infection with another bacterium or protozoan from the tick.

The variety of possible symptoms, all of which can have many other causes, makes diagnosis difficult. In the 1970s and 1980s, Lyme disease was under-diagnosed, because doctors didn't know much about it. The author once had a student bring a friend into class after he taught a lesson on tick-borne diseases. She had a textbook erythema migrans rash on her upper leg, ten days after pulling out an engorged tick. Her doctor didn't recognize the rash and diagnosed flu. Now, however, Lyme disease may be over-diagnosed because of all the publicity. Also, the blood tests are not completely reliable. The **ELISA** test can give a false positive for other infections; and the **western blot** test, given when the ELISA is positive or borderline, does not always detect Lyme disease.

Treatment

If a tick has been feeding on you, and you experience the symptoms of Lyme disease within a month of the bite (whether or not you have a rash), you should be treated with antibiotics. In 1998, a **vaccine** was licensed by Smith Kline Beecham, which was about 76% effective after three injections. It stimulated the production of antibodies that attacked the organism in the gut of the feeding tick. The duration of the vaccine's protection, however, is unknown, and it was withdrawn from the market in 2002 because of declining demand and a class action lawsuit filed against the company.

Bring it back alive

If possible, bring back a tick alive in a sealed ziplock bag containing damp paper toweling if it has fed on someone. The moisture inside will keep the tick alive for testing. Label the bag with the time and date that the tick was embedded and removed. Also note from what part of the body it was retrieved and the location where the tick was encountered. An entomologist can then identify the species and tell you whether it is one that can transmit disease agents to humans. Also, a live tick can be tested in some Public Health Departments for Lyme disease, and the test is more accurate than the ones performed on humans. Even if the tick is infected, it may not have transmitted the infection. However, if it is not infected and you're sure you had no other tick bites, you can save yourself anxiety as well as medical expenses.

Rocky Mountain spotted fever

Rocky Mountain spotted fever was first recognized in the Bitterroot Valley of Montana, toward the end of the 19th century. Howard T. Ricketts, who studied the disease from 1906 to 1910, correctly described it as an infection carried by ticks. The organisms that cause this and many other diseases are named after him – *rickettsiae*. They are very small bacteria that (unlike most bacteria) trick cells into ingesting them. Then they increase and multiply until the cells burst. Since the spotted fever organisms infect cells in the walls of blood vessels, they cause many small hemorrhages. These hemorrhages show as red spots on the skin that do not itch, and usually start on the limbs (2 to 5 days after the onset of fever), then spread to the torso. But the real damage is inside vital organs.

Like viruses, *rickettsiae* are protected from antibodies by their position inside the cells, but aureomycin and tetracycline usually cure Rocky Mountain spotted fever if it is diagnosed and treated in time. Incubation ranges from two days to two weeks. The telltale spots may appear late (in 10% of cases) or not at all, so 2 - 3% of all victims still die, as do 20% of those untreated or treated late. Before antibiotics, mortality in the Bitterroot Valley was 70%. Fortunately, the infection rate in ticks that carry the disease is only 0.1%, but about 2,000 cases per year in the United States are reported to the Centers for Disease Control and Prevention each year, mostly in southern states.

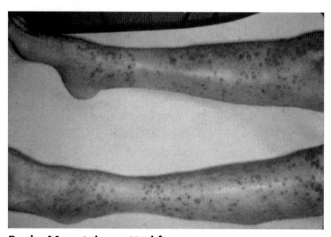

Rocky Mountain spotted fever
Photo courtesy of Ben Schifrin, MD

Signs and symptoms may come on suddenly or after a few days of malaise. They often include a splitting headache and pains in the back, neck, joints, or legs. Light can become painful to the eyes, and a stiff neck can confuse the disease with meningitis. The victim is restless, sleeping poorly, often delirious, and runs a temperature of 104-106°, which is why it is called "fever."

Other tick-borne diseases

Other *rickettsiae* cause **human ehrlichiosis** and **human granulocytic anaplasmosis**, each of which afflict hundreds of people in the United States, mostly in the southeast and central states. Like victims of Lyme disease, they have flu-like symptoms in the early stages: fever, chills, malaise, headache, and muscle pain. Later, the patient may suffer vomiting, coughing,

abdominal pain, diarrhea, swollen lymph glands, and (with anaplasmosis) a rash. They can usually be cured with antibiotics.

Tick paralysis

Some ticks, including the one that carries Rocky Mountain spotted fever (transmitted by the Rocky Mountain wood tick), can inject a toxin that causes a creeping paralysis. This paralysis starts in the hands and feet and moves up the limbs to the face. If it reaches the respiratory muscles, it can kill. In the United States, the paralysis is reversed by removing the tick, as the remaining toxin is cleared out of the system within a day or two. But in Australia, there is a more potent tick toxin, whose effects continue after tick removal.

Tick protection and removal

Using repellents containing DEET or picaridin on the skin and spraying or soaking clothes with permethrin, will help keep ticks off. Wear light-colored clothing so that you can see the dark brown or blackish ticks, and tuck your shirt into your pants. You should also tuck your pants into your socks and wear gaiters. A hat saturated with permethrin will make it harder for ticks to get into your hair. Larvae and nymphs, and some adults, will be on or near the ground and crawl up your legs. Before feeding, adult Ixodes pacificus ticks are about 1/10 of an inch long; nymphs less than half as long; and larvae barely visible.

Do frequent **tick searches** on yourself and your friends, especially before going into the tent for the night. Ticks that have crawled up the legs or body often seek warm, moist places to feed, such as the butt crack or armpit. Ticks that get onto the head when you brush against vegetation may be concealed under hair or behind an ear. A stiff back brush can help remove ticks crawling on your skin when you take a shower. To kill ticks in or on clothing, add borax or permethrin to laundry detergent, and use the hot setting for both washer and dryer.

There are several devices designed to remove ticks, which are less likely than tweezers to break off the body and leave the mouth parts embedded. The Tick Spoon (tickedoff.com) is a small spoon with a V notch that you slide between the tick's body and embedded mouth parts to lever it out. The Tick Key has a keyhole shaped opening. Sawyer Tick Pliers grip the tick from either side but work the same way. Some devices come with a small magnifying glass to help you see what you are doing. You should slowly pull the tick straight out and not twist, to avoid breaking off the mouthparts and leaving them embedded. If the mouthparts remain embedded, remove them as you would a splinter. If they remain embedded, they can cause a secondary bacterial infection at the bite site, because a tick's exoskeleton is covered with bacteria.

Another method of tick removal is to use dental floss or strong thread. Tie a loose overhand knot, slip it over the tick, and gently close it around the tick as close to the skin as possible. Then slowly pull both ends of the floss or thread upward to remove the tick. Be careful not to touch the tick, since the Lyme disease organisms (which may have been released if the tick was damaged in removal) can penetrate unbroken skin.

None of the folklore techniques for removing ticks work. Anointing them with oil, nail polish, or vaseline won't kill them, because they can survive for hours without breathing. Touching them with a hot match head won't do anything except possibly make them regurgitate, which could transmit any infection they may be carrying. If you remove the tick properly, however, you will reduce the chance of infection, even if the tick is carrying Lyme disease, because it takes 24 hours or longer after the tick attaches and starts feeding for the bacteria to migrate from the tick's gut to its salivary glands (but 12 hours or less for the Rocky Mountain spotted fever organism).

Chagas disease

Chagas disease is endemic in South and Central America, where it infects 10 million people. About 30% of them develop life-threatening conditions, especially heart disease – flabby, weakened hearts with abnormal heart rhythms. Chagas disease is transmitted by triatomine bugs, which only acquire wings in the adult stage, after going through 5 wingless nymph stages. They are called kissing bugs because they come out at night, typically crawl on the face and bite around the mouth. They transmit the disease by defecating as they feed. Charles Darwin described the experience in his first book, *The Voyage of the Beagle.*

Triatomine bugs are found in all but the northern states of the U.S., up to about 120° northern latitude.

Recent studies found that 28% of kissing bugs in southern California and 55% in northern California were carrying the parasite, Trypanosoma cruzi; and 57% of the bugs collected in Texas. So in states that have triatomine bugs, it would be prudent to avoid sleeping outside a tent. Treatment (even if Chagas is correctly diagnosed) takes months, and the drugs have to be ordered from the CDC.

Photos by Isias Montilla courtesy of WHO

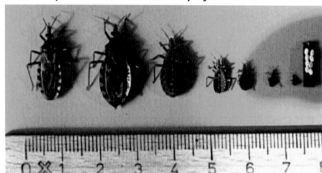

Left to right: Adult male; adult female; nymphs; eggs.

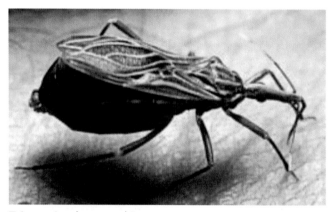

Triatomine bug on skin

Conclusion

Travelers, especially to the tropics, need to get current information from the Centers for Disease Control and Prevention(www.cdc.gov) on diseases carried by mosquitoes and other blood-sucking bugs, and on medications that still give protection.

You can reduce the chance of infection from ticks and blood-sucking flies by wearing protective clothing, using repellent on skin, and spraying permethrin on clothing and mosquito netting. In tick country, you should do frequent tick inspections throughout the day, and remove ticks that have attached before they can transmit any infection they may carry.

Chapter 23. Spiders, bees and wasps

Venom may contain neurotoxins that paralyzes prey or antagonists and enzymes that pre-digest prey before feeding. In humans, venom from bee, wasp, or ant stings usually just causes pain and swelling around the sting. Some spider venom is more potent. A widow spider bite can make the victim very ill for several days. Brown recluse spider venom has such strong digestive enzymes that it can cause serious tissue damage. Victims who have been sensitized to any venom by repeated exposure, however, may suffer an allergic reaction.

Bees and wasps

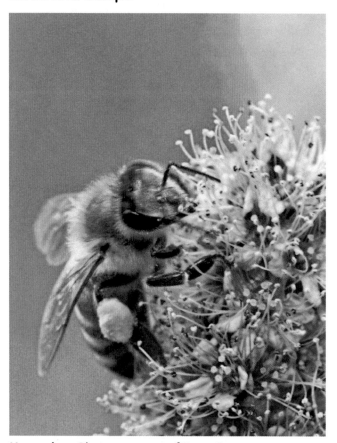

Honey bee *Photo courtesy of Dean Fanara*

Bees and wasps will usually attack only in defense of their nests or territories. The so-called killer bees (African bees imported to Brazil) form larger and more aggressive swarms, and have been spreading northwards at a rate of a few hundred miles per year. But unless they can adapt to a colder climate than they are used to, they will probably be limited to the southernmost of the United States. While wasps can sting repeatedly, honeybees have a barbed stinger that usually cannot be retracted from human skin. The bee leaves the venom sack still pulsing and injecting venom as it pulls away. So it is important to scrape the sack off as quickly as possible with a credit card or whatever is handy.

Allergic reactions

Up to 4% of the United States population is allergic to stings, usually to bee, wasp, or ant venom. A local reaction will cause more pain and swelling than the initial bite, spreading around the sting. A more widespread reaction is the eruption of red and itchy swellings over the body (hives). A full anaphylactic reaction can be fatal. Those who know that they are sensitized can usually develop a blocking antibody response by immunotherapy using purified venom.

The word "anaphylaxis," from the Greek *an* (without) *phylaxis* (protection), is based on a misunderstanding. A researcher in 1913 was testing the effects of insect venom on dogs. He thought that the first dose of venom given to a dog had somehow knocked out the immune system, leaving the dog without protection against the second dose. In fact, just the reverse happens. After repeated exposure, the immune system can over-react to the venom, which causes a much more serious problem than direct effects of the venom. Mast cells release histamines, which cause airways to constrict, swell, and congest, and blood vessels to dilate. The victim's face will swell alarmingly, and circulation will become sluggish as blood pressure drops.

But the narrowing of the air passages is what can kill. The victim will be showing obvious signs of respiratory distress, wheezing, and straining for breath. There is only one treatment – give epinephrine or an equivalent medication, which will reverse the action of the histamines. Epinephrine opens up the air passages and constricts the arteries. Victims who know they are allergic may be carrying a bee-sting kit with an epinephrine auto injector (a hypodermic with a shielded needle that you just have to jab into a muscle).

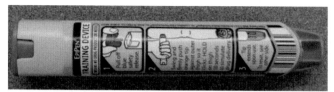

Epipen. The blue safety cap locks the shielded needle

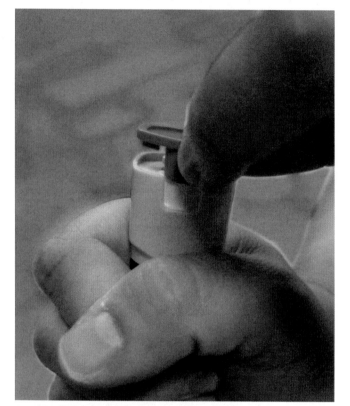

Remove the safety cap to release the needle.

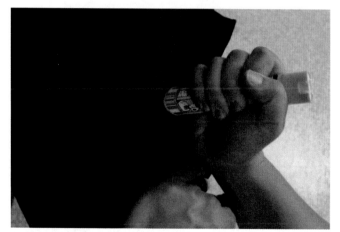

Grip the epipen firmly and jab it into the side of the thigh, midway between hip and knee, so that it goes into muscle. Hold for about 10 seconds. Do NOT put your thumb over the end, in case you have it reversed with the needle pointing outward. Document the time when you administered it.

Another way to give the medication is with an epinephrine inhaler. If the victim still has enough airway open to suck in, the inhaler will get the medication to the receptor sites and open the air passages faster than injection - often within a few minutes. An antihistamine will stop the mast cells from producing more histamines. The fastest route for the antihistamine is under the tongue. If the antihistamine is in a capsule, break the capsule open so that you can sprinkle the medication under the tongue for immediate absorption. You should also give oxygen if you have it.

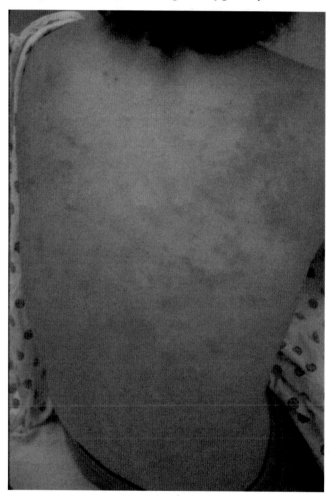

Hives *Photo courtesy of Ben Schifrin, MD*

Scorpions

As desert travelers know, scorpions are nocturnal feeders who seek shelter by day in crevices or under wood or ground debris. They will also crawl into shoes, clothing, and sleeping bags, so it is important to shake these out before putting them on or crawling into them. Worldwide, there are over a million scorpion stings per year, causing over 3,000 deaths. In the U.S., only the Arizona bark scorpion is dangerous to humans, and there have been only four deaths in 11 years (emedicine.medscape.com). But scorpion stings can be very painful, because their venom is acidic, which increases the intensity of pain signals. Scorpions are found in the deserts of the Southwestern United States: California, Nevada, Arizona, New Mexico, and Texas.

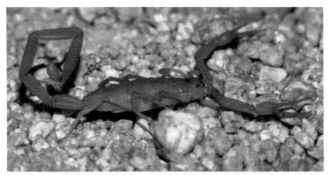

Arizona bark scorpion, *Centrurodes sculpturatus*.
Photo courtesy of Mike Cardwell

Scorpion venoms are neurotoxic. They have no digestive enzymes to cause tissue destruction, so the symptoms are neurological. In a mild envenomation (Grade I), pain and numbness will occur around the sting site, and pain will increase if you tap on the site (**tap test**). If the pain and numbness spreads to other parts of the body, envenomation is more serious (Grade II). In Grade III envenomation, you will see either cranial or somatic skeletal nerve disfunction.

Cranial nerve dysfunction may include jerky eye movements, blurred vision, trouble swallowing, slurred speech, and upper airway problems. Skeletal nerve dysfunction may include restlessness or jerking and shaking of the extremities that can mimic a seizure. If both cranial and skeletal nerves are affected, then the victim has a severe (Grade IV) envenomation.

Treatment for Grade I and II stings is ice packs in cloth (30 minutes every hour) and oral pain killers. For Grades III and IV, the main concern is keeping the airway open and making sure that the patient is breathing normally. An antivenom is available, but it does not relieve the pain. Doctors will usually give it only if the symptoms are life-threatening, because it can cause an anaphylactic reaction.

Spiders

About 30,000 species of spiders are known. Most of them have venom glands, but only a few dozen species are dangerous to humans, because the others either do not have enough venom or can't penetrate human skin. Spiders have fangs, which in most species move horizontally like pincers; but in some hunting spiders are vertical. Their venom sacks are modified salivary glands.

The venom of hunting spiders has both neurotoxin to paralyze the prey, and digestive enzymes to liquefy the prey inside its husk so that the spider can suck it out. Neurotoxins can cause pain, and paralysis of muscles where the venom spreads. The venom of most web spinners is not neurotoxic, because the silk webs immobilize the prey. However, widow spiders are an exception. In a few spiders, such as the recluse, the digestive enzymes are strong enough to destroy cells and cause systemic toxicity in humans. In the United States, five species each of widow spiders and recluse spiders are dangerous to humans.

Widow spiders

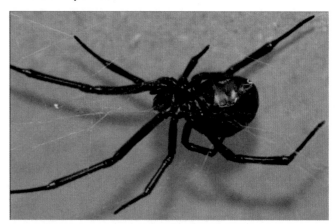

Female Western black widow spider
Photo courtesy of Mike Cardwell.

Every state except Alaska has at least one species of *latrodectus* (Latin "robber" Greek"biter"), also called the widow spider, because it eats the much smaller male after copulation. Their webs are irregular, but the silk is very strong. It was used for many years to make surgical sutures. Widows are shy spiders that are found in sheltered corners of fields and gardens. They are found under stones, logs, vegetation, wood piles, in wall crevices, and even in unoccupied buildings such as garages and barns. Outhouses were a notorious habitat, because they attracted flies. Widow spiders do not leave their webs, but defend them if disturbed, which is why people who used infested outhouses were bitten on the buttocks or genitals.

The females have bulbous bodies about 1 cm long. Black widows are shiny black with a red hourglass marking on the abdomen, but other species are brown or reddish. Their bite is usually painful from the start, though it may feel like a pinprick or cause a burning sensation. But within an hour, it will hurt more and more. Victims with severe envenomation often describe it as the worst pain they ever felt. Skin around the bite may sweat, and body hairs stand up. The neurotoxin causes neurotransmitter release, which can make muscles spasm and blood vessels constrict, increasing blood pressure (hypertension).

Other possible signs and symptoms include:
• abdominal or back pain (58% of victims);
• extremity pain;
• malaise;
• nausea and vomiting;
• headache;
• fever;
• tremor;
• Respiratory muscle weakness (which may cause the victim to stop breathing).

In a pregnant woman, the venom can cause premature contractions and birth. The victim usually recovers within days, but pain may continue for a week or more. Treatment may include cold packs and calcium gluconate injections for the pain, as well as cleaning the wound and checking tetanus immunization to prevent infection. Because of the risk of anaphylaxis, physicians use widow spider antivenom only in case of respiratory arrest, seizure, uncontrolled hypertension or pregnancy.

Recluse spiders

Loxosceles (Greek "with slanting legs") reclusa (Latin "reclusive") spiders are found worldwide in warm climates and are native to the southernmost United States. But they sometimes turn up in colder states as indoor spiders that were transported (unnoticed) to their new homes. They like warm, undisturbed environments such as vacant buildings, storage sheds, closets, and attics. They may nest in stored bed sheets or clothes. Recluse spiders are not aggressive, but may bite when threatened (e.g., when trapped against skin or shaken out of stored sheets).

Females have slender bodies up to 1 cm long, and legs up to 3 cm long. Different species may be fawn to dark brown in color, and they often have a dark, violin-shaped patch on top. This is why they are sometimes called fiddle spiders.

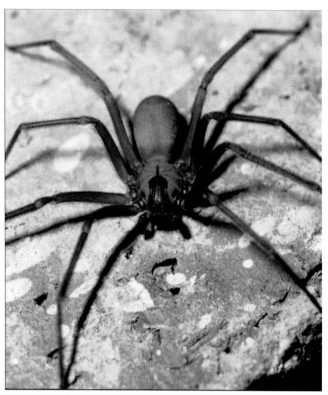

Brown recluse spider
Photo courtesy of Mike Cardwell

Their bite may be felt as a sharp stinging, or be unnoticed. Also, if only a little venom is injected, it may cause only skin irritation. But moderate or severe envenomation causes serious tissue destruction, because the digestive enzymes it contains are so strong. The usual progression is:
• 0-2 hours: blister formation.
• 2-6 hours: blood vessels near bite spasm, cutting off circulation.
• 6-8 hours: stinging stops, aching and itching start.
• 5-12 hours: skin turns white and blue around the red blister, from lack of blood.
• 12 hours on: tissue destruction begins.

Severe envenomation may create an open, ulcerating wound, so it is important to make sure that tetanus immunization is up to date. Other possible effects of envenomation include swelling, elevated skin temperature, joint pain, malaise and nausea. Systemic effects, which are more frequent in children, may include blood in the urine, anemia, weakness, fever, and chills.

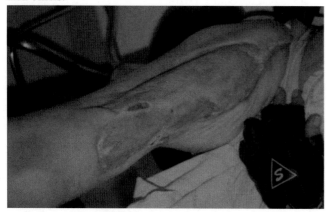

Recluse spider bite. *Photo courtesy Ben Schifrin, MD*

It may help to apply cold compresses, elevate the bitten limb, and immobilize it loosely. Some surgeons tried cutting away damaged tissue, but this is no longer recommended. An antivenom was tried in the 1980s, but with mixed results. One treatment that may help is hyperbaric oxygen – breathing oxygen under higher than normal pressure to force more of it into the tissues and speed healing. Hyperbaric oxygen has been used to treat serious burns.

Other spiders

Many large, hairy spiders are called tarantulas because of the mistaken belief that their venom causes tarantism ("stupor and the desire to dance"). They are nocturnal hunting spiders with vertical fangs that rear back to strike, somewhat like rattlesnakes. Their bites can be painful, but few species are dangerous. In fact, some of them are sold as pets.

The wandering spider (*Phoneutria nigrivin*) can travel with bananas exported from South America, so it is sometimes called the banana spider. Bananas may also have clusters of the wandering spider's eggs attached by spider silk, which look like small patches of white mold with dark spots. In South America, the wandering spider causes about half the hospitalizations from spider bites. If venom is injected, it causes severe pain that radiates up. It can also cause sweating and salivation, nausea and vomiting, vertigo, visual disturbances, and priapism (uncontrolled erection). Victims usually recover in one to two days, though occasionally they die of respiratory paralysis. An antivenom is available in Brazil.

The funnel web spider (*Atrax robustus*), native to Australia, is probably the most venomous spider in the world. Because it is so aggressive, and has such strong fangs, it probably bites more humans than any other spider in the world. But since an antivenom was developed in 1980, nobody has died from it.

Conclusion

With a bee or wasp sting, the main concern is an allergic reaction, which can be life-threatening. The only way to reverse an anaphylactic reaction is with epinephrine or an equivalent medication, either injected or inhaled. Both of the venomous spiders native to the United States are web spinners that bite only when threatened. To avoid them, you need to be aware of their possible habitats and watch for the widow spider's strong, irregular web. Widow spider bites can cause severe pain and neurological problems. If the symptoms are severe, a physician may give antivenom. Recluse spider bites can cause serious tissue damage. Treatment includes pain control, preventing infection, and possibly hyperbaric oxygen to speed healing.

Chapter 24. Venomous snakes

Estimates of fatal snakebites vary – possibly up to 100,000 per year in Asia, for example. But only 10 to 20 people per year die of snakebite in the United States. Yet venomous snakes are found in every contiguous state except Maine. Why do they kill so few people? There are several reasons:

- Most people in the U.S. live in urban areas.
- Mechanized U.S. farming has destroyed snake habitats and driven out venomous species.
- Africa, Asia, Australia, and Latin America have more species of venomous snakes with much deadlier venom than North America.
- Medical care is usually available in the U.S.

Even though snakebite in the United States is seldom fatal, however, it can cause serious tissue damage. About 8,000 bites are reported every year, and probably many more go unreported.

In 1927, almost all reported snakebites in the United States were accidental. Less than 5% were from intentional exposure to snakes and 59% were on the legs or feet. By 1988, 57% of the bites were from intentional exposure and 87% were on the arms or hands. Also, 28% of the victims were intoxicated.

Touch me not

Aside from impaired drinkers, what kinds of people deliberately handle venomous snakes? Some people keep them as pets, although it is not legal in most states to sell front-fanged snakes. Professional snake-catchers, who supply snake farms, zoos, and research institutions and the staff that handle the snakes may be bitten. But people are also exposed to possible bites in the rattlesnake roundups that are popular in some states. There are prizes awarded to those who bring in the greatest poundage of snakes; contests in which snakes are released into a ring and participants try to stuff as many of them as possible into a sack; and stations where spectators can be photographed handling live snakes.

Gods, demons and victims

In Grasshopper Valley, Tennessee (1909), George Went Hensley decided that handling venomous snakes was a test of faith. He based his belief on Mark XVI,

17-18: "They shall take up serpents, and if they drink any deadly thing it shall not hurt them." It is fortunate for his followers that venomous snakebites in the United States are rarely fatal, and any deaths can be attributed to a lack of faith. Hensley himself finally died of rattlesnake poisoning in 1955, but the cult continues, mainly among the laboring class in southern states, who have a hard life. For them the ordeal and excitement of dominating the evil serpent provides an emotional outlet and confirms their faith.

How did snakes acquire such an evil reputation? In the Epic of Gilgamesh, when the hero crosses the waters of death to pluck the plant that will make him immortal, a snake eats it while he sleeps. Hence snakes (according to folklore) became immortal, and ever since have renewed themselves by shedding their skins. In some mythologies, snakes are associated with godly knowledge, and the Aztec god Quetzlcoatl was a giant snake. In ancient Greece, snakes were associated with healing, and snake venom was supposed to have medicinal properties. This tradition survives in the caduceus, which is still the symbol of Medicine – two snakes twined around what was originally the herald's wand. Also, some components of venom from snakes and other animals do have medicinal value. A protein from black mamba venom can be used as an analgesic. A peptide from the saliva of the Gila monster is used to treat type II diabetes. And the international Venomics project (www.venomics.eu) is analyzing the venom from 200 species to test for treatment of diabetes, obesity, and heart failure.

In Genesis, however, the serpent is the tempter, passing on knowledge of life and death that is now forbidden. On that basis, serpents were demonized by Christianity, along with many pagan gods. Saints, however, were supposed to be able to control serpents and to be immune to their bites – a tradition that Hensley revived.

Snakes of the United States

Venomous snakes in the United States hardly deserve their bad reputation. They usually bite humans only in defense, when surprised or threatened, because they can sense that we are too big for them to eat. They feed on small animals, especially rodents, and often play an important role in controlling rodent populations.

Rattlesnakes, cottonmouths, and copperheads account for 98% of human bites in the U.S., because they have long fangs that unfold when they strike, acting like hypodermic needles. It is a very efficient mechanism for injecting venom.

Coral snakes, found only in the South and Southwest, are small, shy snakes with small mouths, and have to chew to inject venom. Their venom is a very potent neurotoxin, which can paralyze and even kill from respiratory or heart failure. They are related to cobras. But they account for less than 1% of snakebites in the United States, and almost all of those bites are to people handling the snakes.

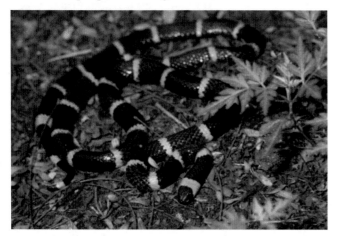

Texas Coral snake. *Photo courtesy of Mike Cardwell*

Cottonmouths are similar to rattlesnakes, but they are found mainly in swampy areas of southern states.

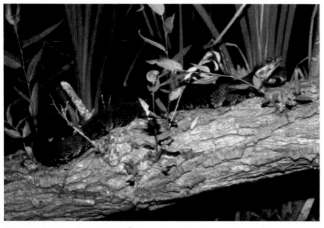

Western cottonmouth.

Photo courtesy of Mike Cardwell

Copperheads are found in central and southeastern states but their bite, though painful, is not very dangerous. Most serious snakebites in the United

States, therefore, come from rattlesnakes, which are found in every contiguous state except Maine.

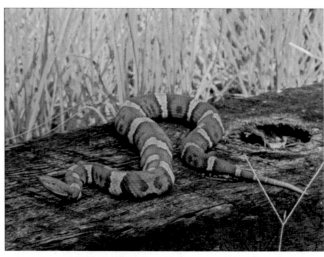

Trans Pecos Copperhead.
Photo courtesy of Mike Cardwell

Rattlesnakes, cottonmouths, and copperheads are called pit vipers because they have heat-sensing pits behind the nostrils that guide their strike at the warm prey. Their sense of smell is augmented when the forked tongue picks up odor molecules from the air and brings them to receptors in the roof of the mouth. They have slit pupils, which can admit more light to adapt them for night hunting. Their eyes are sensitive to motion, but cannot focus sharply because they have no fovea. They also lack external ears, but they can sense ground vibration with the middle ears.

Rattlesnake habitats and behavior

Most forest is too cool for rattlesnakes, but they are found in brushy or rocky hills, grassy meadows, and desert. In the mountains, they may be found up to 9,000 feet and up to 11,000 feet in the California summer. Since they have no sweat glands or internal temperature regulation, the temperature range in which they can function is limited. Rattlesnakes are most active at 80-90° F. Below 61° F, they seek shelter, and at 46° F they are immobilized. In the desert, they often control their temperature by lying across the edge of a shade patch or burying their coils in the insulating sand (which makes them hard to see). At 108° F, they can survive only about 12 minutes.

When the temperature drops, they may coil up on a rock or an asphalt road that is radiating heat. On a warm night, however, they are likely to be out hunting.

They hibernate in winter and are most active in spring. This is because they are hungry after hibernation, and it is mating season. Rattlesnakes do most of their growing in the first two years but can live up to 30 years. They shed their skin one to four times a year, depending on how often they feed. The shed skin bunches at the tail, producing the rattles that give the snakes their name. The number of rattles, however, is not a reliable sign of age, since they may break off; so it is not possible to tell how often a snake has shed.

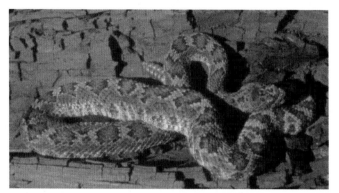

Rattlesnake. *Photo courtesy of Ben Schifrin, MD*

Since rattlesnakes can travel no faster than three miles per hour, they ambush prey by waiting along animal trails, especially at night. They also go down burrows or into rock crevices after prey. When in range they strike, disengage, wait for the prey to die; then find it by scent. They swallow the prey whole, head first. Although the jaws dislocate and the tissues stretch, rattlesnake prey averages only about one-third of their own weight. A full meal lasts them about two weeks, and they can fast up to a year.

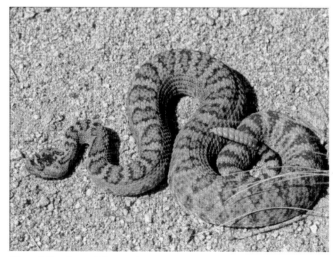

Great Basin rattlesnake.
Photo courtesy of Mike Cardwell

In response to a threat, rattlesnakes may freeze and blend into the surroundings. Some of them can even change color slightly. Or they may retreat, sometimes keeping their heads raised and poised to strike. When cornered, they may go into a striking coil (a vertical spiral), hissing and shaking their rattles in warning - the Hollywood image of a rattlesnake. Unfortunately, many snakes have not seen the films and do not know the Hollywood rules. They can strike from any position, especially if handled, and can snap into a striking coil in an instant to get more range and leverage. From this position, they can strike up to one-half or even three-fourths of their body length.

Fangs and venom

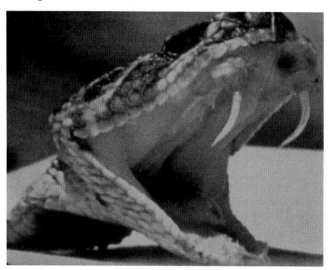

Photo courtesy of Ben Schifrin, MD

A rattlesnake strike is fast (about 8 feet per second), though not quite as fast as a human fist. A 4-foot snake, for example, can strike 2 feet in one-fourth of a second, which leaves little chance to dodge. During the strike, the mouth opens 180°, and the fangs unfold so they are aimed at the prey. In a large rattlesnake, these fangs may be 7/8" long. They are replaced every six to ten weeks, and new fangs are always growing in behind the old. The venom glands and ducts are contracted by the external jaw muscle, independently of the striking and biting action; and the size of the prey or threat (gauged by the heat-sensing pits) determines the amount of venom injected.

In humans, a mature snake may inject 25% to 75% of its venom. Baby rattlesnakes also have venom, so they are also dangerous even though they do not have the striking range and power of mature snakes. Even a mature rattlesnake, however, does not always inject venom when it strikes. A glancing angle or protective clothing may interfere and prevent enough penetration to inject venom. About 20% of rattlesnake bites are dry, with no venom injected, and about 30% inject only a little venom. The remaining 50% of bites inject enough venom to cause moderate to severe damage in humans.

Rattlesnake venom has several functions. It immobilizes and then kills prey; predigests the prey inside its skin; and defends against enemies. Peptides in the venom kill prey by damaging cell membranes and the walls of blood vessels, causing fluid loss and shock. In humans, the dose is almost never enough to kill. Enzymes digest the prey, and in humans can cause swelling, blisters, and serious tissue destruction.

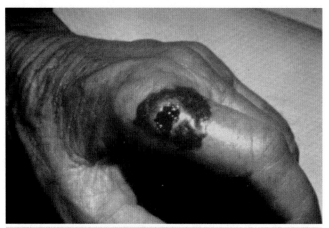

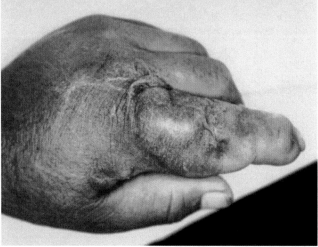

Rattlesnake bite: Progressive swelling and blistering
Photos courtesy of "Ben Schifrin, MD.

Venom of rattlesnakes or other pit vipers can also cause long-term impairment of function, especially in people bitten on a hand or finger. Some components of the venom can cause leakage of red blood cells and

fluid shifts from the blood, lowering the blood pressure (hypotension). Neurotoxins, which paralyze prey, can cause numbness and partial paralysis in humans. Some Mojave rattlesnake venom has especially potent neurotoxins, which can occasionally paralyze the breathing muscles in humans.

Weakness, numbness (usually around the scalp, face and lips) and nausea occur in about three-fourth of rattlesnake bite victims as the venom spreads. Pain and swelling start within minutes, and with severe envenomation, can spread to the whole limb in one hour. Usually, if no pain or swelling occurs after 20 minutes, either the bite was dry or it was not a rattlesnake. About one-fourth of victims develop blood blisters from 6 to 36 hours after the bite, which spread up the limb.

Venomous lizards

Some lizards are also venomous. Gila monsters, native to the Southwestern deserts of the United Sates, inject venom while chewing. They have a very tenacious grip. The venom (as potent as a rattlesnake's) flows along the grooves in its teeth and mixes with saliva. Gila monsters rarely bite humans, however, because they are slow and sluggish.

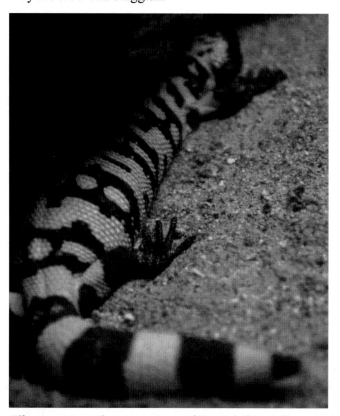

Gila monster. *Photo courtesy of BenSchifrin, MD.*

Treatment: history and folklore

In ancient times, all snakes and lizards were considered dangerous, and harmless snakes are still often mistaken for venomous ones. This gives credibility to innumerable folk remedies – if the victim of the supposedly venomous bite doesn't die, it "proves" that the remedy works. Even if the bite was venomous, in the United States the victims almost never die, no matter what rescuers do to them. In the 18th and 19th century, for example, snakebites were doused with ammonia, cauterized by igniting gunpowder on them, or just treated by amputating the limb. In the Western states, whiskey was considered both prevention and cure and getting drunk was supposed to immunize against the venom. In fact, alcohol causes blood vessels under the skin to dilate, which spreads the venom faster.

Many folklore remedies are unfortunately still repeated and used. For example, the infamous snakebite kits with razor blades have probably done more damage than snakes. Slashing with a razor blade, especially around the hands, wrists and ankles (which are commonly bitten), can cut nerves and tendons as well as blood vessels. Ironically, the little rubber suction cup provided with the blade did not extract any venom. Trying to suck venom out with the mouth is also a bad idea, because in effect it adds a human bite to the snakebite. Human bites are among the most dangerous, because they often become infected.

Applying ice will not do much except possibly cause frostbite, and electric current does not "devitalize" the venom. Shocking the victim with DC current from a stun gun was actually recommended in an article published in a medical journal (*The Lancet*), and widely reported by the popular media. But the article was based on a few dubious, undocumented tests on Ecuadorian Indians. It was debunked by Dr. Paul Auerbach with an obvious laboratory test - running DC current through a vial of venom, then testing the venom to see if it had lost any of its potency. It hadn't.

First aid and medical treatment

For the bites of snakes whose venom is likely to be fatal if it spreads to the heart and other vital organs, such as cobras, bushmasters, and mambas, you should use an elastic bandage to immobilize and compress the entire area over and around the bite, or the entire limb if the bite is to an arm or leg. This will slow the spread of the venom by shutting down the lymph system, allowing more time to reach a hospital with the appropriate antivenom. In North America, however, only coral snake bites (or bites from deadly exotic snakes bought as pets) require the pressure bandage treatment.

For rattlesnake and other pit viper bites, there is no evidence that a pressure bandage would be helpful, and it might increase local tissue damage. Constricting bands (which should only constrict lymph vessels under the skin) are not helpful either, especially if they are too tight, and act like a tourniquet.

If the bite is to the hand or arm, it may help to immobilize the arm loosely and keep it below the heart. For many years, snakebite experts have also recommended using a plastic suction pump to extract some of the venom; and several manufacturers now make them. Intuitively, it seems that they should help, but no published studies support their use, and a recent study done on pigs showed no significant venom extraction or effect on swelling.

Keeping the patient calm and limiting physical activity may help to slow the spread of venom. Drinking fluids (provided that the patient isn't too nauseated) will help to prevent shock. If no pain or swelling occurs within 20 minutes, however, and no other signs or symptoms are found, then probably no venom was injected.

Once you have done the first aid, you should get the patient as quickly as possible to a hospital that has antivenom. For a patient who can walk, that is usually the fastest way to the trailhead, especially if other people in the group can take the patient's load. If you do activities in rattlesnake or cottonmouth country, you should know where the nearest hospital with antivenom is. Call ahead, because they will have to order it to be sent to them by air if it is not stocked, and the sooner it is administered the more effective it will be. Also, describe the effects of the venom (e.g., the hand is swollen to twice its normal size), so that they will believe you. Don't waste time trying to kill or even identify the snake, because the antivenom for all pit vipers is the same. During the evacuation, mark the boundary of the swelling and the time on the patient's skin every 15 minutes with a sharpie pen, to provide a graphic record of the venom's progressive effects.

There is no clear evidence that antivenom prevents tissue damage, unless it is administered within 30 minutes of the bite; but if administered within 24 hours of the bite it can reverse systemic effects such as hypotension, coagulopathy (blood doesn't clot), nausea, and loss of nerve function. The old ACP antivenom, made with serum extracted from horses that had been injected with venom, caused serum sickness in 56-100% of patients, depending on how much was administered; and could trigger a life-threatening anaphylactic reaction. The current CroFab antivenom (for all pit viper envenomation in North America) is safer, and causes serum sickness in only about 10% of patients. But it is expensive, costing the hospital over $2000 per vial, which is only a fraction of what the hospital will bill the patient. For a severe envenomation, a patient may receive a dozen or more vials. For venom that causes coagulopathy, doctors use the 20 minute whole blood clotting test to check whether more antivenom is needed: collect 3 to 5 ml of the patient's blood in a test tube; keep it at room temperature for 20 minutes; then tip the test tube to see if clotting has occurred.

Conclusion

In the United States, people are seldom killed by snakebite; but pit viper venom can do serious damage. If you or someone in your group is bitten, you should get the patient to a hospital with antivenom as soon as possible; and avoid traditional snakebite treatments, which can be harmful as well as ineffective.

Other continents, especially Asia, Africa, and Australia, have much deadlier snakes than North America. So the immediate goal if bitten by one of them is to slow the spread of venom (by wrapping the affected area or limb in an elastic bandage to shut down the lymph system) until the patient can be given the appropriate antivenom.

Chapter 25. Hazardous mammals

Attacks on humans

Whenever a bear injures or kills a human, news stories describe it in gory detail. Yet from 1900 through 1985, a total of only 162 bear-inflicted injuries were reported in all U.S. and Canadian national parks, an average of less than two per year. Since then, about three people per year in North America have been killed by bears, compared to 15 people per year killed by dogs.

Similarly, when a mountain lion (cougar) attacks a human, it makes headlines. However, only 66 attacks on humans were documented from 1750 to 1985, which is an average of less than one every three years. Since just one-third of these attacks were fatal, cougars killed an average of less than one human every nine years in the United States. By contrast, deer kill dozens of people every year by jumping in front of speeding cars. So driving cautiously and watching for deer on back country roads is more likely to save your life on a wilderness trip than a 44 magnum or a can of pepper spray.

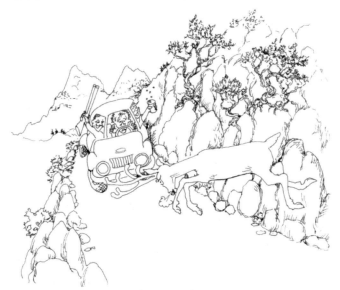

Also, more people in the U.S. are killed or injured by exotic pets (75 deaths and 1610 injuries reported from 1991 to 2011) than by wild predators. State laws on exotic pets vary, but they are advertised for sale on the internet, and some states have large auctions. For example, there are about 5,000 tigers (bought when they were cubs) kept as pets in the U.S. – more than survive in the wild.

Habituation and elimination

Why are there so few bear attacks on humans? Probably because for centuries bears that showed aggression toward humans were killed and eliminated from the gene pool. But bears have learned that humans bring them food. For many years, Yellowstone, Yosemite and other national parks turned open garbage dumps into bear cafeterias. Some of them surrounded the dumps with bleachers and floodlights so that the tourists could watch bears rooting in the garbage at night.

By the time the park system changed its policy, it was too late. Bears in national parks were not only habituated to humans; they also associated humans with food. Moreover, bears that have fed on garbage and backpackers' food may be hundreds of pounds heavier and reach sexual maturity earlier than those that do not. As a result, they have a breeding advantage, and females teach that behavior to their cubs.

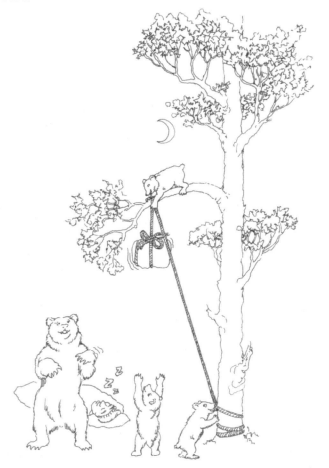

Although parks now provide bear boxes (steel food lockers) and supposedly bear-proof garbage bins in some campgrounds, rent supposedly bear-proof food containers to backpackers, and warn tourists not to leave food in cars or tents, the bears continue to learn faster than the tourists. For example, when tourists leave their car windows open a crack in hot weather, bears can hook their claws over the tops of the windows and pull them down. They are also not afraid to smash closed windows if they smell food or see anything that looks like a food container inside. A large bear can open a car or camper like a tin can. And of course you should never keep food in your tent when there are bears in the neighborhood.

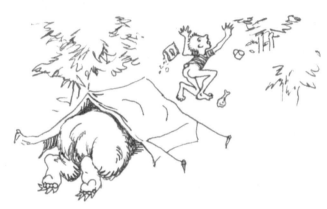

Bear bagging food

Getting between a bear and food is one way to provoke an attack, so effective bear bagging is a good way to stay out of trouble in bear country. Most of the traditional techniques, however, no longer work with the educated bears of heavily trafficked national parks and forests. They have learned how to climb out on limbs from which food is suspended and snag the cord with their claws; or send their cub out if the branch is too thin to support them.

If the cord or rope is tied to the same tree from which the food is suspended, bears can often find the tie, hook their claws under it, and snap it. Using several trees, however, you can hang food more securely. You need two pieces of 1/8" braided nylon cord (400 lbs. breaking strength), each 75 feet long, and three carabiners. Tie loops in both ends of each cord.

To hang the food, find two trees at least 30 feet apart, with limbs at least 20 feet up. Stand between the trees, tie a rock to an end of each cord and throw one over each tree. Now connect the ends of the cords between the trees with a carabiner, and clip the food

bags to it. Go to the other end of a cord, clip a carabiner to it, and walk away with it until the food bags are about 15 feet from the tree limb. Walk sideways now and wrap the cord around another tree until you've used up the slack and can clip the carabiner to the cord. Do the same thing with the cord going over the other tree limb, clipping a belt or piece of webbing into the carabiner as a harness to haul up a heavy load of food. Make sure that the lowest food bag is at least 15 feet up. The bear will not be able to find where the cord is tied, because it is too high to blunder into, and too far from the food trees. So it won't be able to get any leverage to break the cord, and the nylon is too thin for it to get its teeth into.

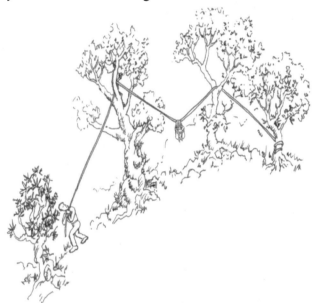

Even this technique may not be completely bear-proof, however. Near Half Dome in Yosemite, the author hung food with new nylon cord. In the morning, the cord was stretched, so that the bottom of the lowest bag (still higher than a person could reach) was ripped open. We re-hung the food higher and were woken up at five o'clock the next morning by a swatting sound. We walked to the food trees and saw a bear with its whole body stretched out on the 1/8" nylon cord, holding on to the tree with the claws of its hind legs.

As we watched, the bear just managed to snag the nearest food bag. Obviously it had tried the same tactic the previous morning and been unable to reach, but its weight had stretched the new cord just enough so that it could leap up and slash the bottom of the lowest bag. This bear wore a red tag in its ear, showing that it had been evicted from Yosemite Valley for stealing food.

Another precaution is to get a bear-resistant food bag called the Ursack (www.ursack.com), which is made of Aramid, the same fabric used for bulletproof vests. These are tested on bears in zoos. Some food-habituated bears in national parks and some persistent rodents have managed to chew through them. However, most bears and other animals give up, especially if the bag is hanging so that they cannot get any leverage.

Bear behavior

Grizzly bears are bigger and generally much more aggressive than the so-called black bears (which on the West Coast are usually brown). Bear experts advise making plenty of noise through grizzly bear territory, especially if you're walking into the wind, in case bears are not warned of your approach by scent. Mothers are especially dangerous if their cubs are around, and most bears will defend carcasses that they have killed or claimed. They will also defend any food taken from backpackers, because once they get their paws on it, the food belongs to them. If you do get too close, the bear may retreat, threaten, or charge. Before taking action, it may rear up to sample the air and find out what you are. While bears have good eyesight, they rely more on their sense of smell to identify you.

Threatening behavior may include huffing, snorting, paw swats, display of teeth, turning sideways to show you how big it is, and making charges that stop short. A large group may respond by trying to dominate the bear – clumping together to look like a very large animal, and making loud noises.

This may not work with an aggressive grizzly, however. Submissive behavior is a safer response, especially if you are alone or in a small group. You should avoid eye contact, look small, and slowly back off. But don't turn and run, because that can trigger prey chasing behavior in the bear. If a bear catches you, most bear experts advise playing dead, and curling up to protect your head and abdomen, unless the bear has been stalking you as prey (which is very unusual). Some people have survived bear attacks by this tactic, though most suffered severe injuries.

Most of the infrequent bear attacks on humans, however, are provoked by human behavior: careless handling and storage of food, getting too close (especially to a mother with cubs), or treating bears as pets. This includes feeding them, poking them, or even trying to shake hands with them. By treating bears with respect, not reinforcing their unfortunate habituation to human presence and food, we should be able to share the wilderness with them, and minimize the chance of hostile encounters.

Rabies

The word means "to do violence," and comes from the Sanskrit "rabhas" by way of Latin. Rabies has a fearsome reputation, and it kills many people in developing countries. In India, for example, an estimated 25,000-50,000 people die of rabies every year. Dogs are the number one vector of rabies worldwide, because they are so common in both urban and rural areas and have frequent contact with humans. In the United States, however, the disease kills only a few people each year, because it has been almost wiped out in domestic dogs by vaccination and quarantine.

Rabies is caused by a virus transmitted in saliva, usually by bites, but sometimes by an aerosol, especially in bat caves where saliva rains down from clusters of bats on the roof. Besides dogs and bats, it is also carried by skunks (number one carrier in the United States), raccoons, cats, monkeys (especially in Asia), foxes, and wolves. The chance of infection from bites depends on their number, severity, and location. Since the virus attacks the nervous system, bites on or close to the head are the most dangerous, because the virus will reach the brain more quickly.

After a bite, the virus may remain in muscle tissue for days or weeks before starting to move up peripheral nerves at a rate of 3 mm per hour. Once the virus reaches the spinal cord or brain, the victim cannot be saved. Incubation periods average 2 to 12 weeks, but may be as short as half a day in a case of severe bites around the head, or as long as several years. Vaccination before exposure is expensive and not completely effective, so it is usually given only to lab workers who handle potentially rabid animals. Given after exposure, the best vaccine (injected into the deltoid muscle in a series of shots) is 100% effective during the incubation period. However, developing countries, where rabies is a major problem, are likely to have older and cheaper vaccines that are not as effective or as safe. So the problem is to recognize and diagnose rabies before it attacks the nervous system. If traveling in countries with a high risk of rabies, you should know where the nearest source of modern vaccine is.

Signs and symptoms vary. Often the victim feels pain and numbness spreading from the bite. Systemic effects as the virus spreads may include malaise, chills, fever, and fatigue. If it attacks the respiratory system, it can cause sore throat, cough, and breathing difficulty. In the digestive system it can cause nausea, vomiting, abdominal pain, diarrhea, and loss of appetite. About one-third of the victims suffer hydrophobia ("fear of water") and difficulty swallowing.

As it attacks the central nervous system, the virus can cause headache, vertigo, irritability, and anxiety. Spasms and convulsions may follow, especially in response to stimuli that can be sights, sounds, smells, or touch. Other signs and symptoms may include disorientation, hallucinations, violent behavior, priapism (uncontrolled erection), insomnia, nightmares, and depression. Only about one-third of victims (animal and human) show hyper-salivation (foaming at the mouth); and 20-30% (usually pre-vaccinated victims infected by vampire bats) have no symptoms except paralysis creeping up from the level of the bite.

Any unnatural behavior in an animal may be caused by rabies, including daytime activity by nocturnal animals and apparently friendly behavior by wild animals. Avoid close encounters. If you are bitten, clean the wound with soap and water, irrigate it thoroughly, and disinfect it with a solution of benzalkonium chloride. Evacuate to a hospital that has modern rabies vaccine as soon as possible.

Hantavirus

In May 1993, a viral disease transmitted by deer mice droppings was recognized in the Four Corners area of Arizona, Colorado, New Mexico, and Utah. Many of the victims, including Native Americans and Forest Service rangers, inhaled the virus while cleaning up cabins infested with deer mice. Hantavirus has now been reported in 31 states, including most of the Western states, as well as Canada and six South American countries. Early signs and symptoms are vague: fever, chills and muscle aches within three to five days. Victims may later suffer headache, nausea, vomiting, abdominal pain, diarrhea and cough.

Hantavirus kills by pulmonary edema (flooding of the lungs), and has a 36% fatality rate. However, according to the Center for Disease Control (www.cdc.gov), the total number of cases reported in the United States from 1993 to 2015 is 659, of which 235 were fatal. And just 18 cases were reported in 2015, of which 4 were fatal. So statistically, the chance of hantavirus infection is very small, but it would be wise to take precautions when cleaning out a cabin infested by rodent droppings. Since Hantavirus infects the lungs when you breathe the contaminated dust, you would need a respirator as well as rubber gloves. You should also wet the droppings down with bleach before cleaning them out.

Conclusion

Bears and other wild mammals kill or injure very few people in the United States, but they have learned to associate people with food; so safe storage of food in the wilderness will help to avoid close encounters. Keeping your distance from any wild mammal is also important for avoiding diseases they may be carrying, such as rabies or plague.

Chapter 26. Marine hazards

Photos not otherwise credited courtesy of Oleg Grachev.

Bacteria that can cause wound infections thrive in the saline medium of the oceans, and are also common in fresh water. The teeth or spines of marine animals that inflict wounds are also usually contaminated with dangerous bacteria. So any wound inflicted in water is likely to become infected, especially if there are foreign bodies or venom in it. It is therefore especially important to clean marine wounds thoroughly. You can also do some simple first aid to alleviate the effects of venomous stings.

Wounds and wound care

Most marine wounds have more mundane causes than attack by a predator (e.g., coral or barnacle cuts). If there is no severe bleeding, then you need to clean the wound thoroughly. Irrigate with clean, fresh water or saline solution, but do not use seawater because it may cause further infection. Use tweezers to remove any visible debris that does not flush out, and scrub a minor wound with soap and water. Do not try to close the wound – cover with a sterile dressing. An ointment such as Bacitracin will form a protective layer under the dressing and help prevent it from sticking, though honey is the most effective topical antibiotic.

Make sure that the patient has a current tetanus immunization, and check the wound regularly for signs of infection such as redness, swelling, pus, heat, and throbbing pain. The same species of bacteria that may infect wounds on land are found in the marine environment – Clostridium, Staphylococcus, and Streptococcus for example. But a marine wound may also be infected with other species that are harder to identify or control. Some species of Vibrio, for example, can cause sepsis with a mortality of 50%.

Sharks and other predators

There are many fearsome marine predators, including sharks and barracuda, but they very seldom attack humans; and injuries from smaller animals are almost always accidental or defensive. For example, a beach wader may step on a stingray or sea urchin; or a diver may brush against a coral reef. So the best way to prevent injuries is to be aware of marine hazards and how to avoid them.

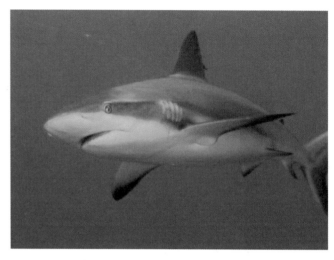

Sharks can inflict terrible wounds with their sharp teeth, and the great white shark can grow to 20 feet, weighing over 2 tons. But only 100-150 shark attacks on humans are reported each year, worldwide, and just 6 to 10 deaths. Chances of being attacked by a shark on the North American coast are about 1 in 5,000,000. Almost all attacks are in shallow water or on the surface. For example, paddling surfers have been attacked by great white sharks - perhaps because their silhouette is similar to that of sea lions, which are a favorite prey of the sharks.

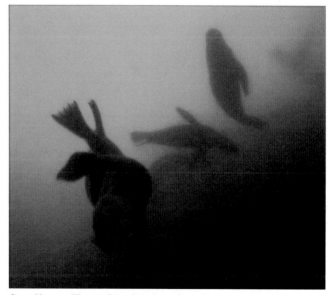

Sea lions: Favorite shark prey

Barracuda are also formidable predators, though they are much smaller than the large sharks, with the great barracuda growing to 6 feet and 100 pounds. Their knife-like teeth can inflict deep wounds, but there are even fewer reported attacks on humans by barracuda than by sharks. In some cases where people were attacked, they were wearing bright metal bracelets or medallions, or bright colored bathing suits, which may have attracted the predator's attention.

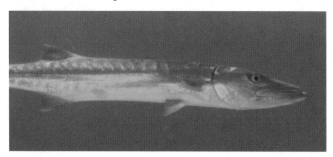

Moray eels can grow to over 10 feet and have powerful, vise-like jaws. But they are bottom-dwellers that wait for their prey in holes or crevices, or under rocks or coral. They typically bite humans only if threatened or startled, e.g., by a diver reaching for a lobster in a hole shared by an eel.

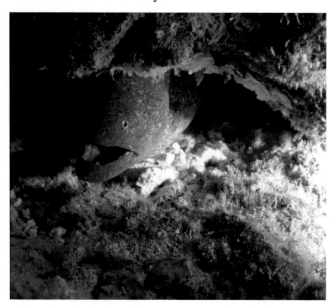

Venomous stings

Stings may cause a pricking sensation or burning pain at first; then itching, numbness, and throbbing pain radiating out from the injury. You may also see blistering, swelling, or wheals. If venom contacted the eye, you may see swollen eyelids or ulcers in the cornea.

Systemic signs and symptoms signal a more serious envenomation. Effects on breathing and circulation are usually from anaphylaxis – an allergic reaction in a sensitized patient who has been stung before. These effects usually begin within 15-30 minutes, though they may be delayed up to 6 hours.

Effects on **breathing** may include:
- tongue and lip swelling;
- bronchospasm (constricting of air passages);
- pulmonary edema (fluid in lungs);
- respiratory failure.

Effects on **circulation** may include:
- spasms of blood vessels (reducing blood flow);
- low blood pressure (impairing circulation);
- blood clots in veins;
- congestive heart failure.

Neurological effects may include:
- headache, vertigo, and loss of balance;
- inability to speak (laryngeal muscles paralyzed);
- impaired sense of touch and temperature;
- numbness or paralysis spreading from the sting;
- seizures or delirium;

Effects on **muscles** may include:
- muscle aches, cramps, or spasms;
- abdominal rigidity;

Effects on the **digestive system** may include nausea, vomiting, and diarrhea.

Fortunately, most marine envenomations are not fatal, except for those by the Australian box jellyfish (which can kill within minutes), Pacific sea snakes, and the stonefish found in coral reefs of the Pacific. But any patient who is getting sick from a sting, especially if there are problems with vital functions, needs to be evacuated quickly.

Treatment of venomous stings

Almost all venomous marine animals are found in warm water, generally in the shallows or around coral reefs. They will usually sting only if disturbed or handled. The goals of treatment for venomous stings (such as those caused by jellyfish or anemones) are to remove any tentacles and stinging cells on the skin and alleviate the effects of the venom.

To remove any adhering jellyfish tentacles or stinging cells, make a paste of baking soda, sand or mud with seawater and scrape them off with a dull knife. Do NOT use fresh water or urine because it will trigger any unfired stinging cells on the skin. Soak the skin with vinegar, which inactivates any stinging cells on the skin that have not yet fired. Re-apply the vinegar soaks for 15 minutes. **After** all the stinging cells are removed, soak the stung part of the body in hot water to break down protein based venom. Then monitor the patient for allergic reactions.

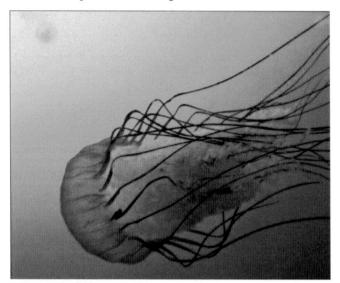

Jellyfish

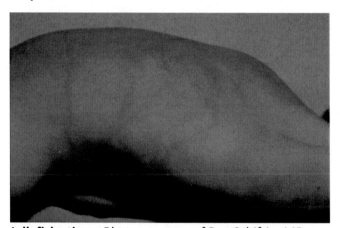

Jellyfish stings *Photo courtesy of Ben Schifrin, MD*

Protection

Some water resistant sunscreen lotions also contain ingredients that seem to protect against jellyfish stings by preventing the tentacles from making good enough contact with skin for stinging and by interfering with the stinging process (see the bibliography for this chapter, reference #9). But covering all exposed skin (including hands and feet) with a wet suit or light weight dive suit will keep jellyfish stinging cells away from your skin.

Stingrays

Stingrays are flat bottom dwellers in warm water shallows that often lie buried in the sand except for their eyes and spiracles. They feed on worms, mollusks, and crustaceans. Species range in size from a few inches across to 12 feet by 6 feet. Their pectoral fins have evolved into wing-like structures that propel them through the water with a flying motion. There are no freshwater species in the United States, though they can enter the freshwater of river mouths from the sea.

Stingrays are the most common cause of fish envenomation, with an estimated 2,000 stinging injuries per year in the United States. Usually the victim was walking in the surf during the spawning season and stepped on the stingray. Its whip-like tail, which has one or more barbed stingers, snaps forward and drives the spike into the victim – usually the foot or leg. The spike can penetrate shoes or a wetsuit and cause a deep puncture or laceration. It often breaks off in the wound.

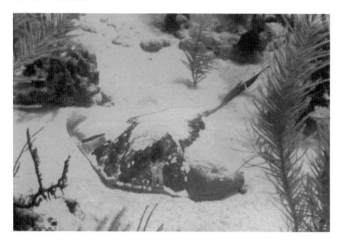

The pain spreads through the extremity and usually peaks in 1-2 hours. The area around the wound will swell, redden, and sometimes turn cyanotic (blue) because of impaired circulation. Systemic effects can include nausea, vomiting, fever, chills, tremors, muscle pain and cramps, weakness, and fainting. To avoid being stung, shuffle your feet in the sand when wading in warm seawater where there may be stingrays.

For venomous puncture wounds, such as those caused by stingrays or sea urchins, you should immerse the extremity in water as hot as the patient can tolerate for 30 to 90 minutes. This should reduce the pain and damage because the protein based venom breaks down when heated. Pull out small spines with tweezers, and use rubber cement to remove fine bristles and spines, just as with cactus spines - let the cement dry, then peel it off. If you don't have rubber cement, sticky tape is a good second choice. Large spines that penetrate deeply must be removed by a doctor – immobilize them with bulky dressings just as you would any impaled object.

Sea urchins

Sea urchins, found in almost all ocean waters, are slow moving invertebrates whose shells are covered with hollow spines that (in some species) are venomous. They may be globular or flattened. Most injuries are to people wading in tidal pools or beaches who step on or handle a sea urchin. The more spines penetrate, the more severe the envenomation. Symptoms of severe envenomation may include muscle aches and weakness, breathing problems, and paralysis. Spines may break off in the skin – remove them with tweezers. Stinging pincers may also remain on the skin – remove them by applying shaving cream or a paste and scraping them off. Starfish have similar spines. Immerse the extremity in hot water to ease the pain.

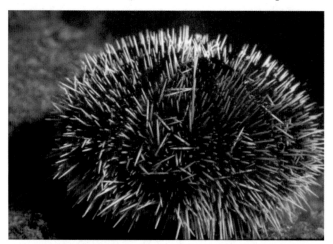

Sea urchin. *Photo courtesy of Paul Auerbach, MD*

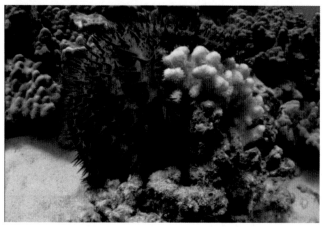

Crown of thorns starfish

Coelenterates ("hollow gut")

Coelenterates are colonies of cells rather than single animals. They include both free-swimmers that float on the surface and trail tentacles, and the stationary sea anemone (named after the terrestrial anemone, "wind flower"). Anemones and some species of coral, as well as jellyfish, have stinging cells called nematocysts. Free swimmers include jellyfish and the Portuguese man-of-war, whose tentacles can trail down 100 feet. At the end of each tentacle are the tiny stinging cells, with coiled tubes that are triggered by contact or a change in osmolality (concentration of ions in the water) – which is why you should not use fresh water to wash tentacles off your skin. Stinging cells of beached jellyfish can remain potent for weeks, even when the tentacles are dried out. The stings usually leave whip-like welts or scattered red blotches that may disappear within hours or a day at most.

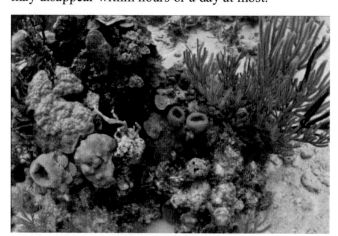

Coral: Look but don't touch.

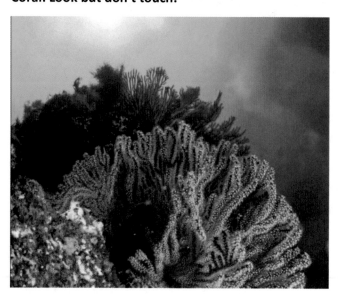

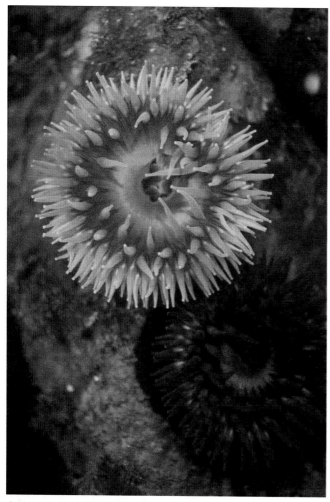
Anemones: Stinging cells

Other hazardous marine animals

Sea snakes are very abundant in the warm waters of the Pacific and Indian oceans. They can grow up to 9 feet, and swim rapidly both backwards and forwards with their paddle-like tails. Their venom, which they inject with 2 or 4 needle-like fangs, is a potent neurotoxin. Sea snakes are not aggressive and have very small mouths, so human envenomation is rare, and usually from snakes caught in fishing nets. In about 75% of sea snake bites, there is no envenomation. But because the venom is so deadly, get the patient to a hospital that has or can get the antivenom – call ahead in case they have to send for it. Meanwhile, wrap the entire limb in an elastic bandage, so as to slow the spread of venom through the lymph system, as with any other potentially deadly snake venom. Symptoms, which usually begin within 3 hours, may include:

- weakness;
- muscle and joint pain;
- blurred vision;
- difficulty speaking and swallowing;
- drooling or vomiting;
- breathing difficulty and paralysis.

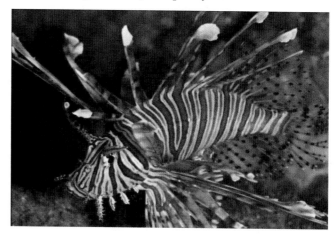

Lionfish, native to the Indian Ocean, are now also found in lagoons and coral reefs on the East Coast of the U.S. and in the Caribbean. They are small but aggressive fish with venomous spines.

Catfish also have spines that can inflict stings. Perhaps the strangest of them is the Amazonian Candiru ("urethra fish"), which is just 1" long and transparent. It can swim into the urethra of someone urinating in the water and lock itself in place by extending its spines. Mega-doses of vitamin C may help to dislodge it. Normally it is a parasite that swims into the gill slits of fish (against the current of the water being forced out) and attaches itself.

Octopuses, despite their Hollywood image, are very shy creatures that have never been known to attack humans unprovoked. The only reported bites have been to people handling them, and the most dangerous species is the tiny Australian blue-ringed octopus, which has the most potent venom.

Conclusion

Contrary to their popular reputation, the large marine predators seldom attack humans. Most marine injuries come from accidental contact with smaller organisms that have spikes or stinging cells, and can be usually avoided. Even minor marine wounds, however, should be promptly cleaned and treated for infection because many wound pathogens thrive in sea water.

Chapter 27. Hazardous plants

If you want to enrich your wilderness diet by gathering edible plants, you should first learn how to identify them (and how to avoid poisonous plants) from an experienced mentor. Trying to match plants to illustrations in a book is risky for several reasons. Not only is it hard for a novice to tell the difference between many edible and poisonous plants, but also plants may grow together, so that you can inadvertently pick up something poisonous with a batch that is edible. For example, the poisonous water hemlock often grows in the same places as the succulent watercress, and immature death cap mushrooms may be confused with delicious puffballs.

You can also poison yourself indirectly, for example, by using oleander sticks as roasting spits or cutting whistles from the hollow elderberry twigs. Many common household and yard plants are poisonous, and small children may chew or eat them. Poinsettias, rhododendrons, mistletoe and boxwood are just a few of many examples. Even if you do not put strange plants in your mouth, you can get a skin irritation or an allergic reaction from substances that rub off onto your skin. You can also be punctured or cut by plants with sharp defenses.

Leaves of three

Three plants in the United States are the most notorious for causing allergic reactions: **poison oak**, **poison ivy** and **poison sumac**. Poison oak grows as a low shrub in the East and South but is found as both a tall shrub and a clinging vine on the Pacific Coast. Poison ivy has many varieties and can grow as a shrub as well as a vine. It is found in wooded areas, and near lakes and streams through most of the United States, though not in the Pacific Coast states. Poison sumac grows as a shrub in swampy areas of the Eastern states.

All of them have an oil called **urushiol** ("milky oil") in their sap. It can rapidly penetrate the skin and combine with skin proteins, so to get it all off you would need to remove it within 10 or 15 minutes. When the plants are in leaf, you can pick up the oil by brushing against them, because the black, sticky sap can accumulate on the surface. It can also seep through clothing, or you can pick it up by handling clothing

that is contaminated. Another way to pick up uroshiol is from a pet. Dogs like to romp in it and can bring it back on their fur. Free ranging pet cats that sleep with you or curl up with you on the sofa can spread it over your whole body.

Mnemonics like "Leaves of three, leave it be" warn us away from poison oak and ivy, because their leaves usually grow in clusters of three – poison sumac has clusters of 12 leaves or more. But urushiol is also found in the stems and roots, so walking through the bare shrubs in late fall and winter can also expose you, if you break any of the twigs or brush against some that are already broken.

If the plant burns, the oil can not only contaminate the skin, but also be inhaled in the smoke. This mechanism has killed forest firefighters and can endanger you if you are close to a forest or range fire. Nearly one-third of the forestry workers and firefighters in the Pacific Northwest, for example, get rashes or lung irritation from poison oak.

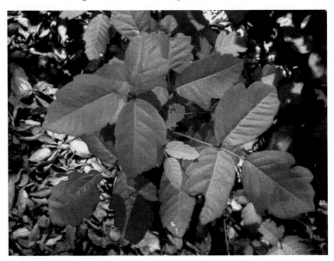

Poison Oak. *Photo courtesy of Linda Garcia*

Protection and treatment

People who are only moderately allergic (perhaps half of the United States population) may have hours to remove unbonded oil from their skin before they get a reaction. However, people who are very sensitive (perhaps 10% of the population) may start reacting in less than an hour. A cool shower with strong soap should get most of it off, though several products are specially designed to remove urushiol, such as Tecnu

Poison Oak and Ivy Cleanser®. You should make sure that no leaves or twigs are still in your clothes or equipment, and isolate clothes that may be contaminated for a separate wash with detergent.

Products that can be sprayed or wiped on the skin before exposure, such as Oak and Ivy Armor and Ivy Block Lotion, form a barrier to the oil. Ivy Block contains bentonite, a clay-like substance that is also used in some cosmetics. It leaves a dry residue on the skin that apparently bonds to urushiol. In clinical trials, it prevented a reaction in 70% of the subjects, all of whom were known to be sensitive to urushiol. Eating the plant, however, far from making you immune, is liable to cause a severe reaction.

The body's over-reaction to urushiol causes the problems – a self-destructive process of shedding tissues contaminated by the oil. Soaks and compresses may help relieve the itching: aluminum acetate solution, dilute potassium permanganate solution, or acetic acid solution. You can also take a tepid bath with baking soda or a packet of Aveeno oatmeal in the water. Calamine lotion may also relieve some of the itching. A local anesthetic, like Prax cream or lotion, is the next step. For a severe reaction with swelling, a doctor can prescribe a corticosteroid, like prednisone, and the sooner you start taking it the more likely that it will relieve the symptoms. Within an hour or two of exposure, it may prevent a reaction; but after 24 hours, it probably won't help. Topical steroid creams and antihistamines usually have little effect.

Plants that sting and stab

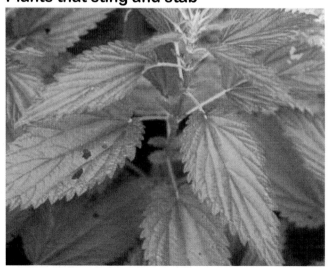

Stinging nettles. *Photo courtesy of Linda Garcia.*

Some plants have stinging hairs on their leaves that can inject irritating substances if you brush against them. In the United States, the most common ones are stinging nettles and spurge nettles. Soaks and cold compresses may relieve the itching, as with exposure to urushiol.

Cactuses protect themselves with spines that may be almost invisibly small, as in the prickly pear, or large enough to cause serious wounds. One way to remove tiny hair-like spines is to lay sticky tape over them and peel it off. You can also coat the area with rubber cement and let it dry before peeling. Industrial strength facial gel from a beauty parlor works even better than rubber cement. Always peel in the direction that body hairs are oriented. Lift up the edge of the dried coating with your fingernails to start it.

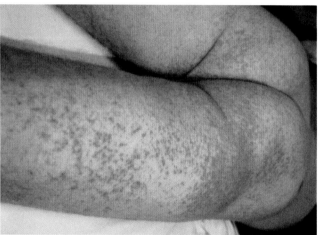
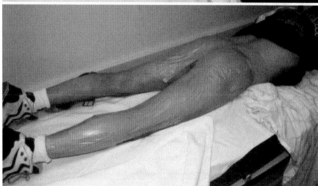

This patient was pincushioned with many small cactus needles. They were removed by covering them with tape, then peeling it off.
Photos courtesy of Ben Schifrin, MD

Large cactus spines that have penetrated deeply may have to be removed surgically, which can be difficult because they may break off under the skin, and they do not always show on x-rays.

Chapter 28. Medical emergencies in the wilderness

On wilderness trips, respiratory ailments are common for several reasons. When people get cold, wet, fatigued, or stressed, their resistance is reduced. Also, if one person has a respiratory infection on a long trip, others in the group are liable to pick it up as they share tents and food. So you need to know how to recognize respiratory illness, how to distinguish the minor types from more serious illness that may require evacuation, and what you can do for the patient.

Respiratory system defenses

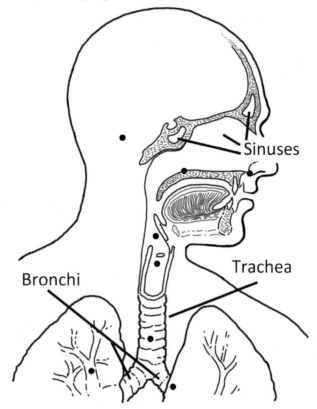

The hairs inside the nostrils are the first line of defense against inhaled dust, which may be contaminated with microorganisms. Then passage into the large sinus (Latin "hollow") behind the nose causes turbulence which tends to carry dust to the sticky mucus membranes. The trachea is also coated with mucus carried slowly upward by the movements of hair-like cilia. There are nerve endings in and behind the nose that trigger a sneeze, and in the airways and lungs that trigger a cough (black dots), when enough mucus accumulates. There are also sneeze triggers in each of the Eustachian tubes between the middle ear and the upper airway. This is a crude reflex for expelling inhaled contaminants. But anything that irritates the walls of the sinuses or air passages, such as cold and dry air, can also trigger mucus production and the sneeze or cough reflex.

Upper respiratory infections

Over-production of mucus in reaction to an infection causes congestion, and swelling of the air passages may further narrow them. This can make it hard to breathe, especially when you lie down to sleep. A decongestant may clear the sinuses, and sleeping in a semi-sitting position may help.

About 200 cold and flu viruses can infect the upper respiratory tract: the air passages and chambers above the neck. They are adapted to the relatively cool environment created by the constant movement of air in and out. The body may react to the infection by raising its temperature (fever). Traditional remedies of staying warm and drinking plenty of fluids may help, and certainly won't do any harm. Unfortunately there is no effective cure for colds and flu, though some medications can reduce symptoms such as congestion. Since they can be spread by aerosol as well as contact with contaminated skin or other surfaces, active respiratory infections are very contagious.

Middle respiratory infections

As long as a respiratory infection is confined to the upper airways, the patient may feel well enough to continue the trip. Any infection of the bronchi, however, is much more serious. These infections are called bronchitis, and 90% of them are caused by viruses, which antibiotics do not affect. Generally, anyone who is coughing (rather than just sneezing) should not be exercising. Typically, the patient has a deep, racking cough that may be dry (especially at high altitude) or may bring up yellow or greenish mucus. With enough congestion, the patient may be struggling for breath. Anyone in this condition should be evacuated.

Pneumonia

The word "pneumonia" means "disease of the lung," and is a blanket term for any inflammation of the lung. While the word "inflammation" comes from the Latin meaning "to set on fire," inflammation is a response of the body that includes diluting fluid, so it can flood the alveoli in which oxygen moves to the blood. The more alveoli are flooded, the less oxygen can move through the lungs. Vomitus aspirated into the lungs can cause pneumonia as well as bacteria and viruses.

Signs and symptoms that distinguish pneumonia from upper respiratory infections may include:

- shaking chills;
- chest pain (sharp rather than dull);
- shortness of breath;
- hot dry skin;
- high temperature.

The patient will probably have a deep, racking cough and should be encouraged to sit up and cough regularly, in order to reduce congestion. An upright position will minimize flooding of the oxygen-exchange surface, because of the shape of the lungs. If the infection is bacterial, a physician may prescribe an oral antibiotic; and the patient may need oxygen. But anyone with pneumonia should be evacuated as rapidly as possible, because it could be fatal in the wilderness.

Asthma

Unlike respiratory infections, asthma (from the Greek word for "gasping or panting") may be triggered by many things including:

- pollen or other allergens;
- dust;
- pollutants;
- sleeping in a moldy tent;
- food or lotion to which the patient is sensitized;
- cold air;
- exercise.

Asthma attacks can be allergic reactions (about 80%), responses to irritants, or reactions to stress. According to the Centers for Disease Control and Prevention (www.cdc.gov), over 24 million people in the United States suffer from asthma, including over 6 million children, and the percentage of people with asthma is increasing more than exposure to air pollution and other irritants can explain. According to the hygiene hypothesis [see bibliography], an overly clean environment in early childhood prevents the immune system from developing normally, so that it over-reacts when it is later exposed to dust or other irritants. Many athletes have asthma, including Mark Spitz (who won several Olympic gold medals in swimming). So asthma need not prevent people from enjoying outdoor activities provided that they carry their medications.

In an asthma attack, the respiratory system over-reacts to an irritant, allergen, or stress. Release of chemicals called histamines causes the air passages to constrict, swell, and congest. As in anaphylaxis, the effect can be dramatic. Since airflow is proportional to the fourth power of the passage's radius, reducing the air passage to one-half of its radius (for example) reduces airflow to one-sixteenth. The victim will be in obvious respiratory distress, wheezing and struggling for breath. Asthma kills 5,000 people per year in the United States, and the number is increasing. If you want to know what it is like to have a severe asthma attack, try breathing through a soda straw.

As with anaphylactic shock, the only way to relieve a severe asthma attack is with a medication that opens the air passages, reversing the effect of the histamines. These prescription medications, such as albuterol, are sold as inhalers. Epinephrine is also a bronchodilator, but it should not be used by asthma patients who are over 45, have heart problems or are pregnant because it is also a vasoconstrictor, and drives up blood pressure. Antihistamines, as the name implies, help suppress the production of more histamines, so they supplement asthma inhalers. If you are leading a wilderness trip, medical screening should include questions about asthma and what medication an asthmatic is carrying.

Chronic respiratory diseases

Over 12 million adults in the United States have Chronic Obstructive Pulmonary Disease (**COPD**), and it is the fourth leading cause of death. Smoking is the biggest risk factor, especially for **emphysema** (Greek *emphysan* "to inflate"). In healthy lungs, the elasticity of lung tissue causes it to recoil and expel air when the respiratory muscles are relaxed after breathing in.

Smoking causes chronic narrowing of the airways by inflammation, which makes it harder to exhale – the increased air pressure stretches the elastic walls of the alveoli (**hyperinflation**). In people with advanced emphysema many alveolar walls are destroyed, so that parts of the lungs become dead air spaces, and the lungs are enlarged. They are sometimes described as having barrel chests, because the chest becomes almost as deep as it is wide. They tend to be chronically short of breath, because the large volume of trapped air reduces the amount of fresh air they can inhale.

Patients with COPD may use **accessory muscles** attached to the clavicles and the top of the sternum to help lift the rib cage – you can see these muscles standing out in the neck when they breathe. You may also see **retractions** when they inhale – indentations above the clavicles and between the ribs. They may sit in the **tripod position** – leaning forward with the arms outstretched and the chin forward so as to use the muscles of the abdomen and the back to help them exhale. As they exhale, they may purse their lips to keep up the air pressure and prevent collapse of the bronchial walls. You may also see jugular vein distension (JVD) when the patient exhales, because the increased pressure in the chest from forceful exhaling compresses the heart and reduces venous return, causing back pressure in the veins.

Smoking or air pollution can also cause **chronic bronchitis** by irritating the trachea and bronchi and stimulating the production of excess mucus as well as swelling that narrows the airways. The patient will be coughing frequently to bring up the mucus and clear the airways. Bronchitis that persists at least three months for two years in a row is called chronic; and in time may destroy the cilia that line the airways – hair-like cells that carry mucus up to where it can be expelled by coughing.

Lung sounds

You can assess a patient's breathing by **auscultation** (Latin *auscultare* "to listen keenly") with your ear against the rib cage. But a stethoscope will amplify the sounds. In a healthy person with no lung or airway problems, the sound of breathing will be soft and low pitched. Any swelling or congestion in the air passages or damage in the alveoli, however, can cause abnormal breathing sounds. There are several free web sites on which you can listen to these sounds and see **phonopneumograms** that show their wave forms:

www.physio-pedia.com/Auscultation; www.easyauscultation.com.

Abnormal lung sounds may be continuous or discontinuous, and high or low pitched. **Crackles** (also called **rales**) are discontinuous, popping lung sounds. The sounds are caused by small airways and alveoli that were sealed by fluid popping open when the patient inhales. Coarse crackles are louder, lower pitched, and last longer. Crackles can be heard at the base of the lungs, near the lowest ribs.

Wheezes are continuous sounds that can be high or low pitched. They are caused by air being forced through narrowed airways. Turbulence makes the airway walls vibrate like the reed in an oboe, creating a sound that is sometimes called musical. Wheezes are heard in the upper part of the chest (over the bronchi and bronchioles), usually when the patient exhales. Very loud, high pitched wheezes that can often be heard without a stethoscope are called **stridor**. They suggest a partial obstruction in or extreme narrowing of the larynx or trachea.

Ronchi are very low pitched wheezes, heard when the patient inhales and exhales. They suggest excess mucus partially obstructing the bronchi.

Using the stethoscope

In the 18th century, Leopold Auenbrugger described his method of tapping on the chest and listening to the sounds it made in order to detect problems in the lungs. If the lungs were congested, tapping produced a dull sound, which he called "morbid". But to hear those sounds, physicians had to press an ear against the patient's chest. In the early 19th century, Rene Laennec discovered that he could hear more sounds in the chest (even without tapping) through a wooden tube; and that the sounds were focused by adding an ear piece. By the end of the 19th century, the wooden tube had been replaced with two rubber tubes (one for each ear), and a chest piece, with a wide diaphragm on one side to amplify higher pitched (lung) sounds and a smaller bell on the other side for lower pitched sounds such as bowel sounds. Some stethoscopes, however, have only a single diaphragm in the chest piece. The ear pieces should be angled slightly forward to fit into the ears.

Stethoscopes can be used to hear sounds of the heart and the digestive system, and to measure blood pressure by auscultation (see Chapter 2). But they are most often used to listen for abnormal breathing sounds. Listening high on the chest can detect sounds in the bronchi and bronchioles. Listening lower on the chest can detect sounds in the alveoli of the lungs. Ask the patient to take deep breaths as you listen, and always compare sounds on each side at the same level. Have the patient sit, hold the chest piece between the index and middle fingers and slip the thumb under the tube so it doesn't rub against the patient's chest.

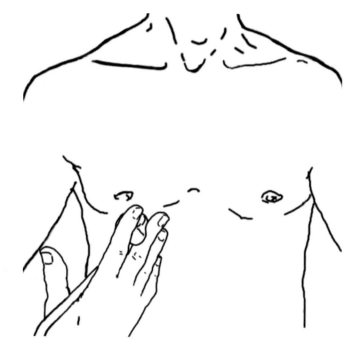

The drawings show some good positions for a quick exam, though you may want to check more locations if there are any signs of breathing problems. On the chest, listen high and low on at least two levels.

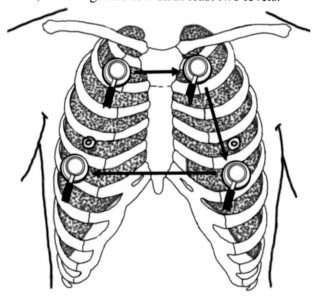

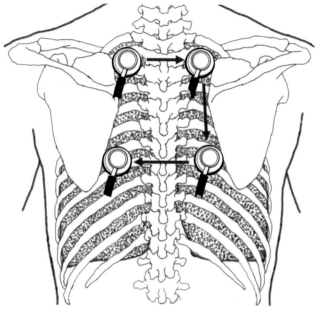

On the back, place the diaphragm of the stethoscope between each scapula (shoulder bone) and the spinal column. The lower positions are in the **triangles of auscultation**, small areas with only one thin layer of muscle over the lungs. You should also listen to the sounds of breathing on either side of the rib cage.

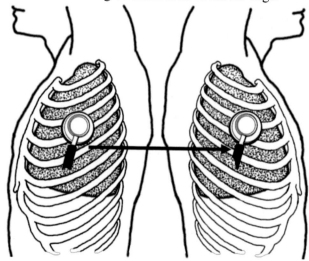

Tuberculosis

According to the Center for Disease Control (www.cdc.gov), one-fourth of the world's population is infected with tuberculosis (TB), which is caused by a bacterium: *Mycobacterium tuberculosis*. These bacteria usually attack the lungs (although they can attack other parts of the body as well), so they spread by aerosol when someone with an active infection coughs, sneezes, or just speaks. In most of those infected, however, TB is latent, and they are not contagious. But any weakening of the immune system can make

185

someone vulnerable to TB infection or allow a latent infection to become active. HIV infection is a risk factor, but so are diabetes, alcoholism, and smoking.

Worldwide, about 8 million active cases of TB are reported each year (though probably many cases are not reported) and about 10,000 are reported in the United States. TB is still the most deadly infectious disease, killing about 2 million people per year. Although there are now drugs for treating TB, multi-drug resistant strains are becoming more common, as patients may stop taking medications when they feel better, but before the infection is completely cleared. Since patients need to take several drugs daily for 4 to 9 months to be cured (even if TB is still latent), it is not surprising that many do not complete the regimen.

TB was for much of its history called consumption, because it seemed to consume the patient. Signs and symptoms include weight loss and anorexia, fatigue, fever, and night sweats as well as coughing and chest pain. Coughing up blood is the classic sign familiar from portrayals of TB in literature and period films. Treatment before effective drugs was a regimen of fresh air and exercise at a sanitarium, supervised by doctors. TB sanitariums, many of them in the mountains, became popular in the second half of the 19th century. Thomas Mann's novel, *The Magic Mountain*, is set in a TB sanitarium.

Health care workers may be required to have a TB test before working in an ambulance or hospital. The tests are only about 80% sensitive, however, which means they do not detect about 20% of TB infections. Also, the skin test can give a false positive for those who have been vaccinated. BCG (bacilli Calmette-Guérin) is a live attenuated vaccine developed at the Pasteur Institute and first administered to humans in 1921. Studies on the safety and efficacy of BCG show very mixed results, however, so it is not recommended except for people who have serious exposure to TB. Protection from infection includes a **HEPA** (High Efficiency Particulate Air) respirator.

Congestive heart failure

In a heart attack, one or more arteries that supply the heart muscle with oxygenated blood are constricted or at least partially obstructed (see **cardiogenic shock** in chapter 4). Oxygenated blood returns to the left side of the heart from the lungs through the pulmonary veins.

If the left ventricle is damaged by a heart attack, back pressure in the pulmonary veins can force fluid into the lungs, which may cause crackles as the patient breathes, a sound that is audible through a stethoscope. A patient in congestive heart failure will usually be most comfortable, and breathe most easily, in a sitting or semi-sitting position. Because of the shape of the lungs, lying down would spread the fluid over much more lung surface and reduce oxygen exchange.

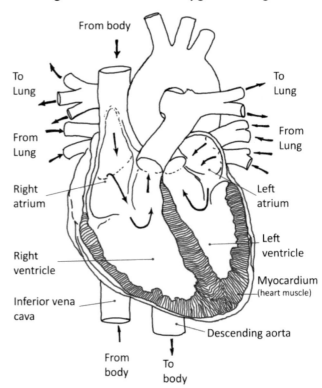

Conclusion

Respiratory illness can be caused by infection, chronic conditions (COPD), or over-reaction of the immune system to irritants (asthma). Someone with an upper respiratory infection may feel able to continue the trip, although the infection could spread to other people in the group, especially if they share tents. But anyone with signs of a bronchial or lung infection should be evacuated.

Gastrointestinal illness

Digestion of food begins in the mouth. An enzyme in saliva begins to break down carbohydrates, and the process continues in the stomach and small intestine. Gastric juices in the stomach begin to break down proteins, but the process of digesting fats does not start until they reach the small intestine. Since the organisms that cause gastrointestinal illness usually colonize the small intestine, carbohydrates will be easiest to tolerate, and fats most difficult to digest.

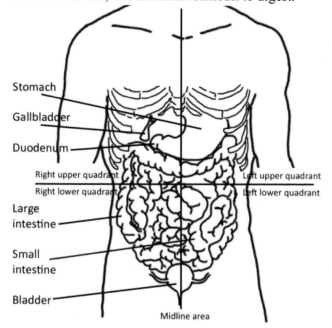

Dysentery (Greek "bad gut") is caused by bacteria that invade dead tissue or open sores (ulcers), usually in the large intestine. It can cause abdominal cramps and blood in the stool, though the victim may not be able to move the stool. **Diarrhea** (Greek "flowing through") is much more common and is usually caused by the body's response to toxins (Latin *toxicum* "poison") released by organisms in food or in the small intestine. The inner surface of the intestine secretes excess fluid, making the stool soft or watery. As a result, the victim becomes dehydrated, and with watery diarrhea, can soon lose enough electrolytes to cause an imbalance. If the toxin is already in the food (food poisoning), then the symptoms may begin the same day. Most organisms that colonize the intestine and produce toxins there take longer to cause symptoms.

Sources of infection

Infected people and animals shed the infecting organisms in the stools, whether any symptoms are shown or not. Some organisms will remain in the stools and continue being shed long after the victim has recovered. These include Giardia and Cryptosporidium as well as some types of E. Coli. The shed organisms may then contaminate water or inadequately washed hands. In the wilderness, contaminated water is a common source of infection. Contaminated or spoiled food can also transmit infection, as well as infected people who handle food or utensils for a group. Ironically, ingested soap from pots and dishes that have not been well rinsed can cause diarrhea. Also, about 7% of the population is sensitive enough to iodine that they may get diarrhea by using it to disinfect water.

Prevention

Water disinfection (described in the chapter on contaminated water) and good camp hygiene are the most important ways to prevent diarrhea in the wilderness. If you swim or bathe in contaminated water, you can accidentally swallow enough to be infected. You should also clean your hands thoroughly with soap and water after defecating and before handling food. If water is scarce, you can use benzalkonium chloride antiseptic wipes. If you carry fresh fruit and vegetables on a wilderness trip, pre-wash and dry them at home, so that you do not risk contaminating them by washing with unsafe water. Dehydrated food is usually safe, because most bacteria that cause gastrointestinal disease cannot grow without water.

Possible signs and symptoms

Anyone with five or more bowel movements per day, or stools that are loose or watery, has diarrhea. Other common signs and symptoms of gastrointestinal disease are nausea, vomiting, gas, and abdominal cramps. A mild case may run its course in a day or two, but if it persists for more than two days, then the victim will probably not be able to continue the trip and should be evacuated. More serious signs and symptoms that also require evacuation are digested blood in the stools (giving it a dark, pitchy appearance), high temperature, swollen abdomen or progressive dehydration in someone who cannot replace fluid loss.

Treatment

For anyone with diarrhea, the most important treatment is fluid replacement. Water or clear fluids such as apple juice, herbal tea and clear broth (with no fat in it) are all good for mild diarrhea. For moderate or severe diarrhea, you need to replace electrolytes as well. You can use a commercial mixture (runner's drink or Oral

Rehydration Salts) or make your own by adding to each liter of water:

- 1/2 teaspoon table salt (sodium chloride);
- 1/2 teaspoon baking soda;
- 1/4 teaspoon salt substitute (potassium chloride)
- sugar or honey to taste (but not too much).

Alternate the electrolyte drink with drinks of plain water. In a hospital, a patient too nauseated to drink or keep fluids down would be given fluids intravenously. If rapid evacuation of such a patient to a hospital is not possible, you may decide to give an anti-motility agent. Check for allergies before giving any medication. Bismuth subsalicylate (Pepto-Bismol), for instance, should not be given to anyone sensitive to products that contain aspirin. Another drug, loperamide (Imodium) should not be given to children.

It is generally not safe to give anti-motility agents for diarrhea if signs and symptoms indicate a severe case, such as an oral temperature over 101° F, swollen abdomen, or blood in the stools. A patient with that serious an illness should be evacuated immediately. Antibiotics are available for many of the organisms that cause diarrhea, but the organisms need to be identified first, which requires laboratory testing. Hydrocortisone cream (1%) can help relieve anal irritation in someone with severe diarrhea.

Recovery diet

Once the patient has started to recover, you can add simple carbohydrates in the form of crackers and toast, gelatin, and hard-boiled eggs (for easily digestible protein) to the fluid diet. When the diarrhea is nearly gone, you can add more carbohydrate foods such as boiled or baked potatoes, plain noodles, rice, bananas, and applesauce. But avoid all fatty foods and milk products as well as fruit and vegetables until the stools are normal, because they are too difficult for an impaired digestive system to digest. When the stools are normal, you can add lean meat, cooked vegetables and yogurt or cottage cheese. You should continue to avoid alcohol, spicy foods and stewed fruit for at least several days to prevent a possible relapse.

Urinary tract infection (UTI)

Urinary tract infections are about 50 times more common in women than in men, because women have shorter urethras. This makes it easier for bacteria to move up the urethra to the urinary bladder. About 90% of UTIs are caused by E. coli bacteria, which are common in the intestines. So prevent UTI by wiping from front to back after urinating or defecating, and then washing the hands thoroughly. **Dehydration** increases the risk of UTI by reducing urine, so that E. coli are not flushed out of the urethra.

The main symptom of UTI is a burning sensation when urinating. Also, the victim feels the need to urinate every five minutes or so, but can only pass a few drops because the bladder is spasming. Over the counter medications such as **Uristat** or **Azo** can suppress the symptoms (pain and urinary frequency) so that the victim can walk out of the wilderness.

If the UTI is caused by E.coli, copious draughts of 100% **cranberry juice** may work by preventing the bacterial from forming attachments to the bladder wall or to each other; but only if it is taken in the very early stages of infection. Physicians usually prescribe antibiotics such as **Septra** or **Keflix**, which pass through the urinary bladder. Most broad spectrum antibiotics, however, don't work for UTI because they are excreted through the large intestine.

Poisoning

If food is contaminated by an organism that has already produced toxins, the toxins may not be inactivated by cooking. They can make you sick in less than seven hours. Some examples of bacteria whose toxins can cause food poisoning are Staphylococcus aureus, Salmonella, Shigella, and Clostridium botulinum. **Staphylococcus** can grow even in food cured with salt, such as ham that has not been kept refrigerated. **Salmonella** is common in poultry and sometimes in eggs, because most poultry feed is augmented with protein from slaughterhouse products. It can also be found in meat and unpasteurized dairy products. The bacteria in poultry intestines contaminate the carcasses and the outside of the eggs. Most adults in the United States probably have some degree of immunity from Salmonella, because the incidence in humans drops very steeply from the age of one to the age of nine. **Shigella** is often transmitted by flies as well as infected food handlers. **Clostridium botulinum** can be found in canned as well as raw food, especially fish. Since it is anaerobic, it does not need oxygen, so it can grow and produce toxin inside a can with contaminated food.

Signs and symptoms

All food poisoning upsets the digestive process and can cause nausea and vomiting as well as diarrhea and sometimes abdominal cramps. With Salmonella toxin, the diarrhea is often foul and watery, and the victim may also get a headache. **Botulism** is especially dangerous, because after several days of gastro-intestinal upset, it can attack the nervous system. The victim may experience dry mouth and hoarseness, difficulty swallowing, facial weakness, sluggish pupils, blurred or double vision, and muscular weakness that can progress into paralysis. If untreated, it is often fatal, but there is an antitoxin for it. So if you suspect botulism, it is important to get the victim to a hospital where it can be diagnosed and treated before it attacks the nervous system.

Other poisoning routes

Most poisons are ingested; but they can also be inhaled, absorbed through skin or mucus membranes, or injected (see chapters 25 and 26 on venomous bites and stings). The word poison comes from the Latin *potio* "potion" by way of the early French *puison*. To the Romans, *potio* also meant a magical drink. In English, a poison is any substance that causes harm when it gets inside the body, by either destroying cells or disrupting their functions. The study of poisons is called **toxicology**, from the Latin word for poison, *toxicum*. Strangely, the Latin word *toxicum* comes from the Greek word for bow (*toxon*), perhaps because some archers coated their arrowheads with poison.

Poisoning information and treatment

Any business that uses potentially toxic chemicals should have **Material Safety Data Sheets** (MSDS) that describe the hazards, how to protect yourself, and what to do if you are exposed. But if you have phone reception, you can call the **American Association of Poison Control Centers** (www.aapcc.org) at their 24-hour hotline: 1-800-222-1222. Their staff give expert advice on what to do after exposure to any poison.

Inducing vomiting is no longer recommended for ingested poisons, because the vomitus can be aspirated into the lungs (especially if the patient is less than fully alert) and corrosive poisons that caused direct damage going down would do even more damage coming up. But **activated charcoal** is recommended for some poisons if the patient is alert enough to swallow safely. It is a fine black powder that adsorbs (binds to) poisons in the stomach and intestines, so that they pass through the digestive system instead of being absorbed into the blood. But it does not work on corrosive poisons (such as drain cleaner) or alcohol.

Ingested and absorbed poisons

Overdosing on drugs, which can be over the counter, prescription, or recreational is a common cause of poisoning. Symptoms (which may be delayed as the drug moves through the digestive system and into the blood) may include abdominal pain, nausea, vomiting, or diarrhea. Overdoses of drugs designed to bring vital functions into the normal range can be especially dangerous. For example, too much of an anti-clotting drug can cause internal bleeding. Overdoses of many medications can affect the heart rate, blood pressure, or breathing as well as the level of responsiveness. Overdoses of depressants (including alcohol, barbiturates and narcotics) can cause respiratory arrest.

Many plants are poisonous, including ornamental plants in gardens and houses as well as those found in the wilderness. Many household products are very poisonous if swallowed. For example, pesticides are designed to kill plants or vermin, so they are very toxic to humans; and cleaning products usually have corrosive ingredients. The oil in poison oak, ivy, and sumac can be absorbed through the skin, and so can any poisons (such as pesticides) that are mixed in liquid solvents.

Inhaled poisons

Volatile chemicals (Latin *volatilis* "flying") have a very low boiling point, so even at room temperature some of the liquid evaporates into fumes. A reaction from mixing chemicals can also produce fumes. For example, mixing ammonia and bleach produces chlorine gas. Some other household products that produce toxic fumes are oven, toilet bowl and drain cleaners; oil-based paint; paint thinner; and bug foggers or sprays. Combustion (burning), a chemical reaction that releases heat, can also release toxic gases as well as particles that cause inhalation injury.

Probably the most common and insidious inhaled poison is carbon monoxide, which is odorless. **Carbon monoxide** is produced by incomplete combustion of any material containing carbon, and is found in the smoke from house and forest fires as well as fumes from cooking with petroleum-based or natural gas fuel. So it is a hazard of cooking in tents and snow caves (see chapter 7). Carbon monoxide is also a component of automobile exhaust and a potential hazard in buildings using natural gas for heating, which should have carbon monoxide detectors with alarms. Carbon monoxide binds to hemoglobin much more strongly than oxygen, so it reduces the oxygen carrying capacity of the blood. **Hydrogen cyanide** is also odorless. It is produced from burning fabrics, paper, plastics and other synthetics that are common in modern buildings. Hydrogen cyanide prevents cells from using oxygen.

Carbon monoxide bound to hemoglobin in the blood can be measured with a pulse CO oximeter, which uses at least 8 wavelengths of light (visible and invisible), compared to 2 wavelengths in a pulse oximeter (see chapter 2). Many fire department and EMS ambulances carry portable pulse CO oximeters. It is an important assessment tool because the symptoms of hypoxia from carbon monoxide poisoning are similar to symptoms of many other conditions: headache, nausea, tachycardia (Greek *tachys* "swift" + *kardia* "heart"), possible seizure, and unconsciousness.

Symptoms of hydrogen cyanide poisoning in low doses may include headache, vertigo, drowsiness, tachycardia, and tachypnea ("swift breathing").

Victims of moderate or high doses may experience tremors, cardiac arrhythmia (irregular heartbeat), convulsions, stupor and paralysis, as well as respiratory depression. Immediate treatment for both carbon monoxide and hydrogen cyanide exposure is oxygen administration. Paramedic level treatment may include intubating to keep the airway of an unresponsive patient open and medications to stabilize the heart and prevent convulsions. Antidotes to cyanide (given in the hospital) are problematic because they temporarily reduce the oxygen carrying capacity of the blood, which may already be reduced by concurrent carbon monoxide poisoning.

Conclusion

Poisoning is possible in the wilderness as well as the home and workplace. If you have phone reception, you should call the Poison Control Center number and be ready to identify the poison. Gastrointestinal illness can be caused by food poisoning, poor hygiene, contaminated water, or simple indigestion. While there are various medications that may relieve some of the symptoms of gastrointestinal illness, prevention is the only way to ensure that your trip will not end in misery. Practice good camp hygiene, because even people with no symptoms may carry and transmit infectious disease. Disinfect water if it may be contaminated. Be prepared to treat diarrhea by keeping the patient hydrated with electrolytes, and recognize when a case is severe enough to require evacuation.

Diabetes

The word diabetes is Greek for "syphon" (*dia* "through" + *baino* "pass", so called because victims seemed to pass water like a syphon. The full name of the disease is diabetes mellitus (Latin "sweetened with honey") because sugar in the urine of diabetics made it taste sweet, and physicians used to diagnose the disease by tasting the patient's urine. Since an estimated 26,000,000 diabetics live in the United States, including many whose disease has not yet been diagnosed, a diabetic emergency is one of the more likely medical problems that you may encounter on a wilderness trip. Even diabetics who control the disease in an urban situation may run out of insulin in the wilderness, or run out of fuel because they underestimate the amount of energy they are expending. So you should know how the disease works, be able to recognize a diabetic emergency, and know what to do about it. If you are leading a wilderness trip, your medical screening of participants should include questions about diabetes, how they control it, and whether they have their insulin or other prescribed diabetic medications with them.

Metabolism and fuel delivery

The digestive system breaks down carbohydrates into a sugar (**glucose**), which is used by the body's cells for fuel. As the amount of glucose in the blood increases, it normally triggers the release of a hormone called **insulin** from the pancreas. Insulin helps transport glucose across the cell membranes and into the cells. Without insulin, glucose accumulates in the blood while the cells run on empty. Body cells have an alternative energy cycle that breaks down fatty acids, though it is much less efficient. But brain cells have no alternative energy cycle, so they need a continual supply of glucose. If the blood glucose level drops to zero, brain cells start to die in 15 seconds.

The pancreas also secretes **glucagon**, which raises and maintains the blood glucose level by converting stored glycogen in the liver to glucose. When the blood sugar level drops, the adrenal glands release **epinephrine**, which stops insulin secretion and increases glucose release from the liver.

If untreated, diabetes causes devastating damage all over the body, because without a dependable supply of fuel, the cells cannot do adequate maintenance and repair. Deterioration of nerves (**diabetic neuropathy**) can cause blindness as well as loss of sensation, starting in the extremities, which in turn can lead to infection of unfelt sores or wounds. So diabetics with this problem need to do frequent foot checks on hikes for blisters that could turn into open sores; and outings leaders should do this for diabetic children. Deterioration of the blood vessels (**diabetic angiopathy**) increases the risk of cardiovascular disease as well as impairing circulation in the extremities. Impaired circulation in the extremities impedes wound healing and increases the risk of infection by reducing delivery of oxygen to the limbs (if not alleviated by hyperbaric oxygen therapy). As a result, diabetics may lose limbs to gangrene.

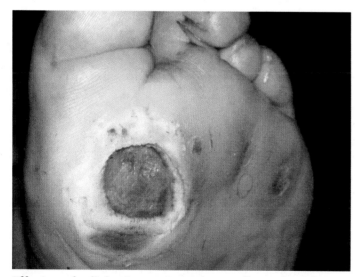

Effects of diabetic neuropathy and angiopathy: Infection of this unfelt blister required amputation of the foot. *Photo courtesy of Linda Garcia.*

Types of diabetes

There are two types of diabetes. In **Type I diabetes**, the body's immune system destroys the insulin-producing cells. Many cases are associated with childhood exposure to a flu virus such as Coxsackie, which has a protein in its shell very similar to a protein on the insulin-producing cells. So antibodies produced against the virus may attack the body's own cells. Type I is called juvenile diabetes, because it usually begins early, and almost always starts in patients under 30. They tend to be thin, with weight loss and muscle wasting; and before insulin was available for medication, they did not live long. There are several types of insulin: short-acting (usually taken before meals); intermediate acting; and long acting (taken once or twice a day). A diabetic may be taking more than one type of insulin as well as other medications.

In **Type II diabetes** (90% of all cases in the United States), the cells become **insulin-resistant**, so that it takes more and more insulin to transport glucose across cell membranes. **Hypothermia** also increases insulin resistance, with similar effects. Regular exercise, on the other hand, reduces insulin resistance. Risk factors for Type II diabetes include:

- high sugar diet;
- sedentary habits;
- obesity (increases peripheral insulin resistance);
- smoking (doubles the risk).

Type II diabetes is usually treated first with diet (especially eliminating high-sugar junk food) and exercise. Cucumbers, dill pickles, and aloe vera juice seem to be helpful in controlling blood sugar. If diet and exercise are not effective, oral medications are prescribed. **Glucophage** (Metformin®) reduces blood sugar by suppressing glucose production in the liver. Glipizide increases insulin production by the pancreas. Rosiglitazone® and Glyburide® reduce insulin resistance in the body's cells. If these medications are not effective, then insulin is prescribed. While Type II diabetes has traditionally been a disease of middle age or old age, it is now appearing in more and more adolescents and children, because junk food dominates their diets. The percentage of obese children in the United States has been increasing rapidly, and about 85% of Type II diabetics are obese.

The Pima Indians of Arizona dramatically illustrate the connection between diabetes and diet. Up until the

1930s, they practiced subsistence agriculture and had a balanced but low-calorie diet to which their bodies were well adapted. Diabetes was unknown among them. Then during the Depression, they gave up their farms and began eating store-bought food that was high in processed sugar and fat. Since then, they have had the highest incidence of diabetes in the world, and it is rare to find a mature adult who is not blind, missing a limb or suffering from cardiovascular disease as a complication of diabetes. Their mortality rate from diabetes is ten times as great as among Caucasians.

Diabetic emergencies

Type II diabetes can often be controlled with a combination of diet and exercise, but in either type of diabetes, the same problems occur when fuel and insulin get out of balance. The most common problem is **hypoglycemia** ("too little sugar"), which means that the patient has run out of fuel. It usually comes on very suddenly. Blood sugar level is low either because it has been too long since the last meal, or because the patient took too much insulin or other diabetic medication.

Even people who are not diabetic can suffer hypoglycemia, though it is much easier for them to restore the fuel and insulin balance. Aerobic athletes call it "hitting the wall," and can experience it either by burning all their stored (and easily metabolized) carbohydrates or by eating too much refined sugar at once and triggering an extreme insulin reaction (**rebound hypoglycemia**).

Treatment is to give a little glucose and see if the patient improves. Then the patient can munch some energy food or sip a sugared drink. You can moisten an unresponsive patient's fingertips, dip them in glucose or honey (which is rich in glucose and fructose) and then place them under the patient's tongue, where the glucose will be absorbed rapidly without risk of choking. Glucose paste (often used by bicycle racers to replenish their fuel on long rides) works well, but should only be given to a responsive patient who is alert enough to swallow safely. Other types of sugar, however, must be swallowed and digested, so they cannot simply be absorbed under the tongue. Diabetics may be carrying glucagon self-injectors, which infuse it directly into the thigh muscle.

Hypoglycemia in a diabetic is sometimes called **insulin shock**, because it can be triggered by too much insulin and resembles shock caused by bleeding or dehydration, though the cause is different. It is also sometimes mistaken for intoxication. Signs and symptoms usually include:

- faintness and dizziness;
- weakness;
- possible tremors.

Breathing and pulse may still be normal, or rapid. The patient may also experience:

- headache;
- double vision;
- seizures;
- apathy or irritability;
- drooling from the mouth;
- tingling or numbness in the hands and feet.

Low blood sugar triggers the release of **epinephrine**, which affects the circulatory system as well as glucose production and release, as part of the fight or flight reaction. Pulse rate may increase (tachycardia), and the skin may become pale, cool and sweaty as blood is withdrawn from the skin.

Unlike other cells in the body, **brain cells** do not have an alternate fuel cycle that uses fatty acids to produce energy. They are completely dependent on a steady supply of glucose, which makes the brain extremely sensitive to hypoglycemia. When blood sugar drops too low, brain cells start to die; which makes severe hypoglycemia life-threatening without an immediate intake of sugar in some form.

In **hyperglycemia**, too much sugar is accumulating in the blood because there is not enough insulin to transport it into the cells, or because the cells are insulin-resistant. People who are hyperglycemic may be undiagnosed diabetics, or known diabetics who did not take their medication. Diabetics who are ill or injured may also become hyperglycemic as the body releases epinephrine, which causes the liver to release more glucose into the system as part of the fight or flight reaction to stress. The patient will eventually lapse into a diabetic coma if you don't treat the problem. Fortunately, it usually comes on slowly over a period of several hours or days. Early signs and symptoms come from the body's dumping of excess glucose in the blood through frequent urination and from lack of glucose in the cells:

- Excessive sweating (sweat may taste sweet);

- Excessive urination (physicians in earlier times diagnosed diabetes by the sweet taste of the urine);
- Excessive thirst (drinking water helps dilute the concentration of glucose in the blood);
- Weakness (from lack of glucose in the cells).

Later signs and symptoms may include:
- intense thirst and dry mouth;
- red, dry and warm skin;
- rapid deep breathing, may be rasping or sighing;
- rapid and weak pulse from dehydration;
- sunken eyes (also from dehydration);
- dim vision;
- fruity or acetone breath odor from ketones (product of less efficient fatty acid metabolism);
- confusion and disorientation;
- vomiting and abdominal pain;

Type II diabetics are less likely to have the fruity breath odor, because the pancreas will still be releasing insulin and enough glucose may still be getting into the insulin-resistant cells to forestall fatty acid metabolism. But the other signs and symptoms will be similar. Treatment is for the patient to rehydrate and take insulin, along with any other prescribed diabetic medications. If insulin is not available, you need to evacuate immediately. Meanwhile, you can reduce the level of sugar in the blood by having the patient drink as much water or unsweetened fluid as possible. However, if you are unsure whether a patient is hypo or hyperglycemic, you should always try giving sugar first. If hypoglycemia is the problem, the patient's condition should improve quickly, and you may save a life. But a little sugar will do no harm even if the patient is hyperglycemic.

Conclusion

Type I diabetics need to take insulin, and possibly other medications, to control the movement of glucose into the cells. Type II diabetics may be taking medications or controlling their condition with diet and exercise. Hypoglycemia is the most common diabetic emergency. It can happen suddenly, and can be fatal if the patient is not given glucose (or another type of sugar) quickly. Hyperglycemia comes on more slowly, as glucose accumulates in the blood for lack of insulin. But when in doubt about a diabetic emergency, giving a small amount of glucose and seeing whether it improves the patient's condition will do no harm.

Seizures

In a seizure, an uncontrolled burst of electrical activity in the brain alters consciousness and may affect muscular control. The word comes from Old French "*seisir*", which means "to take possession of," because people having seizures appeared to be possessed. Seizures range from a momentary lapse of attention or minor muscular twitches (petit mal or "little evil") to a loss of muscular control and unconsciousness.

A petit mal or **absence seizure**, which is most common in children, usually lasts just a few seconds. After a blank stare and possibly some blinking or chewing, the patient becomes alert again, and may not be aware of what happened. A **febrile seizure**, most common in children from 6 months to 6 years old, is caused by high fever, and if the seizure does not quickly subside, you need to cool the patient to prevent brain damage.

In a partial (psychomotor) seizure, which involves one cerebral hemisphere, the patient will be awake but unaware of his or her surroundings. You will see a blank stare, then random activity such as mumbling, chewing, or clumsy movement.

A generalized or grand mal ("big evil") seizure involves both cerebral hemispheres. It may start with a fall and muscular rigidity (**tonus**) that can expel air from the lungs in a loud cry; then continue with violent thrashing (**clonus**). Uncontrolled muscular contractions caused by generalized seizures are called **convulsions** (Latin *convelere*, "to pull together").

A grand mal seizure may last a minute or more. After the convulsions, the patient may lose control of bladder and bowels, may be disoriented, and may sleep for some time afterwards.

Anything that seriously disrupts brain activity can cause a seizure:
- heat stroke;
- out of control fever;
- head injury;
- not enough fuel (diabetes);
- not enough oxygen;
- hypertension;
- meningitis (several types carried by mosquitoes);
- drug or alcohol abuse;
- chronic condition (epilepsy).

Your immediate concerns in a major seizure are to:
- Protect the head and spine as the patient falls.

- Put a cushion under the head if possible.
- Protect the airway if the patient vomits – turn onto the left side and wipe away or suction vomitus.
- Clear away things that the patient could strike.
- Find out the cause, and whether you can do anything about it.

The word **epilepsy** comes from the Greek *epilepsis* "a laying hold of," because it appeared that some force or influence, presumably from the gods, had laid hold of a person having a seizure. The Romans called it *morbus sacer*, "the sacred disease." A patient with epilepsy may be carrying medication (which may not be intended for use immediately after a seizure). Epileptics often learn to recognize the mental changes that precede a generalized seizure, and can take different forms in different people. This sense of an impending seizure is called an **aura** from the Latin word for "a breeze" (which may signal a change in weather). An epileptic may therefore warn you of an impending seizure, and give you the chance to prepare. In Prince Myshkin, the protagonist of Dostoyevsky's novel *The Idiot*, the aura takes the form of a feeling of ecstasy and oneness with the world. Dostoyevsky was an epileptic, so he was writing about seizures from his own experience.

One seizure in a known epileptic needn't end a trip, if the patient recovers well, especially if the patient is carrying medication. But a seizure with any other cause, or an unexplained seizure, usually requires rapid evacuation. A seizure that does not end (status epilepticus), or repeated seizures, will quickly become a medical emergency because the patient cannot breathe effectively when the muscles (including those that control breathing) are spasming uncontrollably.

Stroke

In a stroke, so called because it can be such a sudden affliction, circulation to part of the brain is disrupted by a clot or rupture of a cerebral artery. In an **ischemic stroke** (Greek *ischano*, "I hold in check"), the artery is blocked by a clot. This can happen in two ways:

- An embolus (Greek *embolos* "wedge or plug") forms in the artery.
- A thrombus (Greek *thrombos* "lump or clump") moving from a larger upstream artery jams a smaller branching artery.

In a **hemorrhagic stroke** (Greek *haima* "blood" + *regnumai* "to break forth"), a cerebral artery ruptures. The patient usually gets a sudden and severe headache. With an ischemic stroke caused by a thrombus, the patient may have a headache, because the blockage is sudden; but ischemic strokes from a gradually forming embolus seldom cause a headache. Only 13% of strokes are hemorrhagic, and 87% are ischemic. The distinction is important because clot-busting drugs can clear an obstruction from a cerebral artery, and can prevent brain damage if given within 3 hours of the first symptoms. So time is critical. Hospital treatment begins with a brain scan to tell whether the stroke is ischemic or hemorrhagic.

If you suspect a stroke, ask:
- When did the symptoms begin?
- Did you hit your head recently?
- Have you ever had a stroke before?
- Have you ever had a seizure?
- Do you have a headache?
- Any numbness? One side or both sides?
- Any balance or vision problems?
- Any nausea or incontinence?

To test for a stroke:
- Look for face droop on one side: Ask the patient to smile.
- Listen to the patient's speech: Is it slurred?
- Look for arm drift: Ask the patient to raise both arms; does one arm drop?
- Feel and compare the patient's grip in both hands. Is one side weaker?

Both ischemic strokes and **myocardial infarctions** (heart attacks, described in Chapter 4 as **cardiogenic shock**) are caused by blockage of an artery that supplies tissues in a vital organ; so both afflictions can dramatically impair vital functions. Also, just as a myocardial infarction may have been preceded by recurring angina pectoris ("pain in the chest"), an ischemic stroke may be the climax of a series of **transient ischemic attacks** (TIA), also called ministrokes. In a TIA, the symptoms subside in 24 hours or less as a clot (which may be only partially blocking the artery) is cleared away by the blood flow. But anyone who has experienced a TIA will probably have a stroke someday, without preventive treatment.

Chapter 29. CPR and oxygen in the wilderness

Urban CPR

When citizen CPR training started in 1974, some advocates predicted up to a 60% save rate for out-of-hospital cardiac arrests. Criteria for reporting a successful resuscitation range from arriving at the hospital with a pulse to surviving at least 6 months after being discharged from the hospital. Other factors that affect statistics include ambulance response times. But no matter how the data is collected and interpreted, the success rate has been much lower than pioneers of CPR training hoped. According to a review article published in the American Heart Association journal *Circulation* in 2010 (see Bibliography), the aggregate survival rate for out of hospital cardiac arrest was still only between 6.7% and 8.4%.

CPR alone, even if it is performed effectively, seldom revives a patient in cardiac arrest. But it can keep the brain and other vital organs supplied with enough blood and oxygen to make survival possible, until defibrillation and other forms of life support are available. Every minute that defibrillation is delayed, however, the chance of survival goes down by 10%, so having automated external defibrillators (AEDs) and people trained to use them on site dramatically improves the chance of survival for heart attack victims. Casinos with AEDs have an especially high save rate, because everyone is on camera, so responders with an AED usually reach a customer who collapses within a few minutes.

Wilderness CPR

In the wilderness, no ambulances or defibrillators are likely to be available. If rescuers begin CPR, they will usually have to continue until the victim revives (which is unlikely without prompt defibrillation) or they give up hope. Moreover, wilderness rescuers may be cold or exhausted, and the terrain may be steep or broken, which would make it more difficult to do effective CPR. However:

- Even in the wilderness, CPR could save lives in some situations, e.g. a lightning strike with an unresponsive victim.
- Wilderness guides' responsibility for the safety of others may include a moral and legal obligation to use every reasonable means to save a life, even if the chance of success is small.
- CPR certification is required for many wilderness guides, trip leaders, and wilderness rescuers.
- Wilderness rescuers and guides don't spend all of their time in the back country. In a populated area, CPR training could help them to save a life.

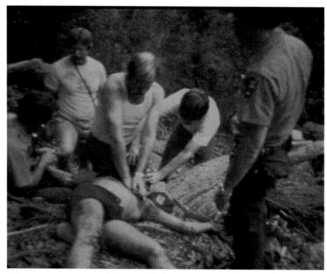

Photo courtesy of Ben Schifrin, MD

How well do rescuers do CPR?

If a victim's pulse is lost because of trauma, the chance of survival is always small; and in a wilderness situation, it is almost zero. A pulseless victim who has suffered a heart attack in the wilderness also has a very small chance of survival. But if people on the scene choose to do CPR, they will almost certainly have to continue it until they give up hope or the victim is loaded into a helicopter. In Hamilton and Paton's survey of mountain rescue teams [see bibliography], the average duration of CPR before the rescuers decided to discontinue it was 36 minutes.

When tested on recording manikins, most experienced EMTs and paramedics do effective compressions (at best) for only the first minute or two. After that, their compressions become so erratic that they are ineffective. And while bad ventilations halve the chance of survival, bad compressions reduce the chance to zero. These studies also contradict the assumption of many EMS professionals that using CPR regularly on real patients will automatically maintain and improve their technique. Only practice with good corrective feedback will do that.

One study is especially relevant to wilderness rescuers, who may have to do CPR in awkward, cramped or unstable situations such as a moving evacuation sled or small helicopter. Braunfels and his colleagues tested the ability of professionals to do CPR in stationary ambulances [see bibliography]. Even in the largest Mercedes Benz ambulance, the percentage of correct compressions dropped from 90 to 77. In the smaller Mercedes Benz, it dropped to 60%; and in the Volkswagon ambulance, it dropped to 38%. In moving ambulances, performance was even worse.

Several studies have tested the ability of both EMS professionals and laypeople trained in CPR to check the carotid pulse. All had similar results: few professionals or lay people can correctly and consistently assess pulse status within the 10 seconds recommended by the *Guidelines*. Some studies were done on manikins with a simulated carotid pulse that could be turned on and off.

By far the most realistic study, however, was done by Eberle and his colleagues, using patients undergoing coronary artery bypass grafting. When these patients were on non-pulsatile cardiopulmonary bypass, they did not have carotid pulses. The authors tested 206 participants, including experienced EMTs and paramedics, EMTs and paramedics in training, and lay people recently trained in CPR. Overall, only 15% correctly found a pulse within the 10 seconds recommended by the guidelines. Even more alarming, only 1 out of 59 correctly assessed pulselessness (in patients who did not have a carotid pulse) within 10 seconds. The median delay in assessment was 24 seconds, and even when they took up to 30 seconds, only 55% of the participants found and identified a pulse when it was there, though 90% eventually verified pulselessness. But taking up to 30 seconds to verify the lack of a pulse would delay starting chest compressions and reduce the chance of patient survival, which is why the *Guidelines* say to take no more than 10 seconds checking the pulse. Interestingly, participants who were still in training, and had recently been through a CPR course, did better as a group than experienced professionals, which suggests that CPR skills deteriorate (even when used on the job) long before CPR certifications expire.

CPR Guidelines

Because of results like these, the 2000 *Guidelines for Cardiopulmonary Resuscitation* eliminated the pulse check from CPR training for lay people, though not from professional level training. Moreover, the 2010 *Guidelines* eliminated the first and second steps of the traditional ABC's for an unresponsive patient: open the airway; look, listen, and feel for breathing. Instead, rescuers should look for signs of breathing (without opening the airway) as they quickly check for responsiveness. Rescuers who are not professionals are trained to start chest compressions immediately on an unresponsive patient who does not appear to be breathing, though professional rescuers are still trained to check the carotid pulse first.

So the mnemonic for the CPR sequence (in the 2010 and 2015 *Guidelines*) is CAB: Compressions; Airway; Breathing. However, this mnemonic applies only to unresponsive patients who do not appear to be breathing. For all patients who are breathing, and for victims of drowning (in which cardiac arrest is almost always caused by hypoxia), the old ABC mnemonic still applies, and reminds us of our priorities.

Choking

Because the openings of the trachea and esophagus are so close together, and both are just behind and under the mouth, choking is a common airway emergency. Coughing is a reflex action to expel whatever is obstructing the airway. If a conscious adult or child who is choking cannot cough, however, you should use an abdominal thrust to expel the obstruction.

First make eye contact and ask: "Are you choking?" Anyone who can say "Yes!" does not have a completely obstructed airway, and should be encouraged to cough. But if the patient cannot speak, and only nods, say "May I help you?" and say it loudly if others are present, so that they do not misunderstand what you are doing. Then say "I'm going behind you." so the patient doesn't turn to keep you in sight. Plant one foot between a standing patient's feet, and the other foot well back, so that you are braced in case the patient goes unconscious. You may have to kneel behind a standing child or sitting adult.

Performing the abdominal thrust pushes the edge of the diaphragm in, causing it to bulge up and compress the lungs. The resulting increase in air pressure usually expels an airway obstruction. To find the right position on the abdomen (between the navel and the rib notch) bring your forearms horizontally against the iliac crests of the patient's pelvis (just below the belt line). Slide your forearms up over the top of the iliac crest. Then make a fist with one hand (thumb straight), and rotate it so that the big knuckle of the thumb is pressing on the patient's abdomen. Wrap your other hand around the fist and press hard, inward and upward. Repeat until the obstruction is expelled.

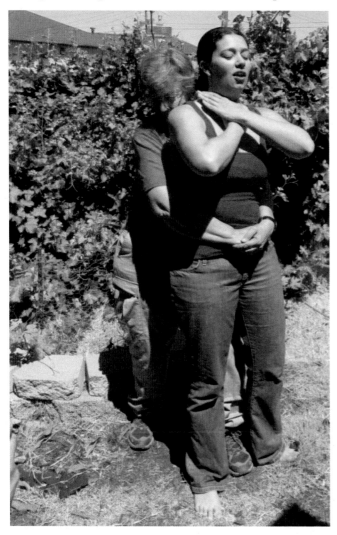

Gently lower a patient who becomes unresponsive onto his or her back, and begin CPR with one addition. Every time you go to the head, open the mouth and look for the obstruction before trying to give breaths. If you see the obstruction, sweep it out with your finger. Otherwise, continue CPR – the chest compressions that move blood in a pulseless patient also compress the lungs, which works to expel an airway obstruction. But use chest thrusts with your arms around the upper chest (rather than abdominal thrusts) on a conscious adult who is pregnant, or too obese for you to reach around the abdomen. On a patient in a wheel chair, after bracing the back of the chair against something so it doesn't tip over, do sternum thrusts from the front with the heel of your hand against the center of the chest.

Breathing problems and ventilation

Anyone who has a pulse but is not breathing needs to be artificially ventilated. Rescue breathing can move enough oxygen into the blood to keep a patient alive, even though exhaled air contains only about 16% oxygen, compared to 21% oxygen in the atmosphere. This was demonstrated in a heroic experiment by Dr. Peter Safar. Medical students volunteered to have their respiratory muscles paralyzed with curare, and were sustained by rescue breathing until the paralysis wore off. A CPR pocket mask with a one-way valve makes rescue breathing more hygienic. At high altitudes, however, rescue breathing is unlikely to be effective because the air is thinner. At 18,000 feet, air and oxygen pressure are just half the pressure at sea level.

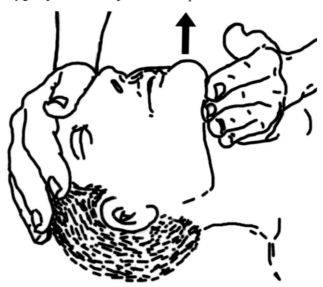

To open the airway for rescue breathing (if there are no signs of cervical spine injury), tilt the head with one hand on the forehead. Fingertips of the other hand push the bony part of the chin up to thrust the jaw forward and help lift the tongue off the airway. If you suspect cervical spine injury, try to pull the jaw up with your fingertips, bracing your thumbs on the cheek bones. But if the patient is not breathing, and the jaw thrust does not work, use the head tilt chin lift because opening the airway is the priority.

A bag valve mask (BVM) is more effective than rescue breathing because it ventilates with fresh air (21% oxygen). But with a BVM, it is all too easy to over-ventilate. The *Guidelines* say to ventilate only with enough air to make the patient's chest rise; and in an adult patient with a pulse, to give one ventilation every 5-6 seconds. But studies of BVM use by EMTs and paramedics show that most of them ventilate too much, too fast. Even if excess air does not go into the stomach and induce vomiting, it will build up pressure in the chest cavity. Pressure on the heart reduces venous return, and thus reduces the amount of oxygenated blood delivered by the circulatory system. So over-ventilating a patient is counter-productive.

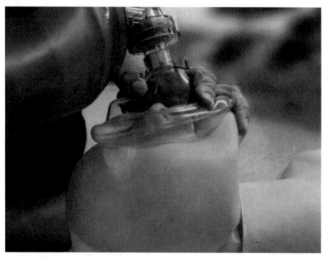

Ventilating with a bag valve mask (BVM)

When using a BVM with a 1 liter bag to ventilate an adult, squeezing out about 2/3 of the air in the bag should make the chest rise. If it does not, re-tilt the patient's head and check the fit of the mask, then try again. The narrow side of the mask goes over the patient's nose and the rounded side between the lower lip and the chin. Your thumb and index finger of one hand encircle the mask and hold it in place. Your other fingers pull the bony part of the chin and the jaw up into the mask and help tilt the head.

If an adult's head is not tilted enough, air from a BVM is liable to go down the esophagus into the stomach (instead of down the trachea) and induce vomiting. In 2-rescuer CPR and in ventilating a patient with a pulse, the best position for using a BVM is kneeling behind the patient's head, and clamping the head between your knees to keep it tilted. You can squeeze the bag between thumb and fingers, or by pressing it against your thigh. Each ventilation should

take a full second (to avoid forcing air into the stomach); and if you are ventilating a patient with a pulse, either use a watch with a second hand or count "One-one thousand, two-one thousand…..five-one thousand" between ventilations.

There are smaller sized BVMs and masks for children and infants. If you have only an adult mask, however, you can use it on a small child or infant by reversing the adult position: the narrow side between lip and chin, and the rounded side on the forehead. Children require less head tilt to open the airway because their heads are proportionately larger; and infants require very little head tilt because they have relatively large heads and short necks. An infant's airway can be blocked by tilting the head too far. Also, it takes very little air to ventilate an infant's tiny lungs, and over-ventilating can actually rupture the lungs.

Performing CPR

After checking the scene for safety, talk to the patient as you tap him on the shoulder. As you check for responsiveness, look for signs of breathing: chest or abdominal movement. The EMT's upright knee next to the patient protects her (and she does not lean too close) in case he was just sleeping or intoxicated, and swings his arms when startled awake.

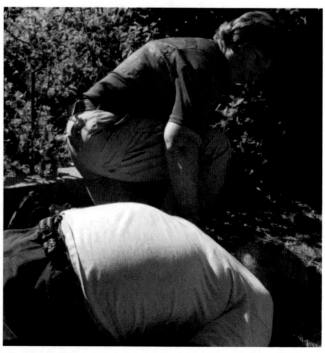

Checking for responsiveness and signs of breathing

Check for the carotid pulse on your side of the neck for up to 10 seconds or until you feel the pulse, while continuing to watch for signs of breathing. Count "One-one-thousand, two-one-thousand…" If you do see signs of breathing (not just a reflex gasp) then you should be able to feel a pulse.

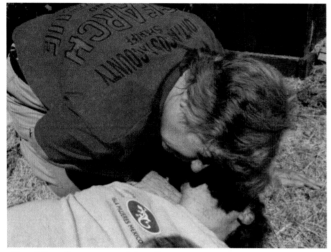

Checking for a carotid pulse

If you don't feel a pulse after 10 seconds, open the clothing, place the heel of one hand in the center of the sternum just below the axillary line (between the armpits). Interlace your fingers or grip the wrist of the compressing hand with the other hand. Lock your elbows; bring your shoulders over the sternum; and push straight down. Use your body weight to push, but come all the way up between compressions to allow the heart to refill with blood. While an adult's chest should depress at least 2 inches according to the *Guidelines*, this is hard to estimate from above; but you should see the center of the chest caving in under the heel of your hand with each compression.

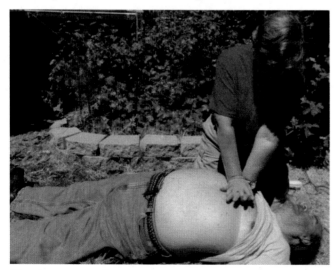

Chest compressions

Do 100 to 120 compressions per minute. The count is "One and two and three and…." up to 30. Count aloud because:

- It helps you keep pace;
- It tells others where you are in the cycles;
- It forces you to breathe.

Do five sets of 30 compressions and two ventilations per cycle, which should take about two minutes. If another rescuer is available, transition to 2-rescuer CPR and change positions after each 2-minute cycle of CPR, to avoid fatigue.

Chest compressions work by using the sternum as a lever to compress the heart and the big blood vessels in the thorax. But even good chest compressions deliver less than 30% as much oxygenated blood to the body as a functioning heart, so inadequate or delayed chest compressions are unlikely to be effective.

According to the 2015 *Guidelines*, it should take no more than 10 seconds to give two ventilations after each set of 30 compressions, but you should be able to do it in 5 or 6 seconds. The longer the interruption, the more compressions it will take to build up pressure in the chest and get the blood moving again.

Give two breaths between sets of compressions. Each breath should take about a second, and be just enough to make the chest rise. Tilt the head as shown (if there are no indications of spinal injury) to open the airway. The EMT has a pocket mask with a one-way valve to protect her from possible infection. You can do compressions only with no ventilations; but they will be effective only until the oxygen already in the patient's blood before cardiac arrest is depleted.

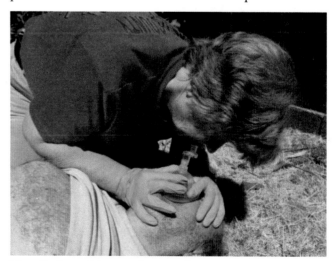

Ventilating with a pocket mask

For adult CPR with one or two rescuers, the ratio of compressions to ventilations is 30:2. For one rescuer infant or child CPR, the ratio is also 30:2. But for infant or child CPR with two rescuers, the ratio is 15:2, because cardiac arrest in infants and children is usually caused by a respiratory problem, which would reduce oxygen saturation in the blood; and infants and children consume oxygen at a faster rate than adults.

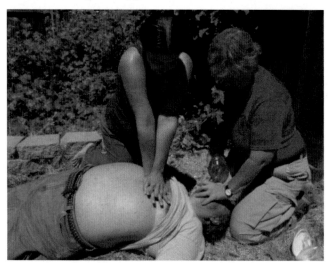

2 rescuer CPR using a BVM for ventilation

Every cycle of CPR starts with compressions and ends with two ventilations. With two rescuers, you should switch positions after 5 cycles of adult CPR, or 10 cycles of child or infant CPR. The person doing compressions calls for a change after the 5th cycle, moves to the head (as the partner moves to the other side of the patient), and positions the BVM or pocket mask as the partner resumes compressions.

Defibrillation

When an automated external defibrillator (AED) is turned on, a recorded voice instructs the user to apply two conducting pads to the patient's chest (pictures on the pads show where they go), and plug in the connector that is wired to the pads.

AEDs are programmed to analyze the rhythm of a pulseless patient's heart, and deliver a shock if the heart still has abnormal electrical activity. There are two shockable rhythms: ventricular fibrillation (uncoordinated twitching of the muscle fibers of the ventricles) and ventricular tachycardia (*Latin* "fast heart") in which the ventricles are contracting very rapidly but too weakly to move blood. If the AED detects either of these rhythms, the recording will say

"Shock advised, charging. Do not touch the patient." Then it will say "Deliver shock now." The shock stops the heart, which may regain its normal rhythm when it restarts, like a re-booted computer. The recording will also remind you not to touch the patient when the AED is analyzing or ready to shock; and whoever is operating the AED must make sure that nobody is touching the patient. If the AED does not detect a shockable rhythm, it will say "Begin CPR" and after two minutes, re-analyze the heart rhythm.

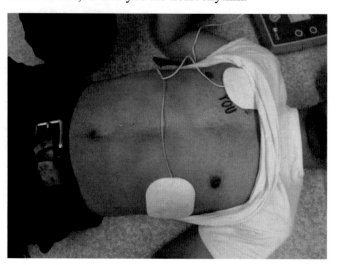

Infant choking and CPR

If an infant appears to be choking but is still conscious, slide one arm under the body until your hand supports the back of the head. Grip the front of the head with your other hand (being careful not to cover the mouth and nose) and clamp the infant between your forearms.

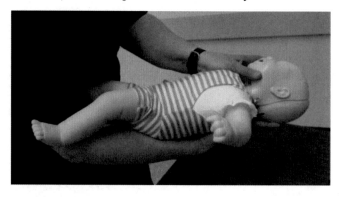

Then rotate the infant face down and brace your forearm on your thigh to give up to 5 back blows. If the infant is squirming or slippery, clamp one of its legs under your armpit. You can also do back blows and sternum thrusts on an infant while seated, but make sure that the head is angled downward so that gravity will help remove the obstruction.

200

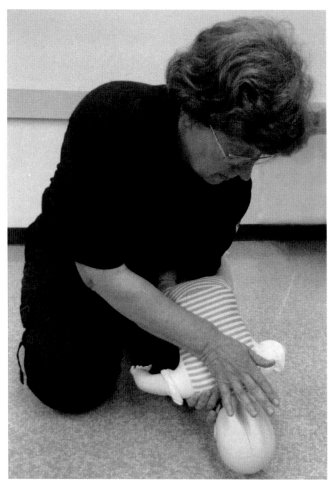

Back blows for a choking infant

Strike 5 times between the shoulder blades with the heel of your hand. Then clamp the infant between your forearms, and rotate him face up. Brace your forearm on your other knee and give 5 sternum thrusts with two finger tips, in the center of the chest just below the axillary line. Keep your hand vertical, with fingers pushing straight down. Otherwise, your fingers can slip, and tear the infant's delicate skin. If the infant becomes limp and unresponsive, begin CPR, with one addition. Before ventilating, look for an airway obstruction, and do a finger sweep if you see it.

To do CPR, place the infant on a firm surface. Tap the bottom of the foot to check for responsiveness as you look for signs of breathing. If the infant is unresponsive, check the brachial pulse on the inside of the upper arm for up to 10 seconds. If you do not detect a pulse, place your fingertips in the center of the chest just below the axillary line (same position as used in first aid for a conscious choking infant) and do 30 sternum thrusts. Push down about 1/3 of the infant's depth of chest, at a rate of 100 to 120 per minute. Then

tilt the head slightly and give two ventilations – just enough air to make the chest rise. Tilting an infant's head too far can block the airway, because the head is so large in proportion to the body. And over-ventilating can rupture the infant's lungs.

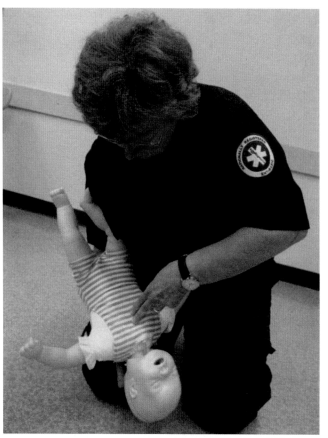

Sternum thrusts for a choking infant

With two rescuers, do compressions by encircling the infant's chest with your hands so that both your thumbs (together) press on the infant's sternum and the fingers reach at least around the shoulder blades. Do 15 compressions per cycle as your partner ventilates with a BVM, and switch after 10 cycles.

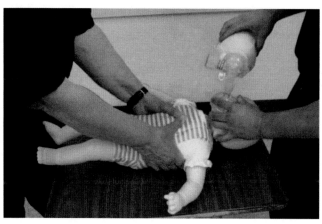

CPR skill summary (2015 *Guidelines*)

Sequence for adult CPR

- Check for responsiveness & breathing.
- Unresponsive? Activate EMS & request AED
- Check carotid pulse on your side of patient for 10 seconds OR until you feel a pulse.
- Continue watching for signs of breathing.
- COUNT as you feel for the pulse "One-one-thousand.....ten-one-thousand."
- No pulse? Start compressions
- Has pulse? Check/assist breathing.

Compressions for adult CPR

- Open clothing to see the patient's chest.
- Place heel of your hand in the center of patient's chest below the armpit line.
- Arms vertical, elbows locked.
- Compress at least 2" deep.
- Push till you SEE center of chest cave in.
- Release pressure between compressions.
- RATIO is 30 compressions: 2 breaths.
- 100 to 120 compressions per minute.
- COUNT aloud: "One and two and three..."

1 rescuer for adult CPR

Use pocket mask for ventilations.

Transition to 2 rescuers

Second rescuer: move to OTHER side of patient, and prepare to start compressions.
First rescuer:
- Give 2 breaths with pocket mask;
- Move above patient's head;
- prepare BVM.

Second rescuer: start compressions.
First rescuer: ventilate with BVM.
Compression to ventilation ratio still 30:2.
Change positions after 5 cycles.
Rescuer at head move to vacant side of patient.

Second rescuer arrives with AED

First, TURN IT ON and LISTEN to the instructions.
First rescuer continue CPR until AED says: "Analyzing heart rhythm, do not touch patient."
Second rescuer: "Clear!" AED: "Shock advised, charging...Deliver shock now."
Second rescuer: "I'm clear, you're clear!" LOOK! Then press shock button and follow instructions.

Infant CPR

Sequence

- Same as adult EXCEPT check brachial pulse.
- Alone? Do 2 minutes of CPR before going to phone to activate EMS for infant or child.

Compressions (1 rescuer)

- Center of chest below armpit line.
- Use 2 finger tips – keep hand VERTICAL.
- 100 to 120 compressions per minute.
- Compress 1/3 chest depth.
- RATIO is 30 compressions: 2 breaths.

Ventilations (1 rescuer)

- Pocket mask or infant BVM for ventilations.
- Just enough air to make chest rise: Over-ventilating can rupture infant's lungs.

Transition to 2 rescuers

First rescuer:
- Give 2 breaths.
- Move above head.
- Prepare infant BVM.

Second rescuer:
- Hands encircle chest, thumbs over sternum.
- Begin chest compressions.

RATIO for 2 rescuer infant or child: 15:2.
CHANGE positions after 10 cycles.

Cardiocerebral resuscitation

Hands only CPR (chest compressions only), recommended by the *Guidelines* for bystanders who do not want to do mouth-to-mouth breathing (especially on a stranger), may be effective if it is started promptly and the patient's blood is still saturated with oxygen after cardiac arrest. Fully oxygenated blood may take up to six minutes to desaturate after cardiac arrest. But hands-only-CPR is unlikely to be effective on a patient whose blood is already depleted of oxygen. Normal breathing brings air into the lungs by expanding the chest cavity. Pushing on the inert chest and recoil does move a small amount of air out of and into the lungs (**passive ventilation**), but not enough to increase oxygen pressure in the lungs and move a significant amount of oxygen into the blood.

However, **cardiocerebral resuscitation**, which combines uninterrupted chest compressions with oxygen administration, has a higher rate of patient survival than cardiopulmonary resuscitation (with pauses for ventilations). In cardiocerebral resuscitation, passive ventilation moves 100% oxygen into the lungs through a nonrebreather mask, instead of the 21% oxygen of atmospheric air.

So patients for whom CPR was delayed, or whose cardiac arrest was caused by a respiratory emergency (usually the case with children), need ventilation if oxygen is not available. And all cardiac arrest patients need ventilation during CPR if supplementary oxygen and advanced life support are delayed.

CPR training

CPR training has become increasingly video-driven, which is feasible because CPR consists of only a few skills that must be done with precision to be effective. The most effective CPR videos first show a whole skill realistically, e.g. adult CPR. Then students practice each component of the skill (such as chest compressions) along with the video. Finally, students practice the whole skill along with the video.

Since student practice is synchronized with the video, and they practice each component before doing the whole skill, it is easy for instructors to spot errors and give corrective feedback – provided that they follow the course plan and use the video, and that there are enough instructors for the number of students. As a result, when students are tested by performing the whole skill with no coaching, they are more likely to

perform the skills correctly, because most errors they were making in the components of the skills will already have been observed and corrected.

Students are also more likely to learn effective CPR on equipment that provides constant feedback, giving them a visual (green light) or audible signal when their compressions are deep and rapid enough to be effective. This also provides a more objective measure of student performance than unassisted instructor observation.

Protecting the airway

A **suction device** can clear fluids or vomitus from the mouth. Suction devices come with several extension tubes: narrow for fluids, wider for vomitus with solid material. Insert the tip in one side of the mouth, then sweep it from side to side as you apply suction and withdraw it. Each sweep should take no more than 10 seconds, timed with a watch or by counting (one-one-thousand, two-one-thousand…).

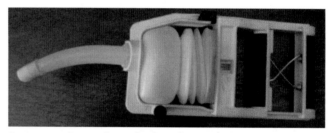

A manual suction device (V-Vac) is operated by squeezing the handle. Ambulances carry battery powered suction devices.

In an unresponsive patient with no gag reflex, an **oropharyngeal airway (OPA)** prevents the tongue from falling back and helps keep the airway open. Patients with a gag reflex may be able to tolerate a **nasopharyngeal airway** (NPA). OPAs and NPAs come in different sizes.

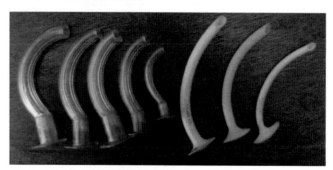

OPAs (left) and NPAs (right)

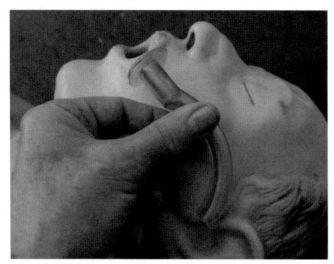

To select an OPA for a patient, measure it against the cheek, from the corner of the mouth to the ear

Insert the OPA half-way with the tip pointed toward the roof or side of the mouth so that it slides over the tongue; then rotate it until it angles downward towards the throat. If the patient gags, quickly remove the OPA and turn the patient on the left side to clear the airway. Use a suction device to clear any vomit.

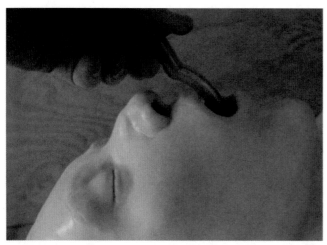

Inserting an OPA

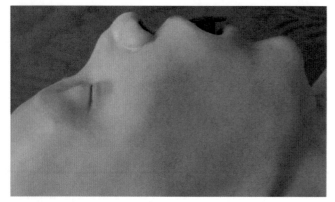

OPA inserted

A **nasopharyngeal airway (NPA)** may be tolerated even by a patient with a gag reflex. Measure it from the base of the nose to the ear. NPAs should come with water-based lubricants, so that they slide in easily.

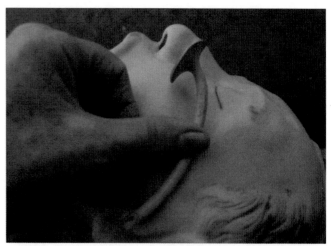

Measuring an NPA: From base of the nose to the ear

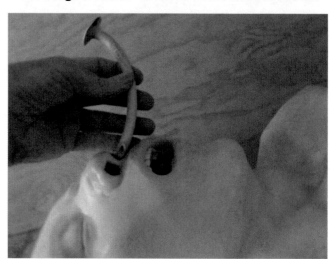

Insert the NPA with the bevel toward the septum (which separates the nostrils). If the NPA is curved toward the top of the head, rotate it 180° as it goes in.

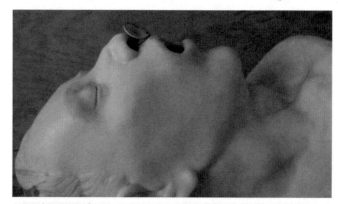

NPA inserted

Oxygen administration

Oxygen can be delivered to a patient's airway through a **non-rebreathing mask** that fits over the patient's face or a **nasal cannula** - two tubes that fit into the nostrils. With a non-rebreathing mask, you can deliver up to 15 liters per minute, and a good seal around the mask will ensure that 90% of it is inhaled by the patient. A nasal cannula can be used for patients who will not tolerate a non-re breathing mask, or who are not seriously hypoxic. At 6 liters per minute (maximum for a nasal cannula), less than half of the oxygen will be inhaled by the patient, and a higher delivery rate would dry out the mucus membranes of the nasopharynx as well as wasting oxygen.

If you have a **pulse oximeter**, check oxygen saturation in the blood to avoid **oxygen toxicity**, which constricts the coronary arteries. A patient with 96% or better oxygen saturation (who has not been exposed to carbon monoxide) does not need 15 liters per minute of oxygen. So adjust the flow rate to the minimum needed to maintain adequate oxygen saturation.

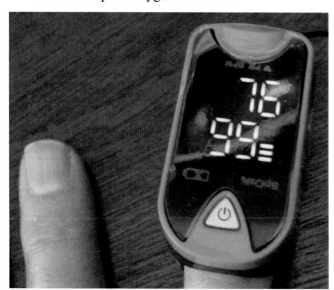

Pulse oximeter showing 99% oxygen saturation and a pulse rate of 76

Oxygen cylinders come in several sizes, and are usually made of aluminum, though some older cylinders are made of steel. Most cylinders meant to be carried to a patient are D size, which hold 350 liters of oxygen when pressurized to 2,000 psi (pounds per square inch). Oxygen cylinders must be hydro-tested every 5 years: pressurized to 5/3 of their normal maximum for testing. If the tank expands more than a safe amount from the pressure, it must be retired.

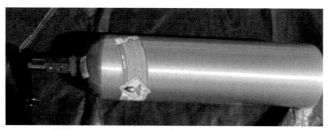

D cylinder with wrench in place

The dials on oxygen regulators, however, show the pressure in the cylinder, not the number of liters of gas. You should not let the pressure go below 200 psi before refilling, to prevent contamination of the oxygen. To calculate how long the oxygen will last, multiply the pressure in a cylinder (minus 200) by 0.16 for D cylinders. Then divide the result by the rate of oxygen delivery. For example, if the dial shows 1000 psi, 800 x 0.16 = 128. 128 divided by 15 liters per minute is 8 1/3 minutes of oxygen. But at 4 liters per minute, you would have 32 minutes of oxygen. For a patient who is not breathing, you can attach the oxygen outlet tubing to a **bag valve mask** and ventilate.

Oxygen and other cylinders for pressurized gases have a threaded opening into which an outlet **valve stem** is screwed. Some outlet valves have a toggle wrench attached at the top. Others require a wrench to open the valve and release the gas.

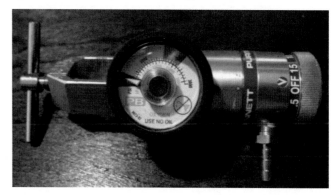

To use an oxygen cylinder, attach a **regulator** to the valve. The regulator reduces the pressure enough so that oxygen can be administered to a patient (40-70 psi) without rupturing the lungs. Regulators have a dial showing the oxygen pressure in the cylinder, and **flow meters** that enable you to select the rate of oxygen delivery in liters per minute.

Before using an oxygen cylinder, open the release valve slightly (turn counter-clockwise) to blow any grit from the outlet hole; then close the valve (clockwise). Set the flow meter on the regulator to zero or OFF, and look to make sure there is a gasket around the oxygen inlet. You will see two pins below the inlet (with gasket) of the regulator, which fit into holes below the outlet on the valve stem of the cylinder.

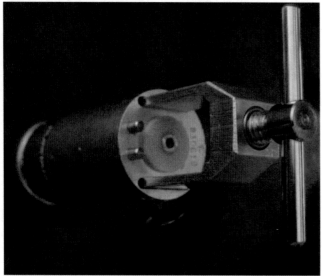

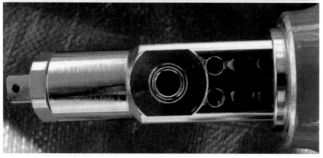

The positions of these pins and their holes on a valve stem are different for each type of pressurized gas, to prevent a regulator from being attached to a cylinder with the wrong kind of gas. Attach the regulator to the valve, making sure that the pins fit into their holes and the regulator is tight. Then lay the cylinder on its side. Keep the cylinder in its bag, especially on a slope, and secure the strap until the cylinder is placed in the litter or sled with the patient. If the bag is insulated, that may also help prevent the oxygen from getting too chilled in cold weather.

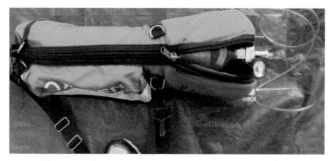

Then attach the tube from the non-rebreathing mask or nasal cannula to the outlet on the regulator. Open the valve of the cylinder one full turn (counter-clockwise), set the flow meter to the desired rate, and hold your thumb over the outlet in the non-rebreathing mask to fill the reservoir bag before placing the mask on the patient's face.

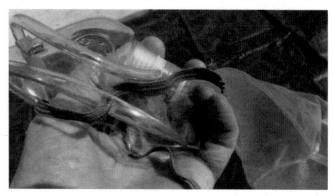

After administering oxygen, remove the mask (or cannula) from the patient before closing the valve on the cylinder and then removing the regulator.

A pressurized cylinder of oxygen (or any other gas) must be handled carefully. If you drop it and break the valve that seals the opening, it will take off like a rocket. So never leave a cylinder upright without supporting it, or in a place where it could fall off.

Conclusion

Any problem that impairs the airway, breathing, or circulation is the highest priority. In an urban situation, a patient with no signs of normal breathing and no perceptible pulse should be given CPR immediately, and connected to an AED if one is available. In a wilderness situation, assessment of vital signs and CPR decisions may be modified based on the patient's body core temperature and the distance from medical care. But techniques for keeping the airway open, and oxygen administration (if oxygen is available) are important for any patient with respiratory problems.

Chapter 30. Pregnancy, wilderness activity, and emergency childbirth

With the technical assistance of Linda Kay Deaton, RN, BSN, and Linda Garcia, NREMT

Pregnant women breathe and circulate blood for two. If they are in good aerobic condition, they will be able to meet these demands more easily. During labor and delivery, when the mother's own demand for blood and oxygen increases, aerobic fitness provides an extra safety margin, which helps keep the baby well oxygenated.

Muscle tone is also important during pregnancy. Pregnant women carry considerable extra weight, whose distribution puts stress on back, abdominal, and leg muscles. Strong and well-exercised muscles make it easier to adapt to this stress. Mothers with good muscle tone are also likely to find labor easier, especially the second stage and the afterbirth, when they use their abdominal muscles to push.

Pregnant women need to guard against two hazards which can bring on pre-term labor: dehydration, and urinary tract infection. Pre-term labor in the first twenty weeks of pregnancy usually results in a miscarriage (spontaneous abortion). From 15% to 30% of known pregnancies end in miscarriage, and up to 50% of all pregnancies, including those too early for pregnancy tests. The most common cause of miscarriage is chromosomal abnormalities in the fetus. Miscarriage can also be caused by uterine or placental problems in the mother and many medical conditions, especially diabetes.

A premature baby born after the twentieth week, however, may survive in an intensive care nursery, so pregnant women should always have a plan for reaching the hospital from the wilderness. Pre-term labor may last for hours to days, so an obstetrician may have time to save the pregnancy, even after a long evacuation.

Vital signs in pregnancy

Plasma volume (the liquid part of the blood) increases by up to 40% which increases blood volume; and the number of red blood cells also increases if the mother's diet includes adequate iron, which increases oxygen carrying capacity. Stroke volume (the amount of blood pushed out of the ventricles with each contraction) increases and the heart beats more rapidly to move more blood through the system each minute. A resting pulse rate of 70 before pregnancy may increase to 100 by the third trimester, and be as high as 120 when the woman goes into labor. Blood pressure, however, should not be increased by pregnancy, and may become somewhat lower by the third trimester. If the blood pressure reading for a pregnant woman seems high, ask what the reading was at her last doctor visit or (if she cannot recall the numbers) whether the doctor considered it normal.

A rise of 30 mm Hg or more in her systolic blood pressure, or 15 mm Hg or more in her diastolic blood pressure, may be a sign of **preeclampsia**, a potentially life-threatening condition that can occur at any time during a pregnancy and up to six weeks after delivery of the baby, though it most often occurs in the third trimester. The word comes from Greek *eklampsis* "a shining forth", perhaps referring to the scintillating flashes of light that may be a symptom of toxemia. In preeclampsia, blood flow to the kidneys is disrupted, causing water and salt retention, so another sign of preeclampsia is edema. Symptoms may include headache, blurred vision, and abdominal pain. Diabetes and pre-existing hypertension seem to be risk factors. A woman with any signs or symptoms of preeclampsia should be evacuated immediately. If it progresses to eclampsia, she may have seizures or become comatose. Eclampsia is often fatal to mother and fetus.

Pregnant women breathe more deeply even at rest, to satisfy the additional oxygen demands of the fetus. Tidal volume (the amount of air moved in and out of the lungs with each breath) increases up to 40% by the third trimester. But the respiratory rate usually does not increase, and an abnormal rate of breathing is cause for concern. Also, if breathing is depressed, it is important to give oxygen promptly because more than one life may be at stake.

Pre-term labor

Signs and symptoms of pre-term labor may include backache, discomfort above the pubis, pain inside the vagina, and menstrual-type cramping. Near the baby's due date, some bleeding is normal as the cervix begins to dilate. Earlier in pregnancy, however, bleeding may be the first sign of a miscarriage (spontaneous abortion). It may also be caused by abnormalities such as a placenta attached to the lower part of the uterus (**placenta previa**); a placenta at least partially separated from the uterus (**abruptio placentae**); or a fetus growing in the fallopian tube (**tubal pregnancy**) instead of the womb.

Vaginal secretions of mucus normally increase during pregnancy. A gush of watery fluid, however, may be from premature rupture of the amniotic membranes (**bag of waters**), which can lead to spontaneous abortion. These fluid-filled membranes protect the growing fetus from trauma to the abdomen.

A woman who feels the symptoms of pre-term labor should lie down on her side while someone goes for help. Even if the symptoms decrease or subside, she is at risk of delivering a premature infant.

Activity and hydration

Since pregnant women are already carrying extra weight, they should carry less weight in their packs. They should also be cautious about activities that require dynamic balancing, such as climbing, because their weight distribution is changed. Sudden corrective movement to recover balance, as well as falling, can cause dangerous stress.

It is easy to become dehydrated during wilderness activity. Pregnant women must be especially careful to drink enough, because dehydration can cause pre-term labor. During pregnancy, they should drink at least two liters of water per day, plus enough to replace what they lose by excess sweating. Severe dehydration decreases blood volume. They must also be careful to take in electrolytes when they are drinking water. Electrolyte imbalance can cause fluid shift out of blood vessels, which will also decrease blood volume.

Infection

Both **urinary tract infection** (UTI) and vaginal infection can cause pre-term labor. **Vaginal infection** may cause itching, which a pregnant woman should report promptly to her obstetrician or midwife. It can be caused by sexually transmitted organisms (e.g., gonorrhea) or by an imbalance in organisms normally present. For **urinary tract infection**, see chapter 28 (Medical emergencies in the wilderness).Pregnant women should have a UTI treated immediately, and if they have a history of UTIs, carry their prescription medication for UTI with them on wilderness trips.

Emergency childbirth: Preparations

If birth is imminent and you cannot get the mother to a hospital, prepare the birth site and organize whatever equipment and supplies are available. A warm quiet place with subdued lighting is best, and a spouse or friend can help by staying with the mother, reassuring her by touch as well as words. You will need: absorbent material to clean up blood and other fluids; a receptacle in which to dispose of them; sterile (or at least clean) nitrile gloves; and two cloth ties for tying off the umbilical cord. If possible, boil the cloth ties in water to sterilize them.

Trim your nails short, clean them, and then wash your hands and arms up to the elbows. Gloves protect you as well as the mother, but if the gloves tear, clean hands are less likely to cause infection. To prevent fluids from spattering into your eyes and mucous membranes, use safety glasses and a mask if you have them. Both blood and amniotic fluid can transmit infectious diseases.

Do not give the mother anything by mouth except clear fluids. The digestive system stops during labor, so the only direction food can go is back up. Find out when the mother last ate, and be prepared for vomiting if she ate recently.

Labor

If the mother wants to lie down, she should be on her side, or in a semi-sitting position with her back comfortably propped up. Lying flat on her back would cause the fetus to press down on the aorta and inferior vena cava, raising the mother's blood pressure and interfering with fetal circulation.

False contractions can occur up to four weeks before delivery, but they are short, irregular, and do not increase in intensity, duration, or frequency. Often they stop with a change in activity. False contractions occur mainly in the lower abdomen and groin, and do not significantly dilate the cervix (opening of the uterus). However, when the blood-tinged plug of mucus that has filled the cervical canal during pregnancy comes out (which the mother may or may not notice), true labor usually begins within a few hours to a few days.

Labor can drive up systolic blood pressure 30 mm Hg during contractions, and 10 mm Hg between contractions. As the name implies, labor is work. The muscles of the uterus cause pain during contractions, but instead of using the negative term "labor pains" when talking to the mother, use "contractions."

True labor contractions are mild at first, 10 to 20 minutes apart, but steadily increase in intensity and frequency. When they are 2 to 3 minutes apart, the baby will probably come soon. The mother may feel pain in the small of her back first, but the pain then spreads to her abdomen, which may become almost board-like during contractions. Involuntary muscles in the bulb (upper part of the uterus) contract and shorten, moving the fetus down into the birth canal. Muscles in the lower uterus and cervix stretch to open the way. This is the first stage of labor.

Labor times vary, averaging 11 hours for a primipara (first time mother) and less for a multipara; so you should ask a mother not only whether she has had children before, but also how long her last labor took, whether there were complications, and what her doctor told her about her present pregnancy.

In the movies, when a woman is giving birth someone usually tells her to "bear down." This is a waste of effort until the baby moves into the birth canal, because the muscles of the uterus are involuntary. When the baby begins to move through the cervix into the pelvis, where the abdominal muscles can assist, the mother will usually sense it and feel the urge to push. This is the second stage of labor.

You can try to distract the mother from her pain by helping her concentrate on her breathing. Encourage her to breathe slowly and deeply, which will help calm her and prevent hyperventilation. Demonstrate the technique and breathe with her.

In the uterus, the baby is enclosed in a fluid-filled bag, the amnion (Greek "the caul", diminutive of *amons* "lamb"), which cushions the fetus in the womb. Usually the bag breaks as the baby comes down the pelvis, and the fluid spurts out. At this time, the mother should be in a birthing position, which can be semi-sitting, lying on her side or back, or squatting with someone supporting her from behind.

Usually, the baby begins its descent facing the mother's side. As the head passes through the pelvis, it rotates so that the smallest diameter (ear-to-ear) fits the narrowest dimension of the pelvis, while the pelvic floor muscles stretch to let the long diameter of the head through. Usually the baby emerges face down (towards the mother's back). The shoulders then rotate to the vertical as they pass though the pelvis, rotating the head so that it faces to the mother's side again.

Delivery

When the baby's head crowns (starts pushing through the vagina), tell the mother to stop pushing and pant to slow delivery until the head is out. Firmly control the top of the baby's head with the fingers of one gloved hand and support the perineum (the area under the vagina) with the other hand.

Otherwise the head may emerge too quickly, which can tear the perineum. In a primipara, the tear may even go through the anal sphincter muscle because the perineum has never been stretched before. This injury is painful and difficult to repair.

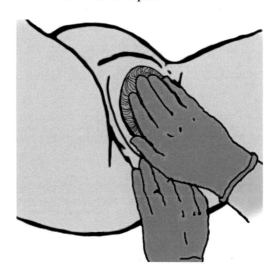

Support the baby's head as it comes out. Clear amniotic fluid, which gushes out after the bag of waters ruptures, will be harmlessly absorbed through the baby's lungs. But a baby that was stressed in the uterus may have excreted **meconium**, a viscous dark green mixture of intestinal secretions and mucosal cells. If the amniotic fluid is greenish or brownish, suction the baby's mouth and nose with a bulb syringe if you have one, or (if you do not) wipe meconium away from mouth and nose with a clean cloth. Aspirating meconium can cause respiratory problems.

If meconium was present, report this to the doctor because a baby that was stressed in the uterus enough to secrete meconium may have other problems.

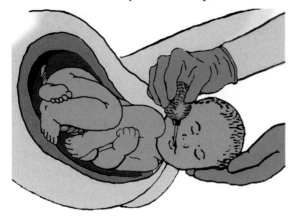

If the baby is born with its bag of waters still around it, tear the membrane with a blunt instrument or a fingernail and peel it away from the face.

Nearly 22% of babies emerge with the umbilical cord looped around the neck. If this occurs, try to free it by easing it over the head with your gloved finger. If it is too tight to pull over the head, slip it over the shoulder. Support the baby's body (which will be slippery) as it comes out but never pull.

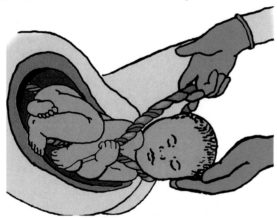

Abnormal deliveries

If the baby emerges butt first, you may have to insert two forked fingers under the face to make breathing room in case the baby starts breathing before the head emerges. But if one limb emerges first, delivery in the field is impossible, so you can only give the mother oxygen (if you have it) and treat for shock while waiting for transport.

Caring for the baby

Wipe the baby dry, and wipe away any residue around the mouth and nose, but do not worry about the white coating (Latin *vernix* "varnish", *caseosa* "cheesy") which acts as a protective coating for the sensitive skin. If the baby doesn't start breathing in a minute or two, stimulate with more vigorous drying, massaging the chest and back, and flicking the bottoms of the feet. If that doesn't work, and the umbilical cord is no longer pulsing, start ventilating the baby. Give just enough air or breath to make the chest rise because it is easy to over-inflate or even rupture a baby's tiny lungs. Also ventilate the baby if the heart rate is less than 100 per minute. Even a baby who is breathing may need oxygen to pink up. If the baby is cyanotic (turning blue), set oxygen flow at 6 liters per minute and hold the outlet near (not on) the baby's face until skin color improves, usually in a few minutes. If the heart rate is less than 60, start CPR.

After the baby starts breathing, it takes a few minutes for the valves controlling blood exchange with the mother to close, and for the baby's circulation to become independent. So until the cord is tied (after it stops pulsing), keep the baby at about the same level as the mother to avoid draining or adding blood. Make the first tie in the cord eight inches from the baby and the second tie a few inches closer. Tighten them slowly and tie with a square knot. There is no need to cut the cord if mother and baby are going to the hospital within an hour.

Delivering the placenta

Usually within a few minutes of the baby's delivery, the placenta (Greek *plakous* "a flat cake") separates from the wall of the uterus. This may cause a gush of blood, because the placenta is the interface between the mother's and the fetus' circulatory systems. When the cord starts coming out again, the placenta is descending, which usually takes 10 minutes or less. The mother can help by gently bearing down with her abdominal muscles. Support the placenta as it emerges, to prevent any of it from tearing and remaining inside, which could promote bleeding and infection. The placenta should be a disk about 7" in diameter, and 1" thick, smooth on one side (and covered with a membrane), rough on the other side. Send the placenta with the mother and baby to the hospital, if practical. If not, examine it carefully, note whether it appears intact, and photograph it if possible.

Suckling

After the placenta is delivered, put the baby on the mother's abdomen, near a breast. Pressing the baby's cheek against the breast triggers the rooting reflex, and the pressure of the nipple against the roof of the mouth triggers the suckling reflex. Suckling bonds the baby to the mother and also helps the mother by stimulating the contraction of the uterus, which reduces bleeding. Keep the baby and the mother warm.

Massaging the fundus

After the placenta is delivered, feel for the top of the uterus (called the fundus) around the mother's navel. If it is still spongy, massage it with a circular motion until it contracts to the size of a grapefruit and becomes firm. This may be uncomfortable for the mother at first, but it stimulates the uterus to contract, which closes placental blood vessels and reduces bleeding.

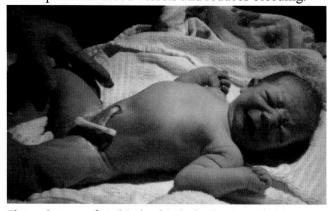

Five minutes after birth, this baby has good skin color, and is moving and crying vigorously for an APGAR score of 10. *Photo courtesy of Lynn Garcia.*

APGAR score

In 1952, Dr. Virginia Apgar described five criteria for evaluating a baby's health after birth. The test is usually performed one minute after birth, to gauge how well the baby has tolerated the experience; and five minutes after birth, to gauge how well the baby is doing on its own. The APGAR score is based on:

- Appearance of skin
- Pulse rate
- Grimace (reflex irritability)
- Activity or muscle tone
- Respiratory effort and breathing rate.

The first letters of each criterion match Dr. Apgar's name, which can then be used as a mnemonic. Grimace

stands for any response to stimulation. For each criterion, the baby gets a score of 0, 1, or 2. A score of 7 to 9 immediately after birth is normal, though a score of 10 is rare because most babies have blue hands and feet until they have been breathing a few minutes. A baby with a score below 7 needs help: clearing the airway, oxygen, or rubbing with a towel to stimulate breathing. A low one-minute score, however, does not necessarily predict poor health provided that the five-minute score is good.

APGAR criteria

Appearance (of skin)
0   Blue-gray (cyanotic) all over
1   Normal except for blue extremities
2   Normal skin color all over

Pulse rate: Stethoscope or feel the brachial pulse
0   No pulse
1   Pulse < 100 per minute
2   Pulse > 100 per minute

Grimace (reflex irritability/response to a pinch)
0   No response
1   Grimace but no sound or movement
2   Also coughs, cries, or pulls away

Activity or muscle tone
0   Muscles loose, no movement
1   Arms and legs flexed
2   Moving/resisting

Respiratory effort
0   Not breathing
1   Breathing slowly (<30 per minute) or irregular
2   Breathing regular, cries strongly

Conclusion

Pregnancy and childbirth are natural processes that usually proceed normally in a healthy mother. Pregnancy does, however, change some vital signs. Dehydration or urinary tract infection can bring on preterm labor, which puts baby and mother at risk.

While emergency childbirth in the wilderness is unlikely today for residents of developed countries, women successfully gave birth for many millennia without hospitals or obstetricians. In an emergency childbirth, our role is to prepare a comfortable environment, support the mother psychologically and physically, assist with delivery, and help take care of the baby during the critical first minutes after birth.

Chapter 31. Survival and evacuation techniques

Photos not otherwise credited are courtesy of Ruth McConnell

Tibetan tuck and penguin huddle

What if you are caught in the open with no shelter or sleeping bag? Then you can use the Tibetan tuck or the penguin huddle to survive. Tibetan pilgrims use these heat-conserving positions to sleep without shelter in sub-freezing, windy mountain passes. To do the Tibetan tuck, face away from the wind and kneel on whatever insulation you have. Put your head on your knees and wrap your hands around your head. Wrap something around your hands and head if possible.

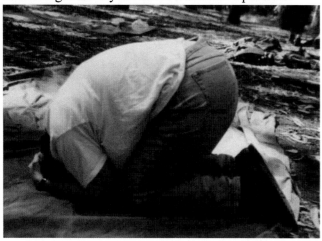

In a group, you can do the penguin huddle. Sit on whatever insulation you have with your back to the wind and your legs comfortably flexed so that only your boot heels are in contact with the ground. Then have the rest of the group sit in front of you between each other's legs, wrapping their arms around each other to conserve body heat. From time to time, the person to windward moves to the downwind side.

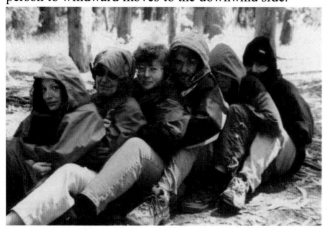

It is wise to carry some lightweight pieces of survival equipment in your daypack, however. This includes a large plastic trash bag, a space blanket, and a sit pad that doubles as a back pad for your day pack. In a fir forest, springy branches laid down in an overlapping pattern can provide ground insulation. Any branches and deadwood leaned against the top of a boulder or large fallen tree trunk can make a lean-to. The plastic bag (or a top-loading pack) can serve as a bivouac sack for your legs. The space blanket can be wrapped around your body after you put on all your clothing. If it is very cold and you don't have much ground insulation, it is best to sit on the little you have, huddled with your arms around your knees, to minimize heat loss into both ground and air.

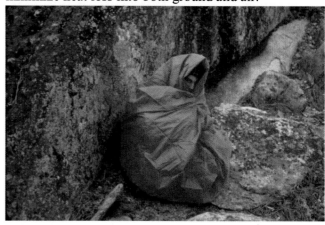

Photo courtesy of Ben Schifrin, M.D.

Bivouacs

To survive an overnight bivouac on a cold night, you must stay warm. To stay warm, you must not only control heat loss with clothing, shelter, and ground insulation, but also generate heat by eating energy food, and drink enough water to maintain circulation and metabolism.

Below the timberline, you can improvise lean-to shelters against fallen trees or rocks, using fallen branches as ground insulation and roofing. In a survival situation, you should plan a shelter that you can construct in about 20 minutes, if possible, so as to conserve energy and minimize exposure. A waterproof tarp and nylon cord are essential to make the shelter wind and rain proof.

Winter shelters

When you are on snow, especially above the timberline, snow shovels and snow saws are the main shelter-building tools, though skis can be used if necessary. **Snow caves** and igloos are possible with firm snow and enough energetic diggers, but a **snow trench** is fastest and simplest, especially if it takes advantage of a natural hollow or windbreak. Just dig a trench large enough to lie in and lean slabs of snow over it to form a peaked roof; or cover it with a tarp, supported by skis and poles.

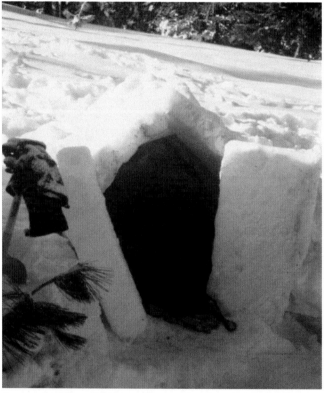

Snow shelter. *Photo courtesy of Ben Schifrin, M.D.*

Another possibility is a tree well that has branches at about the right height to frame the roof of your shelter.

Skis and poles can be used as part of a shelter, or by themselves as the framework of a hasty shelter. Insert the tails of the skis in the snow at about a 45° angle with the tips crossed. Support them with the crossed poles. Use nylon cord or strapping tape (which is reinforced with fiberglass threads) to hold the frame together and secure a tarp around the frame. If you don't have enough ground insulation to lie down, you will have to sit up, with something under the feet to help prevent frostbite. Spare clothing, including mittens, balaclava, and dry socks, can also help you survive the night.

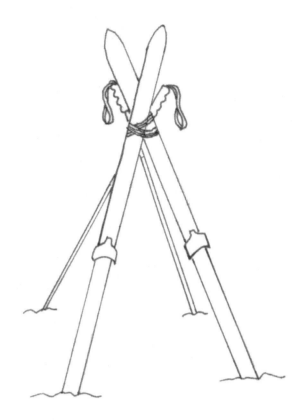

To build a fire

A fire can be a life saver in a cold bivouac, especially if it is built against a heat-reflecting surface. On snow, you need a solid base of logs or heavy branches. Otherwise the fire will quickly sink into the snow. Dry wood can be hard to find in wet weather, but trees often have dead limbs near the ground, sheltered by the living foliage. Branches that snap rather than bend or crumble are good. Fir burns fast, but hardwood such as oak lasts longer.

It is essential to collect enough wood for the night before starting the fire. You don't want to leave it untended, and it is hard to find wood in the dark. Carry several **fire starters**, such as lighters and waterproof, strike-anywhere matches in a sealed container. A strip of survival magnesium, which has a steel insert to strike sparks that ignite the magnesium shavings, is indestructible but harder to use. Flammable paste, sold in squeeze tubes as a fire starter, will usually ignite even damp wood.

Water, water everywhere

In a winter landscape, melting snow is often the only way to get water. Melting snow in the mouth, however, wastes body heat and yields little water, because snow is mostly air. On a warm, sunny day, putting snow in a black, plastic trash bag will at least concentrate it into slush. However, you may still have to burn fuel to make water, and a stove is more dependable than a fire. Hot drinks are pleasant, but do not add significant heat to the body. It is more important to drink as much water as possible if you are dehydrated, rather than spend too much time bringing the water to a boil.

There are several light weight emergency stoves that you can carry as part of your survival kit for day trips that could turn into emergency bivouacs. The Trangia alcohol stove, which weighs about 1/2 lb., is about the size of two small tins of tuna and needs no priming. One filling of alcohol will melt up to two liters of snow in a half-liter aluminum kettle or pot. Esbit stoves burn solid fuel tablets. Compact folding stoves are available that burn twigs and bark.

All stoves produce **carbon monoxide** so they should be used outside the shelter or positioned so that they are well-vented. When inhaled, carbon monoxide bonds to hemoglobin more strongly than oxygen, and does not release for up to eight hours. Even if the dose is not fatal, it reduces the oxygen-carrying capacity of the blood, which can depress the metabolism and make you colder.

Emergency ski repair

If someone in your group is getting cold, depleted, or dehydrated, you may only need to provide water, energy food, or spare clothing to get the reluctant body functioning again. Another common cause of being stranded in the snow, however, is equipment failure of boots, bindings, skis, or poles. A simple repair kit will help you deal with these problems.

To re-attach bindings, for example, carry wooden golf tees, spare screws, a pozidrive screwdriver and a glue stick (used in hot glue guns). Melt glue from the stick with a match or lighter and drip it like wax into the screw hole. Immediately drive in the golf tee (the glue sets in about 10 seconds). Cut off the tee and score an X in the top with the tip of your knife blade to center the screw. Position the binding and drive in the screw. An easier alternative to golf tees are plastic expanding sheaths for screws, sold by ski shops.

Pozidrive screws, which are used on almost all ski bindings, look like Phillips screws. The screw heads both have cross-shaped slots. If you compare a Phillips and a pozidrive screwdriver tip, however, you will notice that the Phillips tip has tapered ridges that come almost to a point; whereas the pozidrive tip has flanges that do not taper. That is why you need to bear down on a Phillips screwdriver to keep it from riding out of the slots, but a pozidrive screwdriver grips more firmly. If you try to use a Phillips tip on the pozidrive screws of a ski binding, it will not grip well and may strip the screw head. Swiss army knives and Leatherman-type tools generally have only Phillips screwdrivers, so for skiing you need to add a pozidrive to your repair kit.

Wire bales are held in Nordic bindings by spring tension. These can be broken or lost, so it is prudent to carry a spare. Sometimes, however, the problem is in the boot. The pinholes in the toe plate can become so blown out that they no longer lock over the three pins of the binding. Sometimes the toe plate itself may break. In either case, you can improvise a cable binding by wrapping strapping tape or wire around the heel of the boot to pull it into the toe of the binding. This also works to replace a broken cable binding.

Broken poles can be splinted with two pieces of angle aluminum 8" long (used for corner molding and found in most hardware stores) and strapping tape. Some patrollers use thin-wall PVC tubing, slit lengthwise to snap over the pole, instead of aluminum. Patrollers also carry spare baskets, since these are sometimes lost or shredded.

Broken skis are more of a challenge. A broken tip can be replaced with a spare plastic tip that jams on and grips the end of the ski with metal teeth. A ski broken in the middle can be jury-rigged in two ways. If it is not completely broken, splints may enable the skier to shuffle out. These can be either aluminum pole-splints or an aluminum plate screwed or tightly taped to the ski. For a ski completely broken in the middle, however, the only solution may be to re-mount the binding on the front segment, using a small hand drill or the auger blade of a Swiss army knife to start the screw holes. A more efficient tool for drilling holes is a gimlet, which you can still find in some woodworking catalogs. Gimlets are drills made from hardened steel wire. One end is machined into a drill bit. The other end is bent into a loop to form a handle, so that you can drill a hole by just rotating and pressing on the gimlet with one hand.

Desert survival

While deserts get cold at night, during the day the main problems are to find or create shade, protect against sunburn, conserve sweat, and carry or find enough water. Much desert water is too alkaline or brackish to be potable, so desert survival books (see bibliography) describe how to make a solar still from a plastic sheet and find water in succulent plants. Wear high boots and gaiters to keep out sand and pebbles, and long sleeved shirts and pants to protect skin from sunburn. Because desert air is so dry, it is perhaps the only wilderness environment where tightly woven cotton is practical.

Emergency carries

Photos courtesy of Ruth McConnell

If you need to carry someone a short distance to a safe or sheltered spot, you can use an emergency carry. The simplest and most stable one-person carry is the piggyback. However, if you have to go very far with it, your arms will soon get tired. To relieve the stress on your arm muscles, make a loop of webbing or a cravat bandage that's about one foot long. Lay it over one wrist before your passenger climbs aboard. Then slip the other wrist through it and twist it until it is snug around both wrists, and hold the connecting length with your hands. This will transfer the weight of the patient to the bones of your arms so that you can relax the muscles, and (if you have strong legs) enable you to carry your passenger a considerable distance. You can also give your patient a looped cravat to help her hold on.

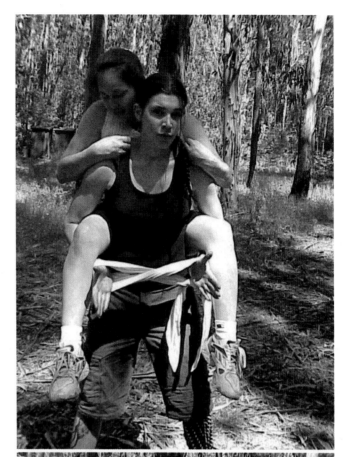

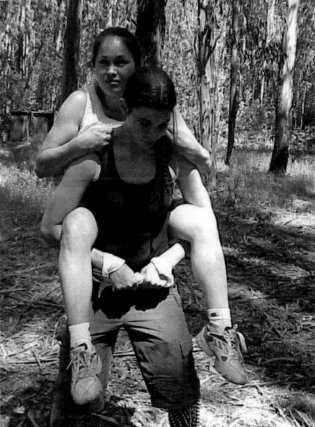

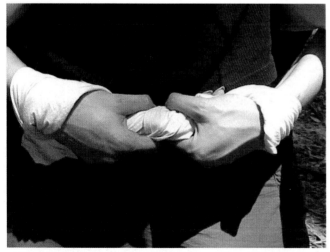

Using a looped cravat to hold the wrists in place instead of arm tension while doing a piggyback carry.

The fireman's carry requires good balance and practice to do safely. If you do it correctly, however, it can enable you to carry someone a long distance, because your passenger is draped over your shoulders and balanced on your upright spine. The disadvantage is that the position is uncomfortable for your passenger and can aggravate injuries; and that if you are alone with a patient who cannot stand, you will have to jerk him upright before pulling him over your shoulders – a potentially hazardous move.

Most books show the rescuer going down on one knee to load the passenger. This makes it easy to get the passenger over your shoulders, but then it will be very difficult to stand up with the muscles of one leg while carrying someone your weight or heavier. An alternative is to squat and step in sideways between the standing patient's legs while pulling the patient over your shoulders. This is actually the first move of a judo throw called kata guruma.

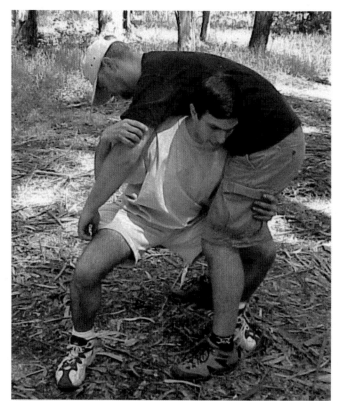

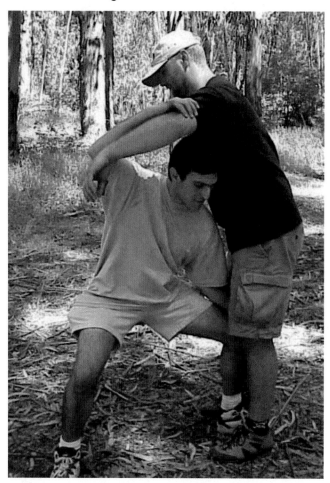

Grip the patient's arm, just above his elbow. Plant your foot between the patient's feet and bend your knees. Look up and keep your back arched.

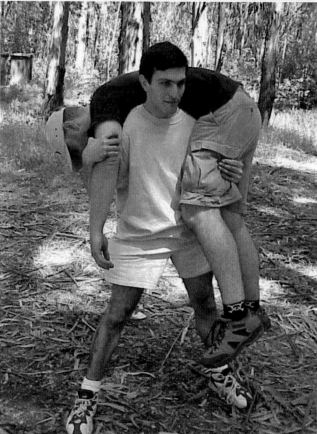

As your right arm reaches between the passenger's legs and your right shoulder serves as a fulcrum, your left arm pulls the passenger across your shoulders.

To do the fore-and-aft carry, one rescuer goes behind the sitting passenger, reaches with both arms under the passenger's armpits, and grips the passenger's forearms.

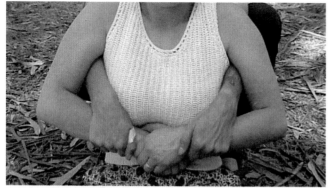

The other rescuer squats between the passenger's legs, facing forward, and picks up the legs, gripping just under the knees.

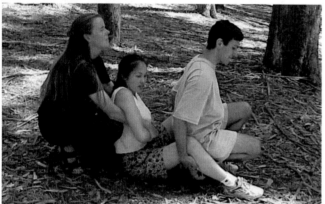

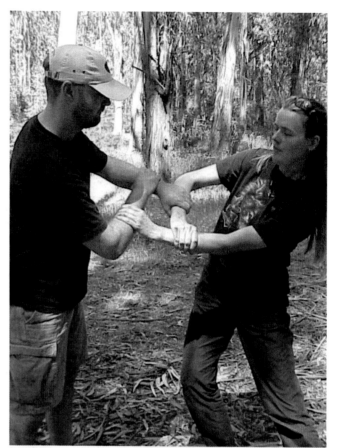

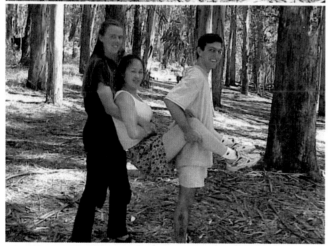

To do the human chair carry, grip your left wrist with your right hand, palm down. Have your partner do the same. Now each of you grip the other's right wrist with your left hand. Squat and have the passenger sit, wrapping both arms around your shoulders. Then stand and carry.

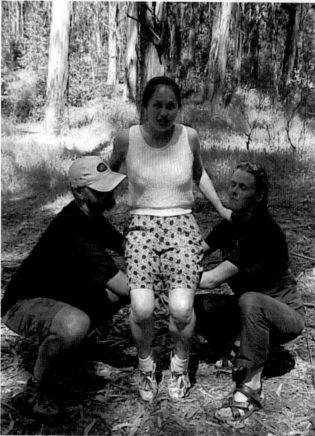

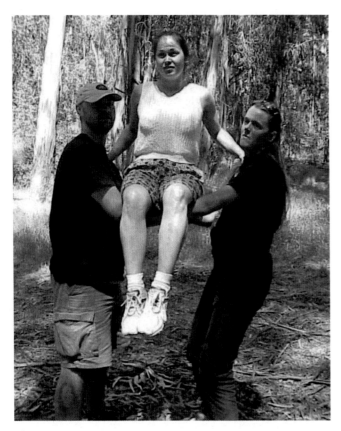

For a passenger who is weak or not very alert, a variation is for you and your partner to face each other and each grip the wrist of the opposing arm. Then have the passenger sit on one pair of linked arms, while the other pair of linked arms forms a back rest.

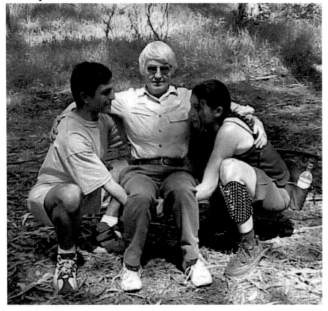

Improvised litters

If you need to carry someone out more than a short distance, you will have to improvise a litter out of poles, packs, or whatever you have. On snow, a sled is a much better option, because you don't have to carry it. On fairly level ground, a travois may work. You pick up the poles at one end and the other ends drag on the ground. A litter designed to be carried is more versatile, but people who have never practiced this technique will seriously underestimate how much time and effort it takes.

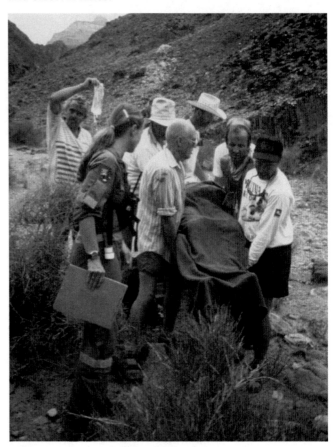

Photo courtesy of Ben Schifrin, M.D.

Generally, you need several teams of six rescuers to take turns carrying the litter, and even on easy terrain, a pace of one mile per hour would be good. So be realistic about how far you can go before dark, check your actual pace, and plan ahead. You don't want to be caught in an exposed place where you cannot safely camp at nightfall. On steep terrain, you would need to be equipped for technical rescue, which requires specialized training.

A rectangular frame of two long, sturdy poles with two shorter poles lashed across near the ends is the simplest design for a litter. You can fill in the space with additional poles lashed across, or a hammock made of rope or webbing. Then lay in foam pads. You can also use spare jackets if the fabric is strong enough. Another possibility is to lash several packs together.

You should secure the patient to the litter if the terrain is steep or uneven. Carrying weight with your hands, however, is not only strenuous; it also drives up the blood pressure. You can rig carrying straps to suspend the weight of the litter from the rescuers' shoulders, as well as equalizing any differences in height. Tie pieces of webbing or rope to the frame of the litter. Then (with the litter empty) give each carrier a sling to use as a bandolier and tie the webbing to it, adjusting the length to equalize height differences. These carrying straps will support the weight of the backboard from the rescuers' shoulders, so that they can use the handgrips to stabilize and control the load.

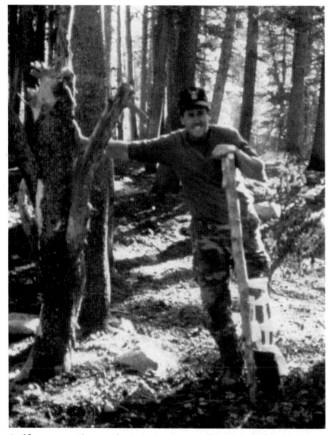

Self evacuation. *Photo courtesy of Ben Schifrin, M.D.*

Improvised sleds

An injured skier who cannot ski will have to be evacuated. Most Nordic evacuation techniques use the patient's skis and poles as the framework for a sled. Lay the skis parallel, just wide enough for the patient to fit between them. Secure the poles to the skis in an X, handles forward, with strapping tape – clear tape reinforced with fiberglass thread. If the skis have metal edges, pad them first with several strips of tape where you plan to wrap. Otherwise the metal edges will cut the tape wrapped around them. Putting climbing skins on the skis will make the toboggan easier to control on hills, but harder to pull on the level.

Shovel handles and other cross pieces (such as removable pack staves) strengthen the sled and give support for the patient. Cord can also be hammocked between cross pieces for additional support. The tow line (20 feet of 7 millimeter rope) must be tied to the bindings, though it should wrap around or pass through the front cross piece to help steer the sled. For downhill, a tail line is also needed. Clip loops of webbing or cravats to the tow line with a carabiner for haul harnesses. Foam pads and insulation go on the frame, and webbing or cravats secure the patient.

For control on slopes, you should add two outriggers of rope or long webbing. Secure them to the bindings, then pass each outrigger across the litter and patient, so that the rescuer on the right side is holding the outrigger anchored on the left side and vice versa. This rigging enables the outriggers to prevent the sled from tipping over when traversing a slope. The outriggers can move forward or back when the sled is not sideways on a slope, to help pull forward or help control the sled when going downhill.

For pulling a patient up a steep slope, it may be necessary to set up a rope system with a mechanical advantage (MA), by running the rope back and forth through pulleys or carabiners. For example, the Z-rig, so called because the rope forms the letter Z, can give a MA of two to one or three to one, depending on how it is rigged. This is a technical skill that is explained in books on mountain rescue [see bibliography].

Conclusion

If you or someone in your group gets stuck in the wilderness, you have two choices: to bivouac and send out for help, or do an emergency evacuation. To survive a bivouac, you need to stay warm and dry. Clothing, shelter, water, food, and fire can all help get you through the night. Evacuation may require no more than equipment repair, but if someone in your group is injured, you may have to do emergency carries or build a sled or litter. You can prepare yourself for these emergencies by carrying some basic repair tools and survival equipment and by learning survival skills.

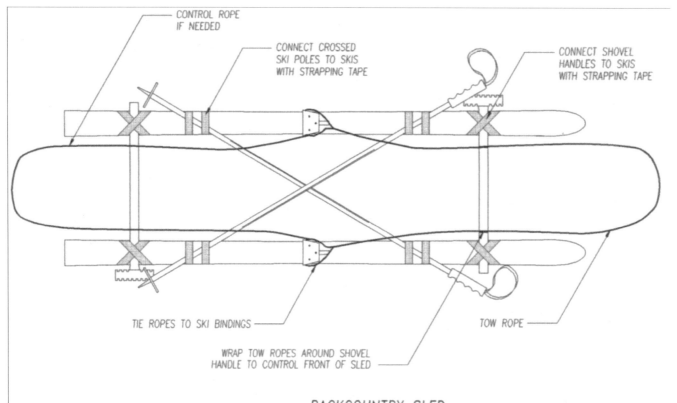

CONTROL ROPE
IF NEEDED

CONNECT CROSSED
SKI POLES TO SKIS
WITH STRAPPING TAPE

CONNECT SHOVEL
HANDLES TO SKIS
WITH STRAPPING TAPE

TIE ROPES TO SKI BINDINGS

TOW ROPE

WRAP TOW ROPES AROUND SHOVEL
HANDLE TO CONTROL FRONT OF SLED

BACKCOUNTRY SLED

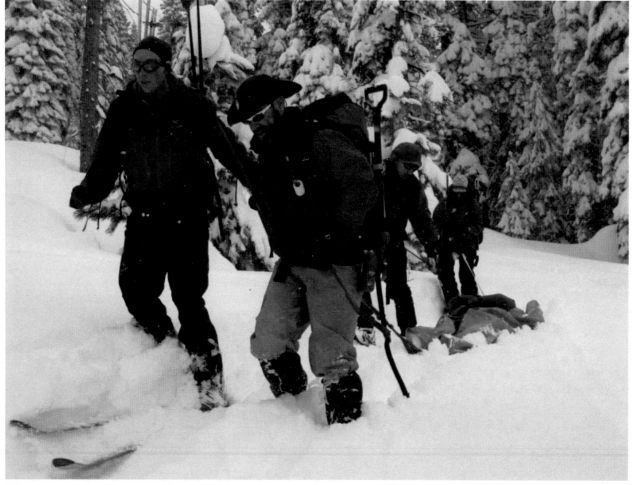

Members of the Pinecrest Nordic Ski Patrol practice hauling a patient in an improvised sled.

Chapter 32. Emergency Medical Services in the wilderness

Photos of wilderness rescue courtesy of Ben Schifrin, M.D.

Emergency Medical Services (EMS) has a long history. Clara Barton, who later became the founder and first President of the American Red Cross, drove wagons full of bandages, blankets, and food to the battlefields of the Civil War to give urgent care to the wounded. This is an early example of one concept on which EMS is based – the golden hour. Victims who are seriously injured or ill need immediate care. Often their survival depends on getting that care within the first hour or so after the injury, before they are transported to a hospital. So the first responders need to provide care at the scene.

Rapid transport to a hospital is the other main concept of EMS. In the United States before 1960, victims were often transported to the hospital in hearses, because those were the only vehicles designed to carry people horizontally. Ambulances became more common in the 1960s, but the drivers were usually trained only to transport or to "swoop and scoop" as it was called. Then in 1973, the **Emergency Medical Services Act** authorized the training of responders to give urgent medical care at the accident scene before transporting patients to the hospital. Responders do so under the authority of a medical director, which is passed on to them by radio contact or standing orders. In the 1970s and 1980s, standards of training and care continued to rise, but each state had its own standards for certification. Even though the **National Registry of Emergency Medical Technicians** (EMTs) offered a written and practical exam for national certification, it was often not recognized by state agencies.

In 1993, The **EMS Education and Training Blueprint** described four levels of EMS training and certification: First Responder, EMT Basic, EMT Intermediate and EMT Paramedic. During the 1990s, the Department of Transportation (DOT) published certification standards and curricula for each of these levels of training. The **National EMS Scope of Practice Model**, published in 2006, revised the standards and curricula and described the four levels as: Emergency Medical Responder (EMR); Emergency Medical Technician (EMT); Advanced Emergency Medical Technician (AEMT); and Paramedic.

Urban EMS

In an urban EMS system, response to an emergency usually has six phases:

1. A citizen or first responder activates EMS, usually by calling 911.
2. A dispatcher sends an ambulance to the scene.
3. The EMTs assess the scene and patients, and call for backup if necessary.
4. They provide urgent pre-hospital care at the scene.
5. They transport the patients rapidly to the hospital, continuing to provide care in the ambulance.
6. The patients are evaluated and treated in the emergency department of the hospital.

To perform all of these functions, an urban EMS system needs:

- public education, so bystanders will activate EMS and care for patients until the ambulance arrives;
- standardized training and medical oversight;
- facilities and equipment including ambulances;
- communication with other agencies as well as dispatch;
- emergency departments in hospitals for urgent care of injuries and life-threatening medical problems.

Wilderness EMS

For Wilderness Emergency Medical Services (WEMS) in the United States, there are no common standards to regulate training, certification or performance at the national or state level. In Canada, wilderness rescue and emergency care are usually run by the military. In Europe, they are usually directed by physicians - the International Union of Alpine Associations (UIAA) publishes criteria for the postgraduate training of physicians in mountain medicine.

Wilderness Medical Society Practice Guidelines for Wilderness Emergency Care, edited by William W. Forgey, M.D. (www.wms.org) is based on a consensus of wilderness medicine experts. These guidelines go beyond urban EMS training in several ways. This is because wilderness responders usually have to take care of their patients for hours or days and protect them (as well as themselves) from harsh weather as well as other environmental hazards. So they need wilderness survival skills, and they may need more advanced medical skills than their urban counterparts. They also may need advanced wilderness skills for technical rescues, such as climbing and mountaineering. Their training may include (among other skills):

- use of airways, intubation, and IVs;
- giving medications;
- field rewarming of patients in hypothermia;
- field reduction of fractures and dislocations;
- radio skills and protocols;
- helicopter and fixed wing protocols;
- use of the incident command system (ICS).

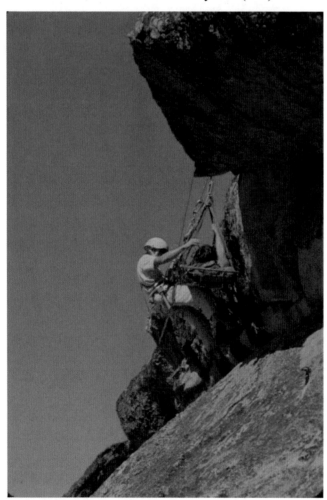

Lowering an injured climber

Incident Command System (ICS)

Many agencies with varied training and certification levels may be involved in wilderness rescue and emergency care. These agencies usually follow the Incident Command System (ICS) to coordinate their efforts. In the ICS, one leader is in charge of the response and delegates responsibilities to other qualified leaders. Usually these responsibilities come under three headings:

- **Operations**: directing rescue staff in the field;
- **Planning and record keeping**: assessing the situation, deciding what resources are needed, and documenting what is done;
- **Logistics**: providing services and support to rescuers, including facilities, food, equipment, and medical supplies;

For a large-scale rescue, the Incident Commander usually stays at the base and communicates with the leaders en route or at the rescue site by radio. If you are involved in a wilderness accident, and you are the most highly qualified person at the scene, you can use the principles of the ICS to organize the group's efforts.

Start system

In an accident where many victims are involved, and you do not have enough resources at hand to care for them, you can use the **START system** to set priorities. The acronym means Simple Triage and Rapid Treatment, and "triage" means sorting out. By quickly assessing each of the victims, the triage leader classifies them into four categories:

- walking wounded who do not need help on scene;
- those who can wait for help;
- those who need help now and evacuation ASAP;
- those who are beyond help.

If you are doing triage, you begin by asking all those who can get up and walk to move to a designated safe area (green tag). Then you quickly check vital functions in the patients who cannot get up and walk. Those whose vital functions are normal and seem stable can wait (yellow tag), no matter what their injuries. Any patient with one or more abnormal vital signs (level of responsiveness, breathing rate, or signs of circulation) needs help immediately (red tag). This initial sorting out should take no more than 30 seconds for each patient.

If a patient does not respond, open the airway and check for breathing. A patient who starts breathing gets a red tag. One who does not start breathing is considered beyond help (black tag), because in the circumstances he or she has little chance of survival, and your resources are better used to help those who are more savable.

Check level of responsiveness (LOR) by talking to the patient. Patients who respond alertly, and can tell you what happened (no lapse of consciousness or memory) have normal LOR. Patients who do not respond, respond only to a pinch, or are disoriented do not have normal LOR. You can also assess breathing by a patient's speech as well as by breathing rate and effort. Frequent pauses between words to breathe are not normal. Capillary refill within two seconds is a quick test of circulation, but difficult to see in poor lighting and not always reliable in older patients. Also, you cannot see capillary refill in nail beds of a patient wearing nail polish. So another way to check circulation is to feel a radial pulse as you talk to the patient or check breathing.

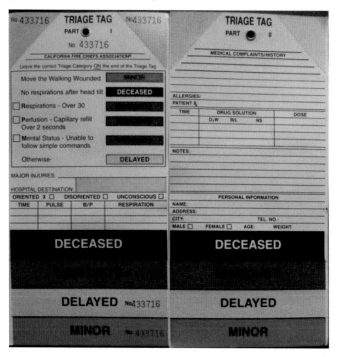

If you are doing initial triage, you quickly fill in Part I of the tag (left) and tear off the colored strips that do not apply. For example, if the patient cannot walk, but has normal and stable vital signs, you tear off the green strip. Whoever is assigned to reassess the patient when triage is complete and emergency responders are available, fills in Part II of the tag, on the reverse side. If the patient's condition worsens, the responder can upgrade the patient's status by tearing off the next colored strip and noting the change. Patients' status can also be downgraded if their condition is seen to be stable, such as a patient whose breathing appeared

abnormally fast because of panic, but is breathing normally when reassessed. If tags are not available, you can sort patients by tying different colored tape around their wrists.

Phases of a wilderness response

A wilderness emergency response usually begins with the decision by a group to get help. Then:

1. One or (preferably) two people go out for help.
2. They activate EMS.
3. The rescue team mobilizes and organizes.
4. They go to the group's location. A hasty team may go first.
5. They locate and assess the patient(s).
6. They provide emergency care, which includes protecting the patient(s) from the environment.
7. They evacuate the patient(s).
8. They turn the patient over to the next level of care.

Before sending anyone out to get help, you should do a thorough patient assessment and record the results in a patient information note, as well as:

- a map with the group's position marked;
- GPS coordinates if possible;
- a list of the group's members;
- a description of the group's situation, equipment, condition, and medical training (if any).

Before starting a trip, it is wise to find out who would be responsible for a wilderness rescue in that area and how to notify them. Some national parks, for example, have their own trained rescue teams. In national forests, however, the local sheriff's department is usually responsible, though often volunteer rescue teams are called out.

Since it usually takes some time to organize and prepare for a wilderness rescue, sometimes a hasty team of fast-moving and highly trained rescuers will go first to treat and stabilize the patient. They may go in on foot or skis, by snowmobile, or by helicopter depending on the situation.

Leadership and teamwork

Although all emergency responders are trained to do a scene size-up as they approach an incident, team leaders take this process several steps further. After checking for hazards, the number of victims, and their status, they:

- Analyze the problems;

- Set priorities;
- Divide the problems into tasks for team members;
- Give clear instructions for performing each task.

When a skilled team leader directs a rescue, it usually goes so smoothly and quickly that it seems rehearsed. Such leaders seem to keep track of everything that is happening, and almost never have to raise their voices. But if we watch more closely, we can usually identify some techniques and traits that make these leaders effective.

- **Courtesy**: Good leaders treat team members with respect, even when they make mistakes. They address people by name, and phrase instructions as requests rather than orders, e.g. "John, would you take another set of vitals for me?' When addressing strangers, they use respectful forms of address such as "sir." They are equally respectful when they address patients, and ensure that team members meet the same standards of courtesy.

- **Clarity**: Good leaders give clear, complete, and unambiguous instructions. For example, instructions for moving a patient should include details such as when, how far, and in which direction, e.g. "two feet to the patient's right," not "two feet to the right."

- **Brevity**: Good leaders do not waste words. They think before they speak and tell team members exactly what they need to know to perform the task. Inexperienced leaders often think aloud, and make several rambling attempts to describe what they want the team to do before they succeed in expressing their intent. In the worst case, a leader's indecision or obscure direction can generate arguments that stall the response and shake patients' confidence in their rescuers. .

- **Logic**: Good leaders anticipate the sequence in which tasks need to be performed, depending on priorities and the mechanics of the techniques the team uses. For example, in cold weather an inadequately clothed patient needs to be protected against hypothermia as soon as it is practical; and for a complex technique such as backboarding or traction splinting, all the equipment needs to be laid out and the patient positioned before the team begins the technique.

- **Delegation**: Good leaders give each team member specific jobs, and make sure that they do their jobs

properly. With an inexperienced team that lacks strong leadership, jobs seem to migrate around the team, with much duplication of effort and some tasks forgotten. Good leaders also select team members for tasks based on their experience and abilities.

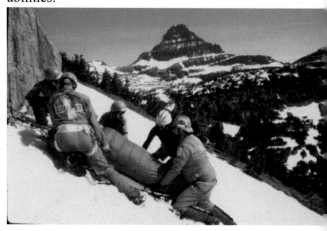

Every team needs exactly one leader. If team members challenge the leader, a rescue response can degenerate into an argument, which will slow the response and make a poor impression on the patient and bystanders. But what if you, as a team member, think that the leader is making mistakes, or not providing adequate direction? There are several ways you can intervene without publicly challenging the leader.

- **Make sure you know your assignment**: If you're not sure what your tasks and responsibilities are, ask the leader to clarify. Don't just make a guess without consulting the leader, unless it is an emergency that requires immediate action.

- **Communicate with the leader**: If you have a concern about what the team is doing, bring it to the leader's attention in a respectful way. Do not start an argument over the patient, since that would embarrass the leader and make a poor impression on the patient and bystanders.

- **Ask don't challenge**: For example, instead of saying "You forgot to apply a cervical collar!" ask the leader "Would you like me [or whoever's responsibility it should be] to apply a cervical collar now?" That way the leader does not lose face, if he or she did neglect to call for a cervical collar, and the team will continue to appear professional in front of the patient and bystanders.

- **Minimize cross-talk**: You sometimes need to communicate with other team members to coordinate your efforts. But such exchanges should not escalate into unnecessary chatter, or a discussion of the operation that could challenge or preempt the leader.

When things go wrong

No matter how skilled and experienced responders may be, events may sometimes threaten to get out of control during a rescue. There are several types of situations that require especially careful handling:

- Failure of leadership;
- Outside team members;
- Uncooperative patients.

Failure of leadership: If discrete support and suggestions from the team are not enough to prevent serious errors by the leader, then the most qualified team member may need to assume leadership. If possible, the transition should be smooth and not confrontational. If the leader is unwilling to step down, then you should try to get him or her away from the group for a private discussion.

Outside team members: You may need assistance from bystanders who are not trained as emergency responders. If you are not sure of their skills, a good way to integrate them into the team is to pair each of them with an experienced emergency responder, who can watch them, model the assigned task, and explain any instructions that may not be clear.

Uncooperative patients: Most people who are injured or ill respond positively to an offer of help, even if they do not think they need evacuation. If a patient refuses care, however (in spite of your best persuasion), then you need to document it with the appropriate form, signed by the patient. A patient who accepts care but is complaining or interfering with the rescue can sometimes be redirected by asking for his or her help, e.g. to hold a dressing or a splint.

Search and Rescue (SAR)

If someone in your party is lost, then you need to activate search and rescue, which requires different skills and usually far more people than a rescue from a known location. According to the United States National SAR Plan (1956), the U.S. Air Force coordinates inland searches, and the U.S. Coast Guard coordinates maritime searches. The Coast Guard (which is under the Department of Homeland Security,

not Defense) probably does more search and rescue operations than any other organization in the world.

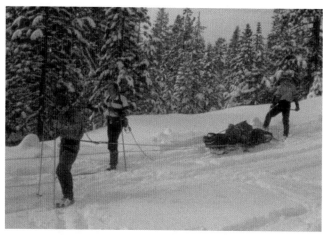

Hauling equipment on a sled that can carry a patient

Inland searches, however, are usually done by the Civil Air Patrol, state police, sheriff's departments, or local volunteer rescue organizations. The Civil Air Patrol, chartered in 1948 as a non-profit organization staffed by volunteers, is an official auxiliary of the Air Force.

Every search should follow the same principles:

- Plan and organize the search.
- Respond fast.
- Confine the search area.
- Search for clues.
- Search by night as well as day.

Usually a hasty team goes in first. They may have rescue dogs trained to follow air scents. A grid search, with lines of people marching through sections of the search area side by side, is the last resort, and usually done only when looking for someone presumed unresponsive or deceased. It is slow, requires many people, is hard to coordinate, and may damage evidence.

You should provide a subject profile to the person in charge of the search. It should include:

- personality;
- physical condition and fitness;
- how the subject might react in different situations;
- medical or mental health problems;
- emotional state;
- clothing and equipment carried;
- circumstances and terrain in which your group lost contact.

Many SAR teams have an interview form that includes all the questions you should ask. If the lost person may have come out alone, then the SAR team will probably do a "bastard search" of likely places first, such as the local bars. But a wilderness search has four phases:
- Locate.
- Access and assess.
- Stabilize.
- Transport.

Locating the lost person requires good navigation and route-finding skills. Getting access may require technical skills and equipment (e.g., for steep rock, caves or mines, white water or snow and ice). Then the searchers need to stabilize their subject, both physically and emotionally, before packaging him or her for transport. Transport may be by sled, litter, snowmobile or helicopter depending on the situation and how urgent the problems are.

Aeromedical transport

In 1870, during the siege of Paris, the French used hot air balloons to evacuate 160 wounded soldiers across the Prussian lines. Then in 1912, during World War I, they converted fighter planes to air ambulances by rigging them to carry litters. The United States began using air ambulances in 1920, and in World War II transported 1,400,000 wounded by air, with only 46 deaths en route. This record owed much to the practice of training flight surgeons, nurses, and medics to give care during air transport.

In 1944, the first casualties were evacuated by helicopter, from Burma. During the Korean War, just 11 Medevac helicopters evacuated 17,700 casualties; and in Vietnam from 1962-1967, helicopters evacuated 94,000. As transportation time decreased, so did mortality. In World War I, it took 18 hours to get the wounded from the battlefield to the hospital, and mortality was 18%. In Vietnam, it took an average of 1 to 2 hours, and mortality dropped to 1.8%.

In 1993, 195 helicopter services were operational in the United States, and 175 of them were affiliated with hospitals or other health care organizations. They transported 172,000 patients. Under the Military Assistance to Safety and Traffic Act (MAST), the military provides helicopters for civilian rescue and transport when requested, if they have the helicopters and staff available, and their budget allows it.

Helicopter capabilities

A helicopter's service ceiling is the highest altitude at which it can climb 100 feet per minute. Different models have ceilings ranging from 13,000 to 20,000 feet. But in the Western United States, they are required to fly at least 2,000 feet above the terrain. Most EMS helicopters can fly at 120 to 150 miles per hour, and different models have ranges of anywhere from 325 to 565 miles, not allowing for wind.

Helicopters are limited by weather and visibility. They cannot safely fly in very high winds or thunderstorms. Most EMS helicopters are not equipped for instrument flight rules (IFR), which are generally used only for airport-to-airport transport. So they will usually only fly on days with visibility of at least three miles. Helicopters are also limited by their load capacity, which must include fuel, equipment, and crew as well as patients.

Landing and safety

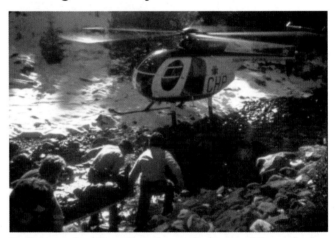

Helicopter landing. People on the ground keep their distance and wait within the vision field of the pilot.

Helicopters need a fairly level landing site at least 75 feet square and 100 feet or more when it is windy. They also need a clear flight path with no trees or other obstacles, since they normally land and take off at a fairly shallow angle. They do not fly straight up and down. They create a tremendous downdraft when landing and taking off, so you should clear away all debris from the landing area and secure all loose equipment as well as the patient. Helicopters land into the wind, so stand at or beyond the front edge of the landing area with your back to the wind, looking at the helicopter as it approaches. If possible, mark the corners of the landing area with smoke.

Once the helicopter has landed, wait for the pilot's hand signal before approaching. Make eye contact to be sure that the pilot sees you and approach from the front or front side only. Duck down as you near the blades, because they can flex quite a bit. If the helicopter is on or near a slope, approach from the downhill side only. Make sure all hats and clothing are secured on yourself and the patient. Carry all equipment below shoulder height.

A helicopter with a winch system may be able to lower a cable with a litter and crew member to extricate a patient from terrain where a landing is not practical. This technique is also used by Coast Guard helicopters to extricate people from the water or a sinking ship, and is shown in the 2006 film, *The Guardian* (made with the help of the Coast Guard).

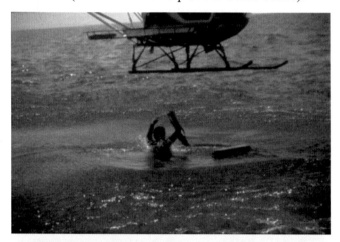

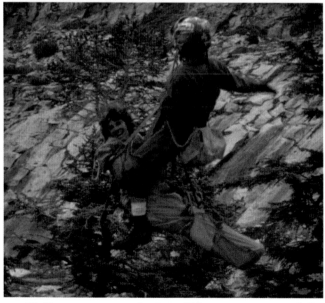

Helicopter rescues in the wilderness are potentially dangerous to the pilot and crew, especially at high altitude and in uncertain weather. So you should not request a helicopter rescue unless it is necessary, because of the condition of the patient or the lack of viable alternatives.

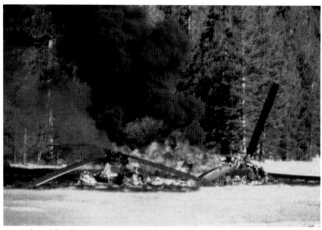

Crashed helicopter burning.

Conclusion

Emergency medical services (EMS), based on the concept of bringing urgent care to patients who need it and transporting them to safety, has a long history in the military. But as a formal and regulated part of the civilian medical system in the United States, EMS began only in the last quarter of the 20th Century. Even in urban situations, the trained responders of the EMS system are sometimes injured or killed trying to help others. Wilderness rescue and emergency care are often much more hazardous, and many of those who perform it are volunteers. So preparation for wilderness activities should include training in safety and self-help; and you should only call for rescue from the wilderness if you really need it.

Chapter 33. Herbal first aid

By Charles Garcia

Director: California School of Traditional Hispanic Herbalism (www.hispanicherbs.com)

No outdoors enthusiast should rely solely on medicinal plants found while backpacking, hiking, or camping for first aid. A well-stocked first aid kit is more convenient in an emergency than grubbing in the rain for medicinal leaves or roots somewhere on the Appalachian Trail or the Pacific Crest Trail.

But you may forget to bring a first aid kit. And even if you do bring it, the contents may not be adequate for dealing with the problems you encounter. Moreover, most of the more potent medications you might need in an emergency require a prescription. So you may need to seek your own remedies in the plants from which many modern medications are derived.

This chapter will introduce you to some of the most common medicinal plants, and how they have been traditionally used. However, you cannot learn to do herbal first aid safely from a book. The next step is to learn and practice identifying the living plants with an experienced herbalist or botanist. Many of these plants are ubiquitous not only in the wilderness, but also in urban patches of greenery. Once you can identify the plants reliably, you can then practice preparing herbal remedies from them.

Terms and warnings

Herbs are most commonly used as **tinctures**--made with an ethyl alcohol base and steeped for three or four weeks before being ready to use as an internal medicine. Herbal remedies made with an isopropyl alcohol base are called **liniments** and are for external use only. In the American wild west, they were called Horse Medicine, used on both horses and people. But they were never drunk (except in the movies).

In an outdoor setting, waiting three or four weeks for an herb to be ready to use is not practical, so the use of herbs outdoors is limited to teas, infusions, decoctions, washes, and poultices.

A **tea** is made by pouring hot or boiling water on leaves, bark, or roots (usually dry) and allowing it to steep for a specified length of time, usually ten to fifteen minutes. If the plant is fresh, it is better to simmer or boil it.

An **infusion** is made by steeping an herb in hot or cold water, for internal or external use.

A **decoction** is made by simmering or boiling leaves, barks, or roots for a specified amount of time. The time varies according to the remedy and the altitude: 15-30 minutes below 1000 feet, and up to an hour at higher elevations.

A **wash** is the external use of either a tea or decoction upon an injured area. The old term for this was a **tisane**.

A **poultice** is the application of mashed herbs or roots directly on an affected area. It can be applied either fresh or slightly warmed. It should NOT be chewed. While that may have been done in the days of the mountain man and is still shown in movies, the mouth is one of the filthiest places in the human body.

Herbs are seldom placed directly on an injury because debris or contaminants may cause infection; a barrier such as a thin piece of cloth allows the oils, juices, or other efficacious parts of the herb to drip directly into the wound. If you lack a suitable barrier, however, and the wound is life threatening, then applying the plant (well rinsed of debris) directly may be the only alternative.

Arnica

Arnica (*Arnica montana*) is also known by the names mountain tobacco and (confusingly) leopard's bane and wolfsbane - two names that it shares with the entirely different plant, aconite. The arnica plant has a lovely bright yellow, daisy-like flower that blooms around July and early August. Found throughout the world, it is often considered a mountain plant, which in the Northern hemisphere can bloom as high as 11,000 feet.

A legend has it that mountain travelers in ancient Europe used to chew the fresh arnica plant to relieve sore, aching muscles and bruises from falls. This might be true, but it is more likely they applied the crushed leaves to their muscles rather than risking the possible reactions from eating this plant, including rapid heartbeat and nausea.

For external use, arnica makes an effective poultice for **sore and cramped muscles**. It quickly decreases pain and helps prevent the **swelling and bruising** associated with sprains, crushed fingers, crushed toes, and broken bones associated with climbing or hiking mountain paths.

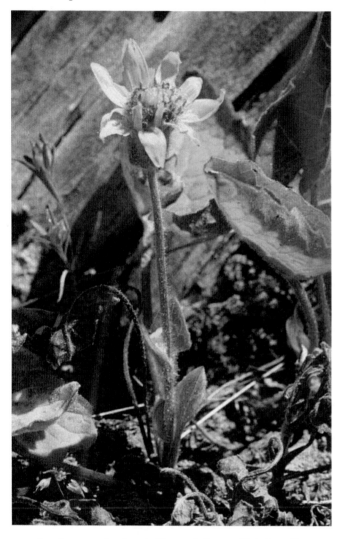

Arnica works best if used immediately after an injury occurs. Americans tend to use the blossoms of the plant for an effective poultice. Europeans prefer the roots. Asian mountaineers tend to favor the leaves. The entire plant is medicinal. A fresh poultice of the plant should be reapplied each hour. Arnica creams and gels are easy to obtain and wouldn't take up too much room in a pack. Athletes have used commercially available arnica for over a generation without ill effect. Clinical trials at Sloan-Kettering have shown it to be effective in the treatment inflammation from osteoarthritis. Other studies have concluded that arnica is completely ineffective for the healing of bruises. I leave it up to the injured to decide.

Blackberry leaf

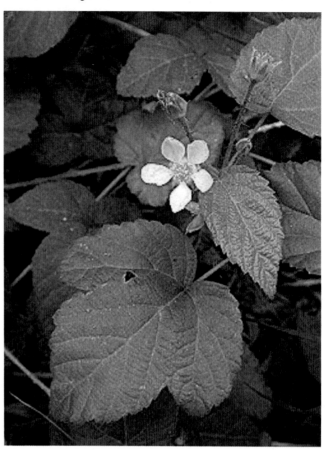

The Runs, Camp Cramps, or Montezuma's Revenge may not be considered life threatening at home, but can be in the wilderness if the sufferer is unable to retain liquids. Common diarrhea is usually treated with OTC medications such Pepto-Bismol. In liquids and tablet form, this pink medication is the remedy of choice for many travelers. In Third World countries, diarrhea is one of the leading causes of death in newborns and young children from rapid dehydration. If rehydration formulas are unavailable, death often follows.

The old name for this problem was **dysentery**. But true dysentery is an inflammatory disorder of the intestine resulting in severe diarrhea (sometimes more than a liter of fluid an hour), containing blood and mucus in the feces and often accompanied with fever and abdominal pain. Up to a century ago, it killed more soldiers and civilians during wartime than gunpowder. If this strikes a backpacking party, it could leave them too weak to reach help. And if it strikes one or two members of the party, it can quickly spread to others.

John Muir, the great naturalist and co-founder of the Sierra Club, noted in his early journals that certain native tribes used a tea made from blackberry leaves

(*Rubus canadensis*) as a remedy for what was then known as the "bloody flux," or dysentery as we know it today. Spanish padres already knew this from first-hand experience over a generation before. Though the native California blackberry is difficult to find these days, its now feral commercial cousin, the **Himalayan blackberry**, can be found in fields, valleys, woodlands, and lower mountain elevations throughout the United States and far into Canada. A decoction of blackberry leaves can ease the symptoms of moderate to severe **dysentery** and **diarrhea**.

To prepare this plant for medicinal use, simmer several leaves for 10 to 15 minutes to produce a light green liquid. If the diarrhea is severe, simmer the blackberry leaves longer until the decoction is brown. Drink two to three cups warm, without sugar or other sweetener. The tea is soothing with a slight celery taste when light green, but bitter when simmered to darker colors. Though not known as an intestinal antispasmodic, it can relieve common stomachache in half-cup doses. I recommend the tea be made only with fresh leaves.

Take care when harvesting the leaves, however, as poison oak often grows alongside blackberry. I suggest taking leaves from blackberry patches at least fifty feet from any visible poison oak. Also remember that blackberry bushes have serious thorns, particularly the Himalayan variety. The thorns on the stems can shred shirts, pants, and gloves.

Many herbal books suggest using the root of a blackberry bush for its medicinal properties, if you can actually get a blackberry root out of the ground without a pick and shovel. Otherwise stick to the upper portions of the plant. The ripe berries are a refreshing and nutritious addition to trail food.

Blueberry

The blueberry (*Vaccinium spp.*) is not only a culinary treat, but also a decent medicinal plant. North America Native Americans have used every part of the plant for medicinal purposes: flowers, fruit, leaves, young shoots, bark and roots. In the 12th century, Saint Hildegard of Bingen, mystic, nun, and the first woman to write on medicinal herbs, wrote that Bilberry (the equally effective European cousin of blueberry) fruits were good for inducing menstruation. Four centuries later, Hieronymus Bock, a German herbalist, claimed

that the berries were useful for the treatment of bladder stones, as well as lung and liver disorders.

In 18th century Germany, blueberries, either fresh or dried, were soaked in water to make infusions or syrups. The infusions were then used in the treatment of coughs, diarrhea, gout, and rheumatism, to relieve symptoms of typhoid fever, as a mouthwash to soothe mouth ulcers, as a diuretic, and to prevent scurvy. While our outdoor recreationalist may have no need to prevent scurvy or typhoid, one can still get mouth ulcers on the trail.

During WW2, improved night vision after eating bilberry jam was reported by British Royal Air Force pilots on bombing missions. These reports led to laboratory and clinical research on the effects of bilberry fruit extracts on the eyes and on the whole vascular system in the 1960's. Researchers concluded that the most effective medicinal use for bilberry or blueberry extract appears to be for improving micro-circulation, which in turn benefits the capillaries serving the eyes, and mucous membranes of the digestive and pulmonary systems.

For **diabetics**, blueberries will help increase insulin production. This can be helpful when the supply of insulin is low, or increased exertion has stressed the body, though it cannot replace insulin injections or other diabetic medications. When used as a tea or decoction, blueberries will lower sugar levels in type II (insulin resistant) diabetics. It is rare that one plant can be used for both types of diabetes.

Because the plant is rich in tannins, it can cause some stomach distress. The leaf is an effective remedy for **diarrhea** while the fresh berries can produce diarrhea in some people and stop it in others. In the far north where mild cases of scurvy can still be found on homesteads, the fruit is used for vitamin C, anemia, and colitis. A decoction of the roots has historically been used for congestive heart failure and urinary stones. Fresh berry juice makes a good gargle for **sore throats** or a mouthwash for **inflamed gums**. Externally, because of the tannic acids, the juice has been used as a wash for **skin eruptions**, **sores**, **wounds**, and **mild burns**. It is an **astringent** and may be mildly anti-fungal, though opinions on this are varied. It could be that the berry has anti-fungal properties only at certain times during its growth.

The most commonly found blueberry is known as the low bush variety (*Vaccinium angustifolium Aiton*) and can be found in bogs, boreal forests, and pine barrens from the Eastern Seaboard, north to the Great Lakes region and into the Pacific northwest.

Chamomile

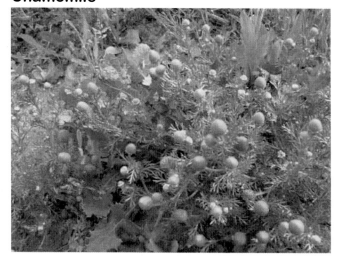

Chamomile is one of the most ancient medicinal herbs known to humankind. It is a member of the daisy (*Asteraceae*) family. Chamomile preparations are used in many cultures for ailments as diverse as fevers, inflammation, muscle spasms, menstrual disorders, insomnia, ulcers, wounds, gastrointestinal disorders, rheumatic pain, and hemorrhoids.

If you visit the battleground of Gettysburg, Pennsylvania, you may notice three medicinal herbs profusely growing in the fields where General Robert E. Lee sent his men into slaughter: yarrow, feverfew, and chamomile grow abundantly where once musket and cannon sounds shattered the summer stillness. In the summer, near the famed clump of trees that marks the limit of the Confederate advance, are thousands of small, white, daisy-like blossoms smelling faintly of apples. No wonder the ancient Greeks named chamomile, "the ground apple." Even the Spanish name for it, manzanilla, means "little apples."

The two most widely used medicinal species are Roman chamomile (*Chamaemelum nobile*) and German chamomile (*Matricuaria recuitita*). Flowering from spring through late summer, chamomile is known primarily as an herb to soothe upset stomachs. Most children are first introduced to chamomile tea by reading Beatrice Potter's Peter Rabbit. The story goes that after eating his way through Farmer Macgregor's garden and barely escaping the wrath of the long suffering farmer, Peter develops a stomach ache and is sent to bed by his mother after drinking a bitter cup of chamomile tea.

Chamomile is recognized as a treatment for a myriad of **stomach ailments** from gastritis to diverticulitis, so Mrs. Rabbit was wise in giving her son the tea for an upset tummy. However, if the tea was bitter, then Mrs. Rabbit let it steep too long. Chamomile is sweet and soothing if steeped for less than fifteen minutes. It will ease the pain of a spasmodic stomach and bring on a comfortable sleep.

Topically, the herb is an excellent anti-inflammatory. A wet poultice of the blossoms and leaves placed directly on inflamed skin will bring quick relief. Carried on camping and backpacking trips as a gentle sleep inducer, the moistened chamomile tea bags can also be placed on swollen eye lids and minor burns.

A simple poultice or wash with the tea is an easy treatment for **contact dermatitis**. The affected area should be thoroughly washed with a strong tea or decoction of the entire plant: blossoms, stems, leaves, and root. To avoid further irritation to the skin, the wash should be no warmer than skin temperature. Keeping the skin moist will speed the anti-inflammatory effects.

While not life threatening, **hemorrhoids** can quickly turn an outdoor adventure into an uncomfortable nightmare. While a wash would be of some comfort, a direct poultice of the blossoms and leaves is more effective. Some backpackers have suggested it is best to use just the blossoms while others favor the full poultice, lightly simmered and allowed to cool. Either will work.

Another uncomfortable problem (that affects only women) is **vaginitis**. A douche of the tea several times a day can ease or eliminate this condition. For douching with the tea, consider using a plastic bag or nitrile glove with a few small pinholes in the appropriate places to allow the tea or decoction to exit under pressure. The sufferer should restrict her movements for two or three days.

There have been a few documented cases of individuals with chamomile allergies. Those who have never used chamomile should do so in a safe environment before they use it in an emergency.

Chamomile should not be taken internally by anyone using the drug Warfarin or any other blood thinner, as it will increase the blood thinning effect.

Still, the most common use of chamomile is as a remedy for upset stomach. So if on your way to a new campsite you happen to eat your way through someone's garden (or stop at one too many fast food joints) take some advice from Mrs. Rabbit and drink a cup or two of chamomile tea.

Charcoal

Although not an herb, charcoal from a campfire can help in cases of food poisoning. This is not recommended for simple stomachache or over-indulgence. But **food poisoning** (or other poisoning) on the trail can be a matter of life and death. If you suspect poisoning, carefully scrape off the outer areas of a piece of wood charcoal (not leftover commercial charcoal briquettes), removing all gray portions. Break into bite size pieces and swallow. If you can't swallow it this way, break it into a fine powder and mix with water. Do this several times and stay well-hydrated.

Chickweed

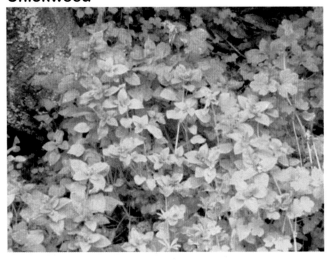

Chickweed (*Stellaria media*) looks like a ground cover when in full bloom. It can be found in shady empty lots, along sidewalks, in moist sections of parks and forest, in older established neighborhoods, riparian areas, and many backyards. It has a very tiny star-shaped flower with five petals. Its leaves are oval in shape and the stems have very fine hairs that sometimes can only be seen in full sunlight.

The hairs are on only one side of the stem. This plant likes a couple of hours of sunlight, but prefers to snooze in cool shade. It is edible, and can be used in salads as well as soups. It should only be cooked for five or ten minutes at most. It has a slightly sweet spinach flavor

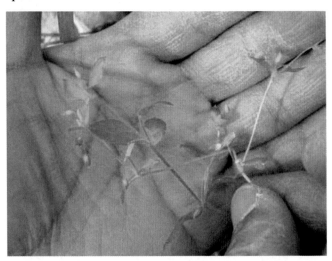

The young leaves have a mild taste, while the older leaves occasionally taste peppery. Chickweed is rich in iron, copper, and vitamin C. Long distance backpackers add this plant to freeze dried meals when they can find it. It has an unusual aroma when cut fresh. Imagine a mild scent of celery and cilantro. Perhaps that's why backpackers value it so highly for wild salads. Like dandelion, however, this plant is mildly **diuretic** and will increase your urinary output. If used at dinner, it is guaranteed to wake you with a full bladder at two or three in the morning.

The fresh plant can be used as an emergency poultice for **burns**. It takes a great deal of the plant to make an effective poultice, but chickweed is extremely prolific. Touching the plant with your bare hands will bring on a cooling sensation. On burns, it may feel almost like ice for several minutes. The crushed plant can be placed against a first or second-degree burn. The fresh juice has slight analgesic properties. Though it will not completely kill the pain, it will make it more bearable. Fresh poultices should be placed on the burn every fifteen to thirty minutes.

Chickweed is also a decent **anti-inflammatory**. It is used topically for swellings. It is especially useful for swellings of the foot, fingers, and hands caused by sprains, arthritis, and gout. Though it is not effective for deep injuries, it will ease most inflammations that appear directly under the skin. This makes it an excellent quick remedy for sunburn.

For **diabetics** who may have a sugar spike and are hoarding their insulin supply, a decoction of chickweed will cause a rapid reduction of glucose in the blood. It should be noted that it is not a sugar stabilizer like dandelion or Devil's Club. It just increases urinary output, which may help reduce glucose concentration in the blood and enable the diabetic to walk out.

Cinnamon

Not found on any hiking trail that I know of, cinnamon has a place in your pack for its medicinal as well as culinary virtues. A strong decoction of the Chinese hard stick variety (*Cinnamomum cassia*) is a remedy for **spasmodic stomach** with projectile vomiting, nausea, and chills. Cinnamon is also an **antifungal** and can be used as a wash. A female herbalist friend has successfully used the same cinnamon decoction as a douche for yeast infections. This could be useful for long distance women backpackers who may develop serious vaginal infections.

Coltsfoot

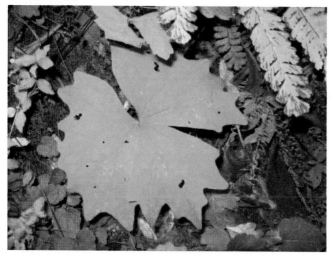

There are two plants called coltsfoot: *Tussilago farfara*, and *Petasites frigidus*, the latter called Western coltsfoot. *T. farfara* is native to several locations in Eastern Europe and Asia where it is believed to have originated. It is a common plant in North and South America where it was introduced, most likely by Spanish settlers, as a medicinal herb. The plant is now often found in waste and disturbed places and along roadsides and paths. In some areas it is considered a weed and is eradicated. The plant spreads by seed and by rhizomes, so dozens can be found clumped together. The blossoms resemble dandelions but appear in spring before the first dandelions show up.

Western coltsfoot, *P. frigidus,* is native to the Northern Hemisphere from the arctic to the temperate area of North America, Europe, and Asia, and is a member of the sunflower family. It does not resemble a dandelion, but has a blossom with white, pink, and sometimes light blue blossoms. The leaves can become quite large, in some circumstances twice as large as a man's hand.

T. farfara was prized by Nicholas Culpepper, who wrote in 1653: "The fresh leaves, or juice, or syrup thereof, is good for a bad dry cough, or wheezing and shortness of breath. The dry leaves are best for those who have their rheums and distillations upon their lungs causing a cough: for which also the dried leaves taken as tobacco, or the root is very good. The distilled water hereof simply or with elder-flowers or nightshade is a singularly good remedy against all agues, to drink 2 oz. at a time and apply cloths wet therein to the head and stomach, which also does much good being applied to any hot swellings or inflammations."

The great Maude Grieve agreed with Culpepper and wrote in 1921: "The botanical name, Tussilago, signifies 'cough dispeller,' and Coltsfoot has justly been termed 'nature's best herb for the lungs and her most eminent thoracic.' The smoking of the leaves for a cough has the recommendation of Dioscorides, Galen, Pliny, Boyle, and other great authorities, both ancient and modern, Linnaeus stating that the Swedes of his time smoked it for that purpose. Pliny recommended the use of both roots and leaves. The leaves are the basis of the British Herb Tobacco, in which Coltsfoot predominates, the other ingredients being Buckbean, Eyebright, Betony, Rosemary, Thyme, Lavender, and Chamomile flowers. This relieves asthma and also the difficult breathing of old bronchitis. Those suffering from asthma, catarrh and other lung troubles derive much benefit from smoking this Herbal Tobacco, the use of which does not entail any of the injurious effects of ordinary tobacco."

Unfortunately for Ms. Grieve, modern science has found that smoking this herb can cause liver damage. So recreational smoking is out. But conscientious herbalists still give small amounts of the tea or the dried leaves to be smoked for out of control **coughing**.

In emergencies it can be used for asthmatic attacks when an inhaler is days away.

P. frigidus was used for the same purposes, especially by the native peoples of the Klamath, up along the Pacific Coast, and into Canada. Although it is not today highly regarded as an edible plant, there are reports that the Western coltsfoot was used by Native Americans as a potherb and medicinal tea. Both eastern and western species were used as a salt substitute, by first rolling the leaves (and petioles) into a ball while still green. After being dried they were placed on top of a very small fire on a rock and burned to obtain a salty flavored ash.

Karuk Indians along the Klamath River in the not so distant past used the roots and rhizomes for the treatment of coughs, colds and chest ailments by making a strong decoction of the plant. The tea is a mild remedy for asthmatic conditions caused by over exertion and sudden shock. Western coltsfoot was often combined with mullein and mugwort as an herbal cigar to help relieve cough, open up bronchial airways, and help ease a person to sleep.

Comfrey

In the same league as arnica, comfrey (*Symphytum officinale*) has been cultivated for at least 2500 years as a healing herb. A large bushy plant with slightly prickly hair on the leaves, comfrey was originally brought to the United States by English settlers as a medicinal plant. It was commonly known as **knitbone**. The name accurately describes its ability to knit cells together. The word comfrey is derived from the Latin word for "grow together."

Common in the mid-West as a fodder plant, comfrey has escaped from family farms to bedevil state agricultural agents for generations. Comfrey supposedly grows best in rich loamy soil and does poorly in most other types. But as with all other herbs, comfrey does not read agriculture manuals. In bad soil and poor weather, the plant may send up small leaves and few blossoms but will still survive until a good rain re-vitalizes it for a few days. Large patches of this plant can be found along the Appalachian Trail as far north as Northern Maryland.

Because the leaves are prickly, when comfrey is used as a poultice for a broken bone, torn ligament, or severe sprain, they should be mashed to green pulp.

Comfrey also has a high water and mucilage content. It can be used effectively on burns for this reason. But be sure to singe off the hairs first or thoroughly mash the leaves into a wet paste. Some individuals suffer minor but irritating contact dermatitis when harvesting the leaves, so wear some sort of protection for your hands.

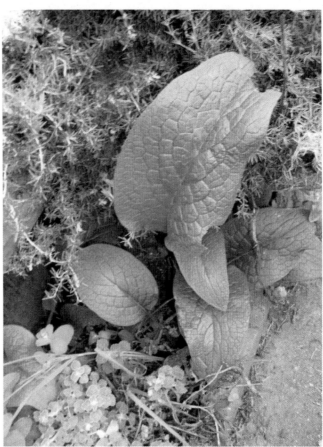

The root is more effective than the leaves for **broken bones**, but can be very difficult to harvest. It should be crushed into a paste and spread onto the injured area. Some herbalists suggest the mash be slightly warmed.

A decoction can be made from the leaves to speed healing from within. Simmer a hand full of cut leaves in two or three cups of water for no more than 10 minutes. Several years ago there was some evidence that comfrey caused cancer in laboratory rats. Use of comfrey as a *fodder* plant was suddenly discontinued. But there is no evidence that drinking an occasional cup of comfrey tea will cause liver cancer in humans.

Although technically not in the anodyne (painkilling) family of herbs, comfrey has been known to alleviate severe pain connected with sores, burns, swollen tissue, back pain, and broken bones. A poultice of well-pulped leaves should be placed directly on the affected area.

Serious **burns** can end any wilderness trip. First cool the burn immediately with water. Then, if a comfrey plant is nearby and rescue is at least 24 hours away, apply the well-mashed leaves as a poultice directly on the skin if necessary. The poultice must be reapplied as many times as possible while waiting for rescue. Anecdotal evidence suggests that comfrey works best with second degree (partial thickness) burns. For minor sunburn, a bandana soaked with the juice of the leaves can be laid onto the skin.

Fennel

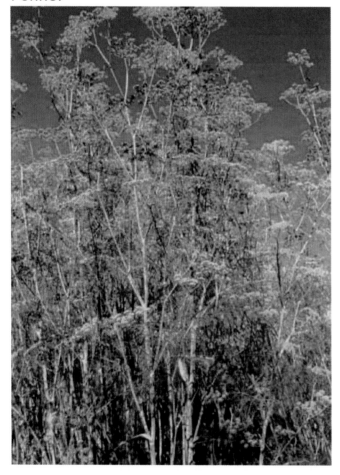

The Spanish padres who originally brought it to the New World called it hinojo. Botanists call it *Foeniculum vulgare*. Kids call it licorice weed. Most herbalists call it fennel. Today fennel is best known as a cooking spice, but this versatile herb also has a long history of therapeutic use as an herbal tea. Since ancient times, fennel has had a rich culinary and medicinal history. The ancient Greeks knew fennel by the name "marathon". The plain where they defeated the Persian army in 490 B.C. was called Marathon, probably because it was overgrown with fennel. In Greek myth, Prometheus delivered fire to man hidden in a fennel stalk. Fennel was revered by the Greeks and Romans for its medicinal and culinary properties.

Culpepper gave the first description of fennel's properties in the English language: "The leaves or seed boiled in barley water and drunk, are good for nurses, to increase their milk and make it more wholesome for the child. The leaves, or rather the seeds, boiled in water, stayeth the hiccup and taketh away nausea or inclination to sickness. The seed and the roots much more help to open obstructions of the liver, spleen, and gall, and thereby relieve the painful and windy swellings of the spleen, and the yellow jaundice, as also the gout and cramp. The seed is of good use in medicines for shortness of breath and wheezing, by stoppings of the lungs. The roots are of most use in physic, drinks and broths that are taken to cleanse the blood, to open obstructions of the liver, to provoke urine, and amend the ill colour of the face after sickness."

Considered a weed through most of the western states, it can be found in semi-desert areas, valleys, and lower mountain elevations. It has a long hollow bright green stem, and yellow umbels of tiny flowers, with thousands of green and string-like leaves.

Fennel "seeds" (actually tiny fruits) have been chewed to help dispel hunger pains during fasts as well as long hikes. Fennel is also a popular flavoring in many beverages and foods, because of its strong licorice taste. One constituent of fennel's volatile oil is anethole, which may be responsible for its reputation as a digestive aid. Anethole assists in the metabolism of fats and aids in a thorough digestion, especially of too many freeze dried dinners and energy bars.

Fennel is a proven **antispasmodic** for the lower intestines. It increases urination and decreases inflammation of the urinary tract. Add this herb to a tea for severe **stomach distress**. You can chew on its string-like leaves to improve digestion, but then spit them out, because they are not easily digested.

Late in the season, fennel seeds can be easily pulled from the dried stems of the plant. A teaspoon of these seeds simmered or boiled briefly in a cup of water will make a sweet licorice flavored tea. One to two cups will ease stomach spasms and dry heaves. In early spring and summer, the plant is lush and leafy. Simmer the greenest part of the stalk and some leaves into a sweet, dark green tea. Drink only in sips.

Both types of tea can be used as a mild anti-inflammatory **eyewash**, which immediately brings a cooling sensation to inflamed eyes. Dip a clean cloth in the tea and wipe the eyes gently for several minutes. This is not a treatment for pink eye, but rather a remedy for tired trail worn eyes.

A **body wash** of fennel tea can soothe soreness and help bring on sleep. It will also rid the body of hikers-hives, that slight irritation caused by too many days in the same clothes.

Wild ginger

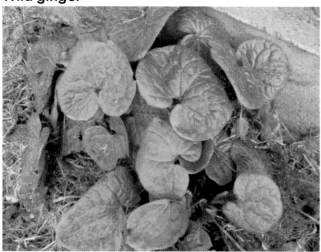

Wild ginger (*Asarum canadense)* has no relation to the ginger found in grocery stores, Asian restaurants, and Chinese markets. Known as snakeroot to natives and early settlers, it is found along the Northern Pacific coast as well as hiking trails in the Hawaiian Islands. Wild ginger grows well hidden in Redwood forests from Santa Cruz County in California to the coastal range of British Columbia. This plant prefers shade, wet weather and redwoods. It is more common at elevations of 3,500 to 7000 feet, but is also found near sea-level in coastal redwoods. The leaves are heart shaped, dark green and leathery, and when crushed give off a strong ginger scent. It has been found as far east as the western mountains of Idaho and Montana, and was once common in the eastern states, where some patches still exist in the cool dark groves of the Appalachian Mountains and Adirondacks.

The North American variety is called *Asarum canadense* because it was first identified in Canada.

European wild ginger *(Asarum europaeum)* was highly regarded by the Egyptians, Greeks and Romans for its medicinal qualities, especially for the application that gave it the name birthwort: assisting a woman in the postpartum discharge of the placenta. *A. europaeum* was cultivated in Europe as an ingredient in a variety of purgatives, as a headache remedy, as a treatment for deafness, and as a palliative for a queasy stomach. It was considered somewhat a panacea, taken in small doses every day to promote general health. To this end, it was one of the ingredients in some types of snuff. It was supposedly used in France as an emetic to induce vomiting after the consumption of an excessive amount of alcohol.

A. canadense was consumed by North American inhabitants as a food additive because of its pleasant, aromatic taste that has been likened to mild pepper and ginger mixed. Early colonists ground the leaves and roots and dried them to produce a powder that was used as a general spice for otherwise bland foods. They probably adopted this practice from Native Americans, who added powdered ginger root to meals made with meat or fish. Ground up ginger root was also added to an Ojibwe dish made from bottom-feeding catfish to offset the taste of mud. The settlers of the Southern Appalachians made candied ginger by boiling the roots and then dipping them in syrup. It was also used as a scent for clothing to cloak the more pungent, earthy smells that lack of frequent washing would cause or, for our purposes, the smell of camp clothing after three weeks on the Pacific Crest Trail.

The leaves are mildly **antiseptic** and anti-microbial and can be used like band aids. They are most effective if slightly steamed or simmered first. If this is not possible, bruising the leaf before placing it on the affected area will help bring out the medicinal qualities of the plant.

The root and rhizomes, when made into a strong tea or decoction, will break up the deepest bronchial **congestion**; but it will not produce coughs (so it is not an expectorant). Forced or chronic coughing will then bring up large amounts of phlegm, allowing for easier breathing.

A decoction made by lightly simmering the leaves provides a tea for difficult or painful **menses**. Two or three cups of the tea provide relief and easier flow during this time.

The tea or decoction can also be used to break fevers by causing copious amounts of sweat. Any time the plant is used for this purpose, the person must be given large amounts of water to replace fluids lost through sweating. Rehydration (or electrolyte) powder can be added to the water in conservative amounts.

A wash made from a decoction of the leaf, root, and rhizomes is a decent **antifungal** for common athlete's foot or the more painful *Tinea cruris*, also known as Jock Itch, Crotch Itch, and Ringworm of the Groin (although it is not ringworm.). This condition is caused by a fungal infection around the groin and can be found on either sex. While not particularly life threatening, it can open up the body to other opportunistic infections such as *Candida albicans*, *Staphylococcus,* and *Cellulitis*. Washing thoroughly with wild ginger and then allowing the groin and other affected areas to dry completely will help with this condition.

Honey

Approved by the Australian and New Zealand medical establishments and the FDA for sale as an **antiseptic**, honey is being used on wounds and second degree burns (as described in the chapter on wound care). The sugar in honey kills bacteria by drawing out their fluid across the cell membranes. Honey is also acidic, which further inhibits bacterial growth. Long used as a food preservative, and long used by herbalists throughout the world, honey is highly effective for topical wounds, surgical wounds, and burns.

An Australian study has verified what folklore healers have long suspected: the darker the honey, the more effective antibacterial properties it has. Lighter grade honeys have higher water content. The darker honeys, from wildflowers and eucalyptus blossoms, not only have a robust flavor. They also have an enzyme (glucose oxidase) producing a low concentration of hydrogen peroxide (not enough to damage tissues) that also inhibits bacterial growth.

Manzanita

When my wife and I attended college together, we often camped out in the foothills of the Sierra Nevada. We had one camping spot near a quarry surrounded by manzanita bushes (*Arctostaphylos manzanita*). Many years later we tried to find the same spot during a visit to our old alma mater. But manzanita had overrun the old path and the camping spot. Considered the Conan the Barbarian of invasive plants, manzanita is loathed by those who must live near or hike through it. Also, the wood contains highly volatile oils. It burns quick and hot. Don't expect to outrun a sudden fire if you are surrounded by manzanita. Manzanita grows at elevations of 2500ft. to 7500 ft. It is a handsome plant, with twisting branches, fairly thick, ovate leaves, and small hanging flowers pollinated by male mosquitoes. And where male mosquitoes are found, the blood-sucking female of the species can't be far behind. The smooth bark is red or orange. It grows as ground hugging shrubs or trees up to 20 feet tall.

The Spanish word "manzanita" means little apple. Though the plant's tart red berry, like cranberry, can be made palatable with lots of sugar, it does not resemble an apple in either in color or taste.

Manzanita is often considered a woman's plant because of its use as a **urinary tract disinfectant**. But this plant is just as effective on males as it is on females. Widely used in the past by native-Americans and early Hispanic settlers, manzanita leaves were made into a tea to ease urinary problems. The tea works best when the urine seems more alkaline or has taken on a sharp odor. Two teaspoons of the leaf to a large cup of water is a common recipe. The tea and decoction are antiseptic, antimicrobial and antibacterial

Because of its high tannin content, some 7 % percent by volume of dried leaf, manzanita is best used as a cold or cooled infusion, followed by several cups of water. The tea can cause nausea and stomach irritation if taken without food or water. If this occurs, drink more water. One cup from three to (at the most) five times a day should be adequate for most urinary bacterial infections. Herbalists consider the dried leaves easier to use as a tea. Fresh leaves should be made into a decoction and allowed to sit until it is tepid. The tea is vile tasting. The decoction is worse.

Because the tea and decoction are astringent, they can also be used topically for **bleeding** or weeping wounds. Some Hispanics have used it for skin eruptions caused by poison oak. This causes the open sores to dry up. It is also a painful, but effective, treatment for hemorrhoids. Soak a clean cloth or bandana in a decoction of the leaves and place it on the offending portion of the body.

Miner's lettuce

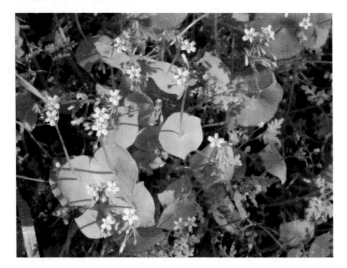

Miner's lettuce (*Claytonia perfolatia*) is often considered a weed in backyards. But for the original 49ers (the gold miners, not the football team) it was an important source of nourishment to ward off scurvy. Found at lower elevations and as high as 2000 feet throughout the Pacific states, this is one of the few American native plants introduced to Europe, where it is called winter purslane and is used for salads and stew seasoning. The leaves of the plant are small, round to oval, with a stem and small white blossom growing from its center. The same leaves can be used as a poultice for minor burns.

While backpackers and long distance hikers enjoy it primarily as a food extender, the California natives ate the fleshy leaves raw or steamed and made a tea from the roots for **constipation**. Though not life threatening, constipation is a common and unpleasant outdoor malady that can be brought on by the change from one's usual diet. The roots can be eaten raw to improve digestion or taken as a tea to improve peristaltic action in the lower intestines. This is a gentle laxative, but will not have immediate results. Two to three cups of the tea should provide relief within a day or two.

Fresh, lightly steamed or sautéed, Miner's Lettuce will improve most backpacker meals. Several Native American tribes of the Eastern Sierra used the plant to help stimulate appetite, so it could be used by long haul hikers who simply can't abide another packet of dehydrated stew.

The Shoshone Indians of Nevada used the crushed plant as a poultice for rheumatic pain. Exactly why this worked is unknown, and the plant is not used as an analgesic by most western herbalists. Although it is used as a poultice for minor burns, the Shoshone and Paiute tribes made large poultices of miner's lettuce and prickly poppy for major burns, but the ratio of plant to plant is unknown.

Mugwort

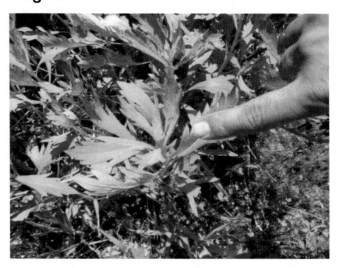

Artemisia douglasiana, known as California mugwort, Douglas's sagewort, Dream Plant, and the no longer politically correct name, Chinaman's herb, is one of many plants called mugwort in the genus Artemisia. The Asian variety has been highly touted as a medicinal plant for a thousand years. *A. douglasiana* is native to Western North America. It thrives in the Western United States and can be found along the coast as far south as Baja California, Mexico. It can almost always be found in cooler shady areas with an abundance of water, or watery meadows. It has been found growing at six thousand feet in the Sierra and lower altitudes in the Cascades.

Its leaves contain the chemicals thujone, which is suspected to have mild psychoactive properties, and cineole, which is **antibacterial** agent. Thujone is toxic in high doses. Chinese apothecaries recognized the plant as a relative to their own mugwort and quickly adapted it to traditional methods of healing. Whether they consulted with Native Americans on their uses is unknown.

Mugwort can be used for various purposes if found by a hiking trail. A mild tea made of the fresh leaves can relieve a sun-induced **headache**. The same tea is effective for **fevers**. A stronger tea or decoction can be used for a sudden **bronchial infection**. The steam has been known to clear congested sinuses, allowing for an easier sleep. The leaves make a decent poultice for sore muscles or a twisted ankle. The anti-inflammatory action has yet to be explained, and is doubted by some scientists and herbalists.

Mullein

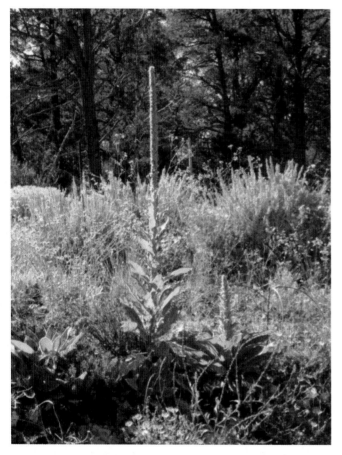

Mullein (*Verbascum thapsus*) grows in fields, burned-out forest areas, along country roadsides, and in waste places, from Maine to Santa Monica. It is easy to recognize with its tall, straight stem, large soft wooly leaves, and its long, dense spike of yellow flowers. Native Americans have used mullein as a health aid for centuries. Applied topically, the bruised or mashed leaves offer some relief for **minor burns**, joint pain from a too heavy backpack, and **hemorrhoids**. Mullein has astringent properties, and is useful in healing **wounds**. The large soft pads can be placed on wounds once the injury is cleaned of debris. The pads can soak up a heavy amount of blood, if necessary. Doubling or tripling the leaves will make a good compress if other materials are unavailable.

An infusion of the yellow flowers steeped in warm olive oil is an old but good remedy for **earaches** and ear infections. Earaches, though not usually serious, can be quite painful. In an outdoor emergency, a teaspoon or two of the flowers or crushed leaves can be simmered for 10 to 15 minutes in olive oil. While still warm to the touch (but not hot), drops can be placed in the affected ear. Cotton, cloth, or paper tissue (soaked in the decoction) can be used to block the ear canal from irritating noises or cold drafts of air.

Mullein is also beneficial when used on **abrasions** (road rash) and soothes irritated skin. On a wildcrafting trip some years past, a student of mine repeatedly wore shorts in a field of drying brush and chaparral. By days end, her legs were scraped and swollen. Luckily, we were in a field with mid-summer mullein. We bruised the leaves and applied them directly to her legs. In the morning, the most severe scratches had healed with hardly a sign.

Mullein also works as an **antispasmodic**. A tea made from the leaves relieves stomach cramps and helps control diarrhea. The same tea can relieve a chronic or asthmatic cough. The tea should be strained before being consumed, as the small soft hairs on the leaves are not digestible. Coffee filters are very effective in straining any type of herbal tea.

The large soft leaves were used by Native American women as **menstrual pads** and can still be used as such. Former students of mine suggest using the largest and softest leaves for this purpose. They can be trimmed as needed. Though not as absorbent as cotton or natural sponge, it is an alternative to soft grasses in an emergency situation.

Oak Bark, Pine Needles, Willow

Although not life threatening, hemorrhoids are embarrassing and debilitating, especially on backpacking and camping trips. Boiling pine needles, oak bark, or small branches of willow or its bark, will make a potent **anti-hemorrhoidal** decoction. Soaking a sock in the still warm decoction and placing it on the offending vein will bring immediate relief. Several applications are recommended.

Oak bark, pine needles, and willow all have astringent properties, which can be used as washes for open wounds. Slightly antibacterial, the tea made from each plant inhibits or slows the growth of bacteria in the worst wounds. The astringency also aids in binding damaged cells, allowing for faster healing. After washing the injury thoroughly, a boiled piece of cloth can be used as a compress.

Although used by natives as a headache remedy, willow branch tea should be avoided. It is bitter and hard on the stomach.

Plantain

Plantain (*Pantago major* and various spp), that ubiquitous weed in your lawn and garden, growing through sidewalks of New York City and at 9000 feet on the flanks of Mt. Whitney, is also called the soldier's herb and **wound wort** because of its historical use after battles. *P. major* (originating in central China) is one of the most abundant and widely distributed medicinal herbs in the world. Poultices of plantain leaves were traditionally applied to **wounds**, stings, and sores in order to facilitate healing and prevent infection. Native Americans call it the white man's footsteps, as it seemed to crop up wherever white settlers went. It was supposedly brought to the United States by Puritan settlers, but this story may be apocryphal.

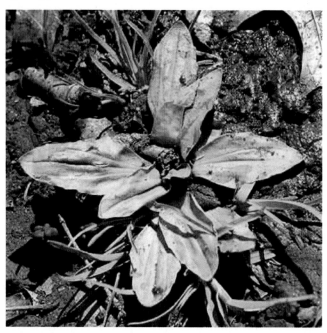

The active chemical constituents are *aucubin* and *allantoin*. *Aucubin* acts as an **anti-microbial** while *allantoin* stimulates **tissue regeneration**. The astringent properties of this invasive visitor are used to treat **diarrhea** and soothe raw internal membranes.

This is done by making a strong tea or decoction. Occasionally the leaves are eaten raw for these treatments.

Broadleaf plantain is also one of those plants touted by wild food enthusiasts as a nutritious wild edible. The taste is akin to kale. The young, tender leaves can be eaten raw, and the older, stringier leaves can be boiled in stews.

When ingested, the aucubin in plantain leaves increases uric acid excretions from the kidneys, forcing its expulsion through the urinary tract. This treatment was used by progressive doctors in dealing with the painful condition of **gout**. America's most famous gout sufferer, Benjamin Franklin, supposedly carried several pounds of this plant on his diplomatic missions to Europe, perhaps unaware that the plant grew in profusion there.

Historically, poultices of the leaves were used for **blood poisoning** caused by wounds from unclean knives, swords, and bayonets. If I ever had doubts about its efficacy for blood poisoning, I put them away the day a well-known Washington state herbalist related this story to me: Three days into a backpacking trip through a primitive reserve in her home state, a friend fell and cut his palm. It subsequently became infected. Within a day, angry black streaks were moving up his arm, the first signs of blood poisoning. They decided to hike out to the trail to reach medical care. She placed plantain poultices on his wounded palm every 20 minutes. At night, she and her husband took shifts, replacing the used poultices with fresh ones. The black streaks began to reverse themselves. By the time they reached their vehicles the wound looked like nothing more than a severe scrape. In the emergency room of the nearest hospital, the attending physician refused to believe the wound had ever been serious…until a day or so later when he was shown photographs of the wound in its earlier stages.

When used to reverse severe infections, this procedure only works if the wound is open. The plantain should be rinsed with clean water and mashed before being placed on the wound, to avoid introducing any more contamination into the damaged area.

A less dramatic use for plantain is for the treatment of mosquito bites. Bruising the leaves, or carefully splitting them, provides a soothing natural band aid for the bite. But first wash the leaves to remove debris.

If on a long multi-month backpacking trip one's gums become inflamed and bloodied, chewing the leaf or root will help strengthen gum tissue and stop bleeding within a day or two. Rubbing the teeth with the ribbed leaf will also help keep them clean. Although not commonly used for **dental emergencies**, the root can be placed on a broken cap or filling to prevent infection.

St. John's wort

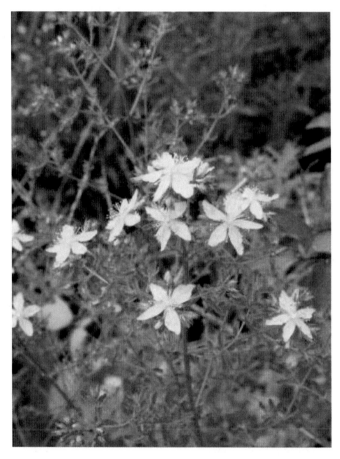

Saint John's wort is an herbal **antidepressant** (among its other uses). *Hypericum perforatum*, is also known as Tipton's weed, rosin rose, goat weed, chase-devil, or Klamath weed. A creeping ground cover variety can be found in the Midwestern states and is known as Aaron's beard. Approximately 370 species of the genus *Hypericum* exist worldwide with a native geographical distribution including temperate and subtropical regions of the world. The blossom of this plant has been historically used as a treatment for a wide variety of nervous disorders. Its name comes from the Greek word meaning "over an apparition", a link to the belief that St. John's wort was such a powerful plant that it could ward off evil apparitions or spirits. It doesn't.

The Crusaders valued Saint John's wort as a cure-all for **wounds** suffered in battle. It is antiviral, antibacterial, antifungal, and has anti-inflammatory properties. Wounds heal faster and with less pain when treated with Saint John's wort. The great English herbalist of the early 20th century, Maude Grieve, considered it effective for pulmonary illness (in this case she meant TB, influenza, and colds), bladder problems including incontinence, dysentery, and a strong topical astringent for wounds. But the last use (as an astringent for wounds) is the only one to which I can personally attest.

While harvesting this lovely plant in the Trinity Mountains of California, I took a fall down a mountainside. I bounced over a small stream when I hit bottom. My palms looked and felt like hamburger. After washing off the dirt particles with water from my canteen, I took the fresh flower petals and pressed them into the wounds. Within minutes I noticed a reduction of pain. I changed the petals three more times that day. By the end of the trip, my palms had healed with no scarring. Little wonder this was the herb of choice for Crusaders heading to the Holy Land.

Unfortunately this plant is not welcome in the modern community as it tends to be an invasive. On farmland, it was ruthlessly eradicated since it was believed to cause sun sensitivity, depression of the central nervous system, and spontaneous abortions in cattle. Other ranchers believed it harmed the taste of milk from cows. Currently Saint John's wort is listed as a noxious weed in over twenty countries. But Saint John's wort survives in wild places with enough moisture and shade to keep it viable.

The blood-red spots on the small yellow blossoms are antibacterial and can be used as a poultice for various injuries. The problem lies in the small number of blossoms growing in any particular spot. If you are lucky enough to find a large patch, you can harvest a few ounces to carry along on your trip. If possible, place the blossoms in an air tight container. The plant can be found in the lower eastern states, especially on the sides of steep hills. Its range extends north into Southern Pennsylvania. In the western states, look for Saint John's wort in the Cascade Range north into Southern Washington, though some hikers claim to have seen it as far north as the Canadian border.

Wild strawberries

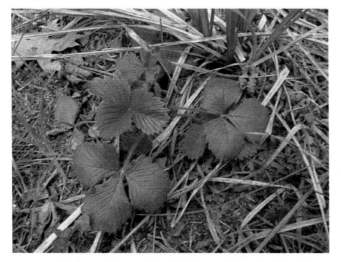

When Sir Francis Drake dropped anchor in California to re-caulk his leaking ship, the Golden Hinde, he also stopped to give his ailing sailors a chance to recover from **scurvy**. According to all accounts, he got along well with the natives, and they brought his ailing men fresh meat and "herbes that eased the bloody flux." Unfortunately, Drake's chaplain, who kept a record of the voyage, was no naturalist. Is it possible the California natives gave them some species of wild strawberry, such as *Fragaria californica*? Two hundred years later another Englishman, Dr. William Butler, wrote: "Doubtless God could have made a better berry, but doubtless God never did."

During that revolutionary winter at Valley Forge, General Washington's troops dug through the snow looking for the still verdant strawberry plants. They ate the raw root or added it to medicinal teas. When in season, the juice from the ripe berry was squeezed into badly inflamed sores. The astringent properties of the plant may have acted as an **anti-inflammatory**. Doctors of the time often combined the juice with water and used it as a wash for badly **irritated eyes**.

General Washington may have also known of its **dental uses**. Mashed into a paste, strawberries can effectively remove tartar, clean teeth, and ease minor toothache (which Washington often suffered). The same mash can be used on sunburn.

Wild strawberries (*Fragaria vesca* and its local variants) can be found throughout the United States, and as far north as the Aleutians. They are often called Alpine strawberries (when found at high altitudes) or Coastal strawberries when found along beaches growing several yards above the high tide line.

Like the blackberry, the Wild Strawberry is a member of the rose family. The leaves of the plant will have three toothed leaflets, much like the Wild Rose, and the blossom has five white petals. The unripe berries are green in color. The ripened red fruit looks and smells similar to the strawberry you will find at your local farmer's market. Most of the fruits are less than 2 cm in diameter. The fruit season varies by location, but usually lasts no more than a month. July to early August are the best times to find the fruit ready to eat or use. It is unmistakable in flavor and aroma, and there are no poisonous look-a-likes on the continent. Though most can be found in open woods, meadows, and seashores, the plant is also found in sub-alpine areas of the Sierra, the Rockies, the Appalachian Mountains, the Adirondacks, in the rainy Northwest coast range, along the Baja peninsula, and the railroad right of ways of the Atchison, Topeka, and Santa Fe. I even found some near the Great Smoky Mountains National Park.

Like other members of the rose family, strawberries are antiscorbutic. High in vitamin C and K, strawberries are easily digested by those suffering from scurvy or other ailments caused by a lack of fresh fruit or an excess of pre-packaged backpacker meals.

A decoction made from the fresh leaves is a gentle and effective remedy for simple **diarrhea** (though not as good as blackberry leaf). Simmer two or three tablespoons of crushed fresh leaves in two cups of water for 10 to 15 minutes, or until the water turns a light green. This remedy can be drunk hot, warm, or cold. The leaves can be purchased commercially and make a nice tea beverage; but for medicinal purposes, use the fresh plant.

A strong decoction of the leaves and roots can be used as a mouthwash and a gargle for **sore throat**. It is also a decent astringent and will help tighten loose gums (good for that occasional case of scurvy or weeks on the trail without a toothbrush). To make this decoction, boil or simmer the entire root and several leaves for ten to fifteen minutes. For a sore throat, gargle the decoction while the water is still warm.

Native American tribes on the East Coast used this same decoction for blood poisoning, kidney pain, dysentery, excessive menstruation, and a host of other problems. While there is anecdotal evidence for the efficacy of these remedies, I suggest it be used primarily for throat, mouth, and gum irritations.

Usnea

Usnea barbata and other spp. have a long history of use by Native Americans, mountain men and early settlers. Currently, it is used in Germany as an alternative for people who do not respond to the popular herbs echinacea and golden seal. A lichen hybrid of fungus and algae, usnea is also known as old man's beard in the Western United States, women's willow in the lower Appalachians and bear's beard in parts of the Northwest for its cascade of green-gray hair-like tendrils that hang from tree trunks and branches. Occasionally, it is misidentified as Spanish moss and other tree mosses. Usnea can be found throughout the world, often attached to oaks, willows, redwoods, cedars and other trees growing along riverbanks and cool shady riparian areas. Usnea is always gray-green in color, even when young.

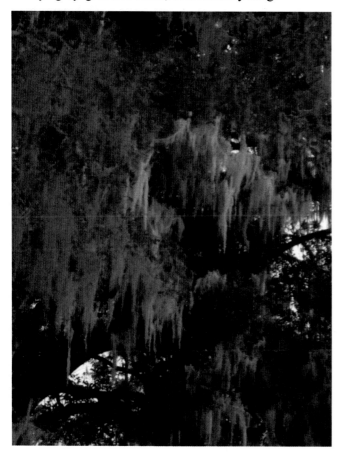

This lichen can grow as a bushy mat or in strands ranging from a few inches to three or four feet long depending on the species. In the wet seasons, it will feel cool and spongy. In years with little rain, it feels dry and coarse. The medicinal species of usnea have an inner core of white material that can be exposed by gently pulling on either end of a strand. The outer coating tears apart to reveal a tough white inner cord. These white-cored species are considered the most medicinally valuable.

Traditional uses of usnea include dusting the dried, powdered herb directly onto open or **infected wounds** or making strong decoctions of the herb and washing the wound. Native Americans used the crushed and powdered plant on knife and arrow wounds, much like WW II medics used sulfa powder on gunshot and shrapnel wounds. This is an excellent outdoor first aid plant for backpackers with open wounds. If the crushed lichen is placed quickly on a wound (and applied often) it can prevent infection.

Although blood will release the usnic acids of the plant, usnea does not yield its healing properties well in water, so a tea is nearly useless. A decoction is somewhat better. To make a decoction of usnea, the lichen must be boiled and boiled well. Using the water and the boiled material on and in a wound is preferable to using the raw plant.

For already established infections of any kind, particularly open wounds, usnea can save your life. This plant has a penicillin-like effect on wounds, but must be replaced several times a day to be effective. If you can't make a decoction, a poultice of the crushed pasta-like interior portion of the lichen is most effective. But if time is short, a crude dressing made from the crushed lichen can be used to cover the wound. Dried usnea works best when crushed and soaked in alcohol, vinegar, or in dire circumstances urine (not recommended unless there is no hope for a quick rescue and a life is at stake).

When made into an alcohol or vinegar based tincture, usnea is a premier cure for severe bladder infections, other than those caused by e-coli. Women tend to get more bladder infections on packbacking trips than men. If you neglected to pack tincture of usnea in your first aid kit, you can still make a strong decoction out of fresh usnea for the affected party. Although usnea is not very water soluble, continued cups of the tea will help eliminate a bladder infection. In a day or two the problem should be controlled.

Usnea is also a specific for pneumonia, strep, and staph infections. Drinking large amounts of the decoctions will help get you back to your car and into an emergency room. For a staph infection on the skin, usnea can be mashed into a powder, made into a watery paste or (better) combined with alcohol or vinegar, then applied on the affected areas. So taking a small bottle of liquor on a backpacking trip might not be such a bad idea (but only for medicinal purposes).

White sage

Found growing wild in various western states and used by all Native Americans with knowledge of it, white sage (*Salvia apiana*) is antibiotic, antibacterial, antimicrobial, and may have antiviral properties. It has a gray stem, blue blossoms, and blue-green leaves. The plant stem can easily reach six to seven feet in height.

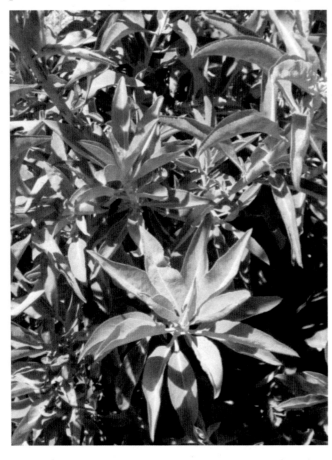

Many hikers in the Southwest mistake the plant Artemisia (often called sagebrush or silver sage.) for white sage. Sagebrush is strongly aromatic and bitter to the taste. These "sages" are often gray to grayish white in color and do not have the large prominent opposite leaves of the Salvia family.

White sage is found from the Great Basin to Southeastern Washington, and throughout the southwest to Sonora Mexico and down the coast of Baja. The limits of its range are not clear as it can grow in both arid and wet climates.

White sage has become one of the most popular herbal medicines in the United States. It can be made into a tea that reduces mucous secretions of the sinuses, bronchi and throat during **allergy attacks**, **colds** and **influenza**. Drunk hot, an infusion of the leaves stimulates perspiration, thus lowering fevers. The cold tea is often used to help digestion, while a warmer tea is a good **sore throat remedy**. The leaves (brewed into a strong uterine hemostatic tea) have been used by Native American women for hundreds of years as a remedy for heavy and painful **menstruation**. But nursing mothers are advised by doctors not to use it since it reduces lactation (unless that effect is desired).

Although white sage is not currently used as a culinary herb, Southwest and California Indians made porridge by the grinding the seeds into flour while the leaves were made into flavoring ingredients for cooking. The leaves of this plant were also smoked, eaten, and used as a prime remedy for colds and fever.

White sage is an effective remedy for some eye ailments, including **Pink Eye** (conjunctivitis). A strong decoction made from the leaves and used as an eye wash will quickly eliminate this problem. Boil the plant material, along with several cloths or bandanas, allow it to cool and carefully bathe the eyes with this wash. Repeat frequently for several hours. Sleep with a decoction infused cloth on the eyes. This should alleviate the problem in 48 hours.

S. apiana can be used for self-grooming, especially outdoors, by crushing the leaves and mixing with water to create an herbal hair shampoo, hair-straightener and dye. You can also rid your body of foul odor by washing with the mixture, or rubbing the crushed leaves all over your skin.

A tea or decoction of white sage can be used for topical and internal **infections**. If necessary, the leaves can be mashed into a poultice and placed on wounds. As a specific for bronchial ailments, white sage was once smoked to ease the pain of infected lungs and sinuses. Though smoking is no longer recommended, a steam made from the leaves can have the same effect along with breaking up congestion. The leaves and stems can quickly be boiled in a Sierra Cup and the steam inhaled.

The leaves of white sage (and many other varieties of sage) are a potent **antiseptic**, used for abrasions, skin inflammations, douches to treat Candida, washes for staph infections and teas for sore throats, colds, and lung infections.

Burning the leaves is a traditional **smudge against insects** that have taken up residence in tipis, hogans, hooches, lean-tos and, (more recently) tents and clothing. The rich, fragrant, aromatic smoke must penetrate all the nooks and crannies of camp life to be completely effective – but take care not to let hot bits of the burning plant escape and contact the fabric of tent, sleeping bags, or clothing.

Yarrow

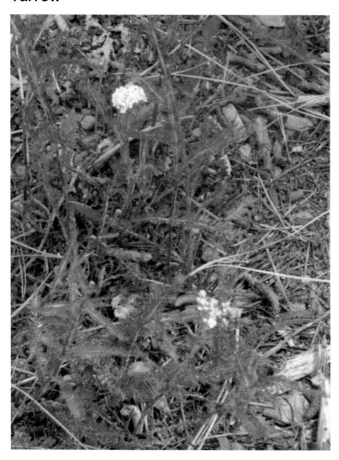

Cuts are among the most common camping and backpacking injuries. Yarrow (*Achilliea millefolium*), will **stop bleeding** in mild to severe wounds. The legendary warrior Achilles, in Homer's Iliad, uses yarrow to treat the wounds of his soldiers. Early Greek physicians used this herb to stop hemorrhage and fevers. Yarrow was mentioned in Culpepper's Complete Herbal in 1553; forty-three years later in Gerard's herbal in 1597; and in many herbals thereafter to this day.

Yarrow was commonly used by Native American tribes for bleeding, wounds, pain, headache, and infections. It is used in Ayurvedic medicine, and traditional Chinese medicine for its ability to affect ailments of the spleen, liver, kidney, and bladder.

The constituents in yarrow make it a fine herb for accelerating healing of cuts and severe bruising. Some people in Europe still call it **knight's milfoil**, a reference to yarrow's ability to stop bleeding and promote healing of wounds from combat or jousting.

The yarrow plant is recognizable by its white blossom clusters and feathery leaves. If applying direct pressure does not stem the bleeding, the blossoms and leaves (quickly rinse off dust and dirt) can halt the bleeding in minutes, if not seconds. Crush the blossoms and leaves and place them on the wound, or if absolutely necessary into the wound. This should only be done if the wound is life threatening. If the plant is not in blossom, scrape off the dirt and the outer layer of the root skin bark, then rinse the root in clean water. Yarrow is purported to have antiseptic properties, but this has not been verified, and infection is likely if the plant is not thoroughly scrubbed or rinsed before application.

Yarrow blossoms are very effective on slashed hands and knees. A quick poultice of the rinsed and crushed plant can be placed directly on the bleeding wound. If there is time, a quickly *boiled* poultice of the root, leaves and blossoms can be made and placed on the injury. The entire mass can be dipped into boiling water for one minute and used as soon as the plant is warm to the touch but not steaming. If available, place a thin clean cloth between the poultice and the injury.

Yarrow supposedly grows best at lower elevations. I have seen fields of yarrow in Pennsylvania, Maryland, Virginia, south into Mississippi and all along the Eastern Seaboard. In mid-summer, it grows in clumps throughout the battlefields of Gettysburg. It tends to grow below six thousand feet. But I have found fields of it on both sides of the high Sierra at nine thousand feet, as well as in and around lower Yosemite National Park. It is common throughout the conifer regions of Nevada, all of Oregon and Washington, throughout Western Canada and as far north as Alaska. The blossoms give off a slight sweet scent reminiscent of chamomile. Though occasionally mistaken for water hemlock, on close examination the plant will not have the purple spots on its stems. Nor will it have the musty smell of hemlock flowers.

Yarrow is also effective against moderate to high **fevers**. A tea or decoction of the blossoms and leaves tends to be most efficacious for this purpose. A teaspoon of yarrow in a cup of boiling water, steeped for 10 minutes, and drunk warm, will begin to ease fevers. As this remedy will cause sweating, liquid intake must be increased. If rehydration drinks are used for this purpose, they should be diluted by two thirds with water. For exceptionally high fevers, simmering or boiling the root for five to ten minutes will be more effective. Yarrow can be taken with a pinch of sugar, and salt to maintain electrolyte balances if rehydration powders are not available. The taste of yarrow tea can be sweet, with a hint of bitterness. The more the tea is steeped, the bitterer it becomes. For headaches, the stronger the bitter taste the stronger the pain relieving properties of the salicylic acids in the plant.

Another use of yarrow is specific to women's needs. Two or three cups of a tea or decoction made from the plant will stop the bleeding from an off-date period or between-cycle spotting, and will also help **ease menstrual pain**.

Yarrow increases urinary output, so a tea of dried or fresh leaves can help alleviate sudden **diabetic sugar spikes** by excreting glucose. Lowering the glucose level in the blood will help a diabetic who has run out of or lost the medications needed to control blood sugar. The yarrow tea should be continued until the diabetic again has access to prescribed medications.

For a **toothache**, carefully placing the crushed root on the affected tooth or gum area will bring complete numbness within 45 minutes. The taste is not pleasant and it does cause excessive drooling. But the side effects are more tolerable than the throbbing of an infected tooth.

Yerba mansa

Anemopsis californica is a true American and botanical original as it is the only type in its genus. With the common names of Yerba mansa or lizard's tail, it was used by native tribes for a multitude of ailments, including sore muscles, bronchitis, influenza, open

sores, wasting diseases, and vaginal problems such as vaginal candidiasis. Yerba mansa is used by modern herbalists as an **antimicrobial**, **antibacterial**, and more importantly as an **immune stimulant** on a par with echinacea and golden seal.

This is a water loving plant once common in California and the wetter areas of the southwest. It can still be found growing along rivers, creeks and ponds, but unlike many herbs it is alkaline tolerant. The white flowers resemble those of a huge plantain. It is lovely in springtime and into early summer. The leaves and blossoms die back and turn brown or black in the fall. The root can still be utilized as a medicinal during this time as it is not dead, but merely dormant.

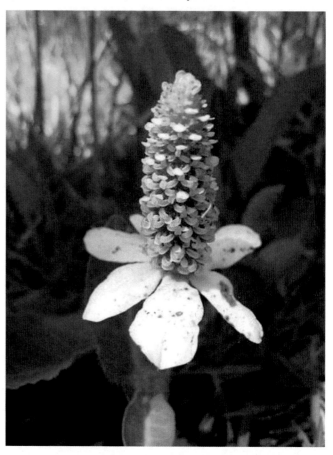

The leaves and roots of this semi-aquatic plant are used in the treatment of inflamed mucous membranes, sore throat and inflamed gums. A warm tea or decoction used as a **mouthwash** will tighten the gums and relieve pain within hours. An infusion of the roots can be taken as a **diuretic** to treat diseases like **gout** by ridding the body of excess uric acid crystals, which causes painful inflammation of the joints. This infusion can also be used for any painful rheumatic condition causing swelling. Yerba mansa also helps prevent the buildup of **kidney stones**. A powder of the dried root sprinkled on affected areas alleviates athlete's foot, jock itch, and diaper rash.

Anemopsis californica tolerates alkaline soil, sand, clay, no drainage and seasonal flooding. It is difficult if not impossible to over harvest Yerba mansa as the remaining rhizomes will create several more viable plants in the following year. However, the plant should NOT be used if there is any chance of heavy metals in the water supply. This plant will clean out a pond or meadow of heavy metals given enough time.

Yerba santa

Yerba santa (*Eriodictyon californica*), also known as mountain balm, consumptive's weed and bear's weed, is an aromatic herb with long, sticky, lance shaped leaves. It is not unusual to find bushes 7 to 8 feet high. The leaves have a resinous look to them, as if they have been shellacked. These plants are found on hillsides and ridges throughout California, the Tahoe Basin, and parts of Northern Baja. It ranges from high desert areas to the lower Sierra Nevada foothills up to 5000 feet.

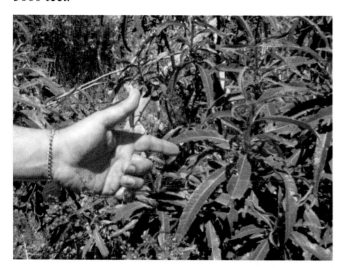

Yerba santa is a powerful **expectorant** and, when used with Wild Ginger, will expel the worst impacted phlegm. As well as a **decongestant** and **bronchial dilator**, it useful for respiratory congestion from colds, flu, bronchitis and hay fever. It has been used to help relieve asthma symptoms but is not considered as effective as mullein. It can be used to treat mild urinary tract infections, and helps to reduce inflammation and decrease excess fluid. Externally, the fresh leaves of Yerba santa can be made into a poultice and applied to

treat **abrasions**, **cuts**, **bruises** and sore muscles. Native American woman supposedly tied Yerba santa to their bodies to keep snakes away, but most herbalists do not share their belief in that effect.

Yerba santa's anti-inflammatory property also makes it useful as an external treatment for **poison oak rash**. A simple poison oak remedy can be made by combining one cup of a strong infusion of Yerba santa, a half cup of vinegar and one and a half tablespoons of salt. Other herbs such as mugwort, grindelia, and horsetail can be included in the infusion.

For internal use, make a tea by infusing a rounded tablespoon of the crushed, dried leaves in a cup of boiling water, let steep for at least ten minutes, and strain. Yerba santa can also be made into an alcohol tincture, which is usually taken by adding 10-30 drops to a glass of water.

The fresh leaves of Yerba Santa can be chewed. They have a strongly pungent, spicy flavor with a sweet aftertaste.

A cure-all herb to the natives of California, this plant was quickly adopted by the Spanish settlers for bronchitis, influenza and asthma. It can be made into a drinkable decoction or used as a steam to help clear nasal passages or phlegm filled bronchial passages. A handful of the leaves tossed into a steaming pot of water will provide relief from cough, congestion, and occasionally, dust-induced asthma.

A tea made the same way can be used for stomachaches and fevers. The mashed and slightly steamed leaf can be used as a poultice for wounds, swellings, and broken bones. Hikers, backpackers, and campers have found it an effective wash against the torture of mosquito bites. It is also used for bee stings but tends to be less effective unless it is applied immediately.

Conclusion

While herbal remedies are not a substitute for standard medical care, proper use of these plants can alleviate many discomforts, and in an emergency might save your life.

Sources

I use over a hundred and twenty herbals in my own practice and courses. Three excellent sources on medicinal plants, their uses, and locations are by famed herbalist Michael Moore. They are: *Medicinal Plants of the Mountains West, Medicinal Plants of the Desert and Canyon West*, and *Medicinal Plants of the Pacific West*. A valuable field guide on the location and use of western state plants is *Edible and Medicinal Plants of the West*, by Gregory L. Tilford.

Tom Brown's Guide to Wild and Medicinal Plant by Tom Brown Jr. is not precisely an herbal; it describes the uses of many plants found in the eastern states that he learned from a Native American elder.

For the traditional uses of medicinal plants, *California Herbal Remedies* by LoLo Westrich, and *Wise Woman Herbal: Healing Wise* by Susun S. Weed are well written and practical.

The Complete Medicinal Herbal by Penelope Ody, is one of the best herbals for beginning enthusiasts. Its photographs of plants and clear instructions for herb preparations alone are worth the price of the book.

Recommended Reading

Wilderness Medicine, 7th[th] Ed. Elsevier, Inc. 2017 (www.elsevierhealth.com). Ed. P.S. Auerbach. Now in two volumes, this is the only comprehensive book on the subject, with over 5,000 large, double-column pages, lavishly illustrated. Its 126 chapters (some of them as long as small books) discuss hazards, injuries, and medical problems in all outdoor environments, from the mountains to the ocean, and from the arctic to the jungle. There are also chapters on survival in and rescue from different environments; children, women, and elders in the wilderness; improvisation; the changing environment; helpful and harmful plants; and ethics of wilderness medicine. Discussion of field medical treatment is thorough. This is a one-volume library for wilderness responders and instructors, written by experts, with all the details that other books omit; and it now comes with access to a dedicated web site for references and other resources. I have used all six previous editions of this book extensively in my teaching and writing for many years.

Wilderness Medical Society: Practice Guidelines for Wilderness Emergency Care, 5th Ed., ed. William W. Forgey. Guilford: Falcon Guides, 2006. This concise book is a consensus of wilderness medicine experts on how to assess and treat injuries and medical problems in the wilderness. Most instructors of wilderness emergency care courses use it for reference. I am a contributor and peer reviewer. Updated guidelines are published in issues and supplements of the WMS journal, *Wilderness & Environmental Medicine*, available online at www.wms.org.

Medicine for Mountaineering and Other Wilderness Activities, 6th Ed, ed. James A. Wilkerson. The Mountaineers, 2010. Since 1935, mountaineering physicians have been teaching backcountry first aid and medicine to other mountaineers in Washington, and this book evolved from their lessons. As the title suggests, it is mostly for mountaineers, though this edition adds more on other environments.

Medicine for the Outdoors: The Essential Guide to First Aid and Medical Emergencies, 5th Ed. Paul S. Auerbach, M.D. Mosby, 2009. Dr. Auerbach's book includes detailed information about tropical, desert, and underwater environments – he is an enthusiastic scuba diver. It has sections on wild plant poisoning, marine hazards, and dealing with diseases in the backcountry as well as injuries and wilderness hazards. Dense with information and advice, it is designed more for reference than for continuous reading.

Wilderness Medicine: Beyond First Aid, 6th Ed. William Forgey, M.D. Falcon Guides, 2012. This 288-page book is designed for reference. Each chapter is divided into short sections with headlines that give clear explanations of problems and practical advice for dealing with them. Dr. Forgey describes many medical techniques, including minor surgery and administering prescription drugs. However, you should make sure that you are trained to use these techniques safely before attempting them in a real emergency.

Outdoor Emergency Care, 5th Ed. Edward C. McNamara, Editor. Brady, 2012. Unlike the 4th Edition of the National Ski Patrol's OEC textbook, which was an augmented version of a standard EMT textbook, the 5th Edition was written and edited by members and staff of the NSP. It includes more on outdoor situations and their hazards, especially the winter environment. The 1264 pages include many color photos and illustrations, as well as skill guides, drills, and scenarios. Although the OEC book shows a few improvised techniques, almost all of the sections on patient care assume that rescuers will have professional quality equipment, as alpine ski patrollers usually do.

Southmayd W, Hoffman M: *Sports Health: The Complete Book of Athletic Injuries*. New York. G.P. Putnam's Sons, 1981. This is still probably the best book on athletic injuries. It explains in plain English how they happen, how to prevent them, and how to rehabilitate yourself if they happen to you.

Hypothermia, Frostbite and other Cold Injuries, 2nd Ed. G.G.Giesbrecht, J.A. Wilkerson. The Mountaineers, 2006. This book explains cold injuries clearly, and packs a lot of practical information into its 160 pages. It includes vivid color photos of frostbite and a discussion of cold-weather clothing.

Hypothermia: Death by Exposure, Wm. W. Forgey, M.D., ICS Books, Inc., 1985. Based on his many cold-weather expeditions as well as a critical review of the literature, Dr. Forgey's book is full of facts, figures, and forthright opinions. His analysis of cold-weather clothing is especially interesting.

Going Higher: Oxygen, Man, and Mountains, 4th ed. Charles S. Houston, M.D. Little, Brown & Co., 1999. Dr. Houston studied the effects of altitude for over 60 years. *Going High* (1981) distilled a lifetime of research, experience, and enthusiasm into a lively and well-illustrated book, which the author revised and expanded for the third time in 1999. He also tells the fascinating story of human experience with altitude and the attempts to explain its effects.

High Altitude Medicine, Herb Hultgren, M.D. Hultgren Publications, 827 San Francisco Court, Stanford, CA 94305-1021, 1997. $70. Everything you could ever want to know about the effects of high altitude on human beings, in 550 pages. Dr. Hultgren, a cardiologist who was one of the world's leading altitude researchers for many decades, completed this book just before his death. He explains the physiology of altitude - its effects on all the vital systems - as well as the different forms of altitude illness. Incredibly thorough, but his style is clear and straightforward. Many graphs and tables give you the experimental data on which his discussions are based.

Rattlesnakes: Their Habits, Life Histories, & Influence on Mankind, Abridged Edition, Laurence M. Klauber. Berkeley: University of California Press, 1982. This classic will probably tell you everything you ever wanted to know about rattlesnakes. Klauber was an electrical engineer who became interested in snakes at the age of 40, volunteered to be the first Curator of Reptiles at the San Diego Zoo, and started publishing scientific papers on them. His writing is clear and unpretentious, and his book is full of historical anecdotes and personal observation as well as scientific description and explanation.

Snake Venom Poisoning, Findlay E. Russell. Great Neck: Scholium International Inc., 1983. Russell cites Klauber's book frequently, but he goes into great detail about snake venoms and what they can do to you. Since he meant his book mainly for physicians, he also describes snakebite treatment thoroughly.

Bear Attacks: Their Causes and Avoidance, Stephen Herrero. Lyons & Burford, 1985. Herrero has a Ph.D. in animal behavior, and has spent much of his career studying bears. In his book, he tells us what he has learned and quotes many first-hand stories of encounters with bears.

The Malaria Capers: Tales of Parasites and People, Robert S. Desowitz. New York: W.W. Norton & Company, Inc., 1991. Robert Desowitz was a professor of tropical medicine and microbiology at the University of Hawaii, but he spent much of his life in the field, investigating tropical diseases. In this lively and entertaining book, he takes you through the history of malaria and its effects on humans, including the politics as well as the science.

Tropical Diseases, Robert S. Desowitz. London: HarperCollins, 1997. Once again, Desowitz makes a book on the history of diseases more entertaining than most novels. This time, he introduces you to all the major tropical diseases (for most of which humans are just part of their life cycle) and to the researchers who discovered how these diseases are transmitted – sometimes at the cost of their own lives.

Plagues and Peoples, William H. McNeill. This book tells the story of how epidemic diseases have evolved and affected human society from its beginnings. McNeill was an historian – professor of history at the University of Chicago. His writing is clear and unpretentious, but his depth of historical knowledge and scrupulous sifting of evidence distinguish this book from more popular ones on the subject, which seem superficial and careless by comparison.

Rats, Lice, and History: A Study in Biography, Hans Zinsser. New York: Little, Brown & Company, 1935. This was probably the first book of its kind, relating the biographies of infectious diseases and their effects on history. Zinsser wrote it "at odd moments as a relaxation from studies of typhus fever in the laboratory and in the field."

Civilization and Disease, Henry E. Sigerist. University of Chicago Press, 1943. Dr. Sigerist was a professor of the history of medicine at Johns Hopkins University. The section titles will give an idea of his approach: Civilization as a factor in the genesis of disease; Disease and economics; Disease and social life; Disease and the law; Disease and history; Disease and religion; Disease and philosophy; Disease and science; Disease and literature; Disease and art; Disease and music; Civilization against disease. He planned to write a comprehensive history of medicine, but unfortunately completed only the first two volumes: *Primitive and Archaic Medicine*, and *Early Greek, Hindu, and Persian Medicine*.

Passions and Tempers: A History of the Humours, Noga Arikha. New York: HarperCollins, 2007. For over 2000 years, medicine in Western civilization was based on the theory that human health and temperament depended on the balance of four humours (Latin *humorem* "fluid") in the human body: black bile, yellow bile, phlegm, and blood. So doctors treated any illness by bleeding, sweating, or purging the patient to restore this balance, which killed many of their patients. The humoural theory of medicine has left its traces in the words for the four temperaments: melancholic, choleric, phlegmatic, and sanguine. But although modern medicine is based on a much more complex view of how the human body works, it is still one of the leading causes of death in the United States. So perhaps many current medical procedures will seem as strange to future generations as Roman and medieval medicine does to us.

The Worst of Evils: The Fight Against Pain, Thomas Dormandy. Dr. Dormandy is a retired professor of chemical pathology and a consulting pathologist, but he has written a cultural as well as medical history of the attempts to understand and deal with pain. He

obviously had a classical education, since he quotes from Greek and Latin authors, but he wears his scholarship lightly. Some of the chapter titles will give an idea of his approach: A gift of the gods; The grape and the poppy; Pain denied; Pain ignored; The heresies; Healing and holiness; Pain exalted; Animal magnetism; The terror of the knife; Hospital disease; Chloroform; The shape of dreams; The rights of pain. Dormandy also wrote *The White Death: A History of Tuberculosis*, which (like *The Worst of Evils*) is cultural as well as medical history.

Wilderness Search and Rescue, Tim J. Setnicka. Appalachian Mountain Club, 1981. More than 600 pages long, this book gives clear and practical instructions for performing rescues in all types of wilderness situations. The author is a park ranger who started his Search and Rescue career doing big wall rescues in Yosemite. His book is also available as a Kindle edition.

CIBA Collection of Medical Illustrations and *Atlas of Human Anatomy*: The structure of the human body and what can go wrong with it revealed in full color by the king of medical illustrators, Dr. Frank Netter. CIBA-GEIGY Corporation, Medical Education Division.

Medical Meanings: A Glossary of Word Origins. William S. Haubrich, M.D. San Diego: Harcourt Brace Jovanovich, 1984. Haubrich explains where medical terms come from, and how they acquired or were assigned their present sense. His writing is clear and entertaining, reflecting his 35-year fascination with word definitions and origins.

Wilderness & Environmental Medicine, the quarterly journal of the Wilderness Medical Society features technical articles based on original research, review articles, book reviews, and abstracts of relevant articles from other journals. It is a peer-reviewed medical journal referenced by Index Medicus and Medline. I edit a regular column for it called The Wilderness Instructor. All issues except the current one are freely accessible online at the Society's web site: www.wms.org.

Bibliography:
Books and articles used for specific chapters

Training for Wilderness Emergencies
1. Salvesen LC. Psychologic responses to accidents. In: Wilkerson JA, ed. *Medicine for Mountaineering*, 4th Ed. Seattle: The Mountaineers, 1992.
2. Donelan S. Classroom and reality: lessons from real emergencies. *Wilderness & Environmental Medicine* 11(2):122-124, Summer 2000

Patient Assessment
Books
1. American Geriatrics Society. *Geriatric Education for Emergency Medical Services,* 2nd Edition. Jones & Bartlett Learning, 2014.
2. American Academy of Pediatrics. *Pediatric Education for Prehospital Professionals*, 3rd Edition. Jones & Bartlett Learning, 2013.
3. Dormandy T. *The Worst of Evils: The Fight Against Pain*. Yale University Press, 2006.

Articles & chapters
1. Smith M. The birth of M.A.N. *Journal of Emergency Medical Services* 22(6):34, June 1997.
2. Klein JR. Children in the wilderness. In: Auerbach P, ed. *Wilderness Medicine*, 6th Ed. Philadelphia: Mosby, 2012.
3. Urb DB, Shimizu US. Elders in the wilderness. In: Auerbach P, ed. *Wilderness Medicine*, 6th Ed. Philadelphia: Mosby, 2012.
4. Olson s, Moore LA. Persons with special needs and disabilities. In: Auerbach P, ed. *Wilderness Medicine*, 6th Ed. Philadelphia: Mosby, 2012.

Wilderness First Aid Kits
1. Tonna JE, Lewin MR. Wilderness preparation, equipment, and medical supplies. In: Auerbach P, ed. *Wilderness Medicine*, 6th Ed. Philadelphia: Mosby, 2012.

Shock
1. Johnson S, Henderson SO. Myth: The Trendelenburg position improves circulation in cases of shock. *Canadian Journal Emergency Medicine* 6(1): 48-49, 2004.
2. Halm MA. Trendelenburg position: "put to bed" or angled toward use in your unit? *American Journal of Critical Care* 21(6): 449-452, November 2012.
3. Gross KR et al. Wilderness trauma and surgical emergencies. In: Auerbach P, ed. *Wilderness Medicine*, 6th Ed. Philadelphia: Mosby, 2012.

Wound Care
Books
1. American Red Cross. *Advanced First Aid & Emergency Care*, 2nd Edition. New York: Doubleday & Company, Inc. 1979.
2. Majno G. *The Healing Hand: Man and Wound in the Ancient World*. Cambridge: Harvard University Press, 1975.
3. Auerbach PS. *Medicine for the Outdoors: A Guide to Emergency Medical Procedures and First Aid*, rev. ed. Boston: Little, Brown & Co., 1991.
4. Davis GG. *The Principles and Practice of Bandaging*. Philadelphia: P. Blackiston's Son & Co, 1902.
5. Forgey WW. *Wilderness Medicine*, 4th Ed. Merrillville: ICS Books, 1994.

Articles & chapters: General
1. Iserson KV, Donner HJ. Improvised medicine in the wilderness. In: Auerbach P, ed. *Wilderness Medicine*, 6th Ed. Philadelphia: Mosby, 2012.
2. Radwin MI, Keyes L, Simons I. Wild animal bite wound irrigation simplified by the use of a modified water filter. *Wilderness & Environmental Medicine* 12(1):53, 2001.
3. Quinn RH et al. Wilderness Medical Society practice guidelines for basic wound management in an austere environment: 2014 update. *Wilderness & Environmental Medicine* 25(3): S118-S133, 2014.

4. Jamshidi R. Wound management. In: Auerbach P, ed. *Wilderness Medicine*, 6th Ed. Philadelphia: Mosby, 2012.

5. Smack DP et al. Infection and allergy incidence in ambulatory surgical patients using white petrolatum vs. bacitracin ointment: a randomized controlled trial. *JAMA* 276:972-7, 1996.

6. Criss EA. Latex allergies. *JEMS* 25(10):42-49, October 2000.

Bleeding control

1. Littlejohn L, Bennett BL, Drew B. Application of current hemorrhage control techniques for backcountry care: Part one, Tourniquets and hemorrhage control adjuncts. *Wilderness & Environmental Medicine* 26(2): 236-245, 2015.

2. Littlejohn L, Bennett BL, Drew B. Application of current hemorrhage control techniques for backcountry care: Part two, hemostatic dressings and other adjuncts. *Wilderness & Environmental Medicine* 26(2): 246-254, 2015.

3. Pusateri A et al. Making sense of the preclinical literature on advanced hemostatic products. *Journal of Trauma: Injury, Infection, and Critical Care* 60(3): 674-682, March 2006.

4. Wedmore I et al. A special report on the chitosan-based hemostatic dressing: experience in current combat situations. *Op. cit.* 655-658.

Honey

1. Cooper P, Molan PC, Harding KG. Antibacterial activity of honey against strains of Staphylococcus aureus from infected wounds. *Journal of the Royal Society of Medicine* 92(6):283-5, June 1999.

2. Al-Waili NS, Saloom KY. Effects of topical honey on post-operative wound infections due to gram positive and gram negative bacteria following caesarian sections and hysterectomies. *European Journal of Medical Research* 4(3):126-130, march 26, 1999.

3. Molan PC, Cooper RA. Honey and sugar as a dressing for wounds and ulcers. *Tropical Doctor* 30(4):249-50, October 2000.

4. Vardi A et al. Local application of honey for treatment of neonatal postoperative wound infection. *Acta Paediatrica* 87(4):429-32, April 1998.

5. Molan PC. The role of honey in the management of wounds. *Journal of Wound Care* 8(8):415-8, September 1999.

6. Postmas T, van den Bogaard AE, Hazen M. The sterilization of honey with cobalt 60 gamma radiation: a study of honey spiked with spores of Clostridium botulinum and Bacillus sub tilis. *Experientia* 51(9-10):986-9, September 29, 1995.

7. Cooper R, Molan P. The use of honey as an antiseptic in managing pseudomonas infection. *Journal of Wound Care* 8(4):161-4, April 1999.

Blisters

Vonhof J. Fixing Your Feet Blog. www.fixingyourfeet.com

Burns

Books

1. Auerbach PS. *Medicine for the Outdoors: A Guide to Emergency Medical Procedures and First Aid*, rev. ed. Boston: Little, Brown & Co., 1991.

2. Forgey W. *Wilderness Medicine*, 4th Ed. Merrillville: ICS Books, 1994.

Articles & chapters

1. Leigh-Smith S. Carbon monoxide poisoning in tents: A review. *Wilderness & Environmental Medicine* 15(3):157-163, Fall 2004.

2. Mosier MJ, Heimbach D. Emergency care of the burned victim. In: Auerbach P, ed. *Wilderness Medicine*, 6th Ed. Philadelphia: Mosby, 2012.

3. Subrahmanyam M. A prospective randomized and histological study of superficial burn wound healing with honey and silver sulfadiazine. *Burns* 24(2):157-61, March 1998.

4. Alexander ME et al. Wildland fires: Dangers and survival. In: Auerbach P, ed. *Wilderness Medicine*, 6th Ed. Philadelphia: Mosby, 2012.

Bone Injuries and Splinting

Books

1. *American Red Cross First Aid Textbook* (Revised). Philadelphia: The Blakiston Company, 1937.

2. Watson F. *The Life of Sir Robert Jones*. London: Hodder & Stoughton Ltd., 1934.

3. Garrick JG, Webb DR: *Sports Injuries: Diagnosis and Management*. Philadelphia. W.B. Saunders Company, 1990.
4. Sinclair M. *The Thomas Splint and its Modifications in the Treatment of Fractures*. Preface by Sir Robert Jones. London: Oxford University Press, 1927.

Articles & chapters

1. Williams H. Hugh Owen Thomas. In: *Doctors Differ*. Springfield: Charles C. Thomas, 1946.
2. Borschneck AG, Wayne MA. Sager emergency traction splint: A new splinting device for lower limb fractures. *EMS Magazine* 2004. WWW.emsmagazine.com.
3. Bledsoe BE, Barnes D. Traction splint: An EMS relic? *JEMS* 29(8):64-78, August 2004.
4. Weiss EA, Donner HJ. Wilderness improvisation. In: Auerbach PS, ed. *Wilderness Medicine*, 4th Ed. St. Louis: Mosby, 2001.
5. Switzer JA, Bovard RS. Wilderness orthopedics. In: Auerbach P, ed. *Wilderness Medicine*, 6th Ed. Philadelphia: Mosby, 2012.

Athletic Injuries

Books

1. Vaughn CL, et al: *Biomechanics of Sports*. Boca Raton. CRC Press, Inc., 1989.
2. Caillet R. *Foot and Ankle Pain*. Philadelphia: F.A. Davis Company, 1976.
3. Southmayd W, Hoffman M: *Sports Health: The Complete Book of Athletic Injuries*. New York. G.P. Putnam's Sons, 1981.
4. Garrick JG, Webb DR: *Sports Injuries: Diagnosis and Management*. Philadelphia. W.B. Saunders Company, 1990.
5. Nieman DC: *The Sports Medicine Fitness Course*. Palo Alto. Bull Publishing Company, 1986.

Chapter

Eckert WR, Stehlik J: Alpine and nordic ski injuries. *Management of Wilderness and Environmental Emergencies*, 1st Edition. New York. Macmillan Publishing Co., 1983.

Head Injuries

1. Auerbach PS. *Medicine for the Outdoors: A Guide to Emergency Medical Procedures and First Aid*, rev. ed. Boston: Little, Brown & Co., 1991.
2. Toschlog EA, Morris JA. Wilderness trauma and surgical emergencies. In: Auerbach PS, ed. *Wilderness Medicine*,4th Ed. St. Louis: Mosby, 2001.

Eye and Face Injuries

Books

1. Auerbach PS. *Medicine for the Outdoors: A Guide to Emergency Medical Procedures and First Aid*, rev. ed. Boston: Little, Brown & Co., 1991.
2. Forgey WW. *Wilderness Medicine*, 4th Ed. Merrillville: ICS Books, 1994.

Articles & chapters

1. Butler FK. The eye in the wilderness. In: Auerbach P, ed. *Wilderness Medicine*, 6th Ed. Philadelphia: Mosby, 2012.
2. Mazzorana V. Management of facial injuries. In: Auerbach P, ed. *Wilderness Medicine*, 6th Ed. Philadelphia: Mosby, 2012.
3. Dickson AE. Nosebleeds in the wilderness. *Wilderness Medicine Letter* 18(2):1-3, Spring 2001.
4. Bledsoe BE, Ho B. Sight-threatening eye injuries. *JEMS* 29(10):95-106, Oct. 2004.
5. Paterson R et al. Wilderness Medical Society practice guidelines for treatment of eye injuries and illnesses in the wilderness: 2014 update. *Wilderness & Environmental Medicine* 25(1): S19-S29, 2014.

Dental Emergencies

1. Herrmann HJ. Dental and facial emergencies. In: Auerbach PS, ed. *Wilderness Medicine*, 4th Ed. St. Louis: Mosby, 2001.
2. Morganti S. Tooth avulsion: a treatment update. *Ski Patrol Magazine* 12(2):62-63, Winter 1996.
3. Herrmann HJ, Idzik-Starr HL. Wilderness dentistry. In: Auerbach P, ed. *Wilderness Medicine*, 6th Ed. Philadelphia: Mosby, 2012.

Managing Spinal Injuries

Books

1. Caroline, N.L. *Emergency Care in the Streets*, 4th Ed. Boston: Little, Brown & Co., 1991.
2. Netter, F.H. *The Musculoskeletal System*. The CIBA Collection of Medical Illustrations, Vol. 8, Part I. Summit, NJ: The CIBA-GEIGY Corporation, 1987.
3. McNamara EC, Johe DH, ed. Outdoor Emergency Care, 5th Edition. Brady, 2012.
4. Garrick JG, Webb DR: *Sports Injuries: Diagnosis and Management*. Philadelphia. W.B. Saunders Company, 1990.
5. Casey JC, et al: *Winter Sports Medicine*. Philadelphia. F.A. Davis Company, 1990.

Download

White CC, Domaier RM, Millin MG. EMS spinal precautions and the use of the long backboard: resource document to the position statement of the National Association of EMS Physicians and the American College of Surgeons Committee on Trauma. Available as a free pdf download at www.naemsp.org/Documents/Position Papers/EMS Spinal Precautions and the use of the Long Backboard_Resource Document.pdf

Chest and Abdominal Injuries

Book

Auerbach PS. *Medicine for the Outdoors*: A Guide to Emergency Medical Procedures and First Aid, rev. ed. Boston: Little, Brown & Co., 1991.

Chapter

Toschlog EA, Moris JA, Jr. Wilderness trauma and surgical emergencies. In: Auerbach PS, ed. *Wilderness Medicine*, 4th Ed. St. Louis: Mosby, 2001.

Hyperthermia: How to Beat the Heat

1. Nelson AG. Body cooling and response to heat – a commentary. *Wilderness & Environmental Medicine* 12(1):32-34, 2001.
2. O'Brien KK, Leon LR, Kenefick RW. Clinical management of heat-related illnesses. In: Auerbach P, ed. *Wilderness Medicine*, 6th Ed. Philadelphia: Mosby, 2012.
3. Kenefick RW et al. Dehydration, rehydration, and hyperhydration. In: Auerbach P, ed. *Wilderness Medicine*, 6th Ed. Philadelphia: Mosby, 2012.
4. Rogers IR. Fluid and electrolyte balance and endurance exercise: What can we learn from recent research? *Wilderness Medicine Letter* 18(3):2-4, Spring 2001.
5. Leon LR, Kenefick RW. Pathophysiology of heat-related illnesses. In: Auerbach P, ed. *Wilderness Medicine*, 6th Ed. Philadelphia: Mosby, 2012.
6. Crawshaw LI et al. Thermoregulation. In: Auerbach P, ed. *Wilderness Medicine*, 6th Ed. Philadelphia: Mosby, 2012.
7. Bennett BL et al. Wilderness Medical Society practice guidelines for the treatment of exercise-associated hyponatremia: 2014 update. Wilderness & Environmental Medicine 25(1): S30-S42, 2014.

Hypothermia, Frostbite and Raynaud's Disease

Books

1. Forgey WW, *Death by Exposure: Hypothermia*. ICS Books, Inc., 1985.
2. Wilkerson JA, Bangs CC, Hayward JS. *Hypothermia, Frostbite and other Cold Injuries*: Seattle, The Mountaineers, 1986.

Articles & chapters: Hypothermia

3. Danzl DF. Accidental hypothermia. In: Auerbach P, ed. *Wilderness Medicine*, 6th Ed. Philadelphia: Mosby, 2012.
4. Hamilton RS, Paton BC. The diagnosis and treatment of hypothermia by mountain rescue teams: a survey. *Wilderness & Environmental Medicine* 7(1):28-37, Feb. 1996.
5. Larrey Baron DJ. Hypothermia and warfare: Napoleon's retreat from Moscow, 1812. Selection by B. Paton in *Wilderness Medicine Letter* 12(1):12, Winter 1995.
6. Giesbrecht GG, Steinman AM. Immersion into cold water. In: Auerbach P, ed. *Wilderness Medicine*, 6th Ed. Philadelphia: Mosby, 2012.
7. Giesbrecht GG. Prehospital treatment of hypothermia. *Wilderness & Environmental Medicine* 12(1):24-31, 2001.
8. Roberts M. 2 sisters saved from fatal freeze in snow. *Redwood City Tribune*, Jan. 2, 1979.

9. Additional information is drawn from an unpublished report by John Kretschmann for the Pinecrest Nordic Ski Patrol and the U.S. Forest Service, Stanislaus National Forest, Feb. 24, 1993.
10. Zafren K et al. Wilderness Medical Society practice guidelines for the out-of-hospital evaluation and treatment of accidental hypothermia. Wilderness & Environmental Medicine 25(1): S66-S85, 2014.

Frostbite

1. Freer L, Imray CHE. Frostbite. In: Auerbach P, ed. *Wilderness Medicine*, 6th Ed. Philadelphia: Mosby, 2012.
2. O'Brien C, Frickmen PN. Peripheral responses to cold: Case studies from an arctic expedition. *Wilderness & Environmental Medicine* 14(2):112-119, Summer 2003.
3. McIntosh SE et al. Wilderness Medical Society practice guidelines for the prevention and treatment of frostbite: 2014 update. *Wilderness & Environmental Medicine* 25: S43-S54, 2014.

Other cold injuries

1. Imray CHE, Castellani JW. Nonfreezing cold-induced injuries. In: Auerbach P, ed. *Wilderness Medicine*, 6th Ed. Philadelphia: Mosby, 2012.
2. Hamlet M. Raynaud's disease: a simple approach to management. *The Physician and Sportsmedicine* 18(3):129-132, March 1990.
3. Zafren K. Hyponatremia in a cold environment. *Wilderness & Environmental Medicine* 9(1):54-55, 1998.

Video

Giesbrecht GG. Cold water boot camp. Video. https://www.youtube.com/watch?v=J1xohI3B4Uc

Dressing for Survival

1. Bowman WD, Kummerfeldt P. Essentials of wilderness survival. In: Auerbach P, ed. *Wilderness Medicine*, 6th Ed. Philadelphia: Mosby, 2012.
2. Dow J, McDevitt MC. Outdoor clothing for the wilderness professional. In: Auerbach P, ed. *Wilderness Medicine*, 6th Ed. Philadelphia: Mosby, 2012.

3. Hamlet DM. The science of clothing for the outdoors. *Wilderness Medicine Letter* 17(1):1-2,4-5,14, Winter 2000.

Altitude Illness

Books

1. Houston CS. *Going Higher: Oxygen, Man, and Mountains*, 4th ed. Little, Brown & Co., 1999.
2. Hultgren H. *High Altitude Medicine*. Hultgren Publications, 827 San Francisco Court, Stanford, CA 94305-1021, 1997.
3. Hackett PH. *Mountain Sickness*. American Alpine Club, 1980.

Articles & chapters : Altitude illness

1. Swenson ER, MacDonald A, Vatheuer M, et al. Acute mountain sickness is not altered by a high carbohydrate diet nor associated with elevated circulating cytokines. *Aviation, Space, and Environmental Medicine* 68(6):499-503, June 1997.
2. Hackett PH, Roach RC. High-altitude medicine and physiology. In: Auerbach P, ed. *Wilderness Medicine*, 6th Ed. Philadelphia: Mosby, 2012.
3. Scherer U, Vollenweider L, Delabays A, et al. Inhaled nitric oxide for high altitude pulmonary edema. *New England Journal of Medicine* 334(10):624-629, March 7, 1996.
4. Grissom CK, Elstad MR. The pathophysiology of high altitude pulmonary edema. *Wilderness & Environmental Medicine* 10(2):88-92, Summer 1999.
5. Luks AM et al. Wilderness Medical Society practice guidelines for the prevention and treatment of acute altitude illness: 2014 update. *Wilderness & Environmental Medicine* 25 (1): S4-S14, 2014.

Prevention

1. Askew EW. Food for high-altitude expeditions: Pugh got it right in 1954. *Wilderness & Environmental Medicine* 15(1):121-124, 2004.
2. Moraga FA, Flores A, Serra J, Esnaola C, Barriento C. Gingko biloba decreases acute mountain sickness in people ascending to high altitude at Ollague (3696 meters) in Northern

Chile. *Wilderness & Environmental Medicine* 18(4): 251-257, Winter 2007.

3. Maakestad K, Leadbette G, Olson S, Hackett P. Ginkgo Biloba reduces incidence and severity of acute mountain sickness [Abstract from the annual scientific meeting of the Wilderness Medical Society]. *Wilderness & Environmental Medicine* 12(1):51, Spring 2001.

4. Pugh LGC. Himalayan rations with special reference to the 1953 expedition to Mount Everest. *Wilderness & Environmental Medicine* 15(1):125-134, 2004.

5. Askew EW. Nutrition at altitude. *Wilderness Medicine Letter* 18(3):9-12, Spring 2001.

6. Berg JT, Ramanathan S, Swenson ER. Inhibitors of hypoxic pulmonary vasoconstriction prevent high altitude pulmonary edema in rats. *Wilderness & Environmental Medicine* 15(1): 32-37, 2004.

Vision & altitude

1. Mader TH, White LJ, Johnson DS, Barth FC. The ascent of Mount Everest following radial keratotomy. *Wilderness & Environmental Medicine* 13(1):53-54, Spring 2002.

2. Mader TH, White LJ. High altitude mountain climbing after radial keratotomy. *Wilderness and Environmental Medicine* 7(1):77-78, February 1996.

3. Dimming J, et al. Lasik on Mount Everest. *J. of Refractive Surgery* 19:48-51, 2003.

Lightning Strike

1. Lichtenberg R, et al. Cardiovascular effects of lightning strikes. *J. Amer. Coll. Card.* 21(2):531-536, Feb. 1993.

2. Ehrlich G. I have been struck by lightning and I am alive. *Hippocrates*, June 1994.

3. Cooper MA et al. Lightning injuries. In: Auerbach P, ed. *Wilderness Medicine*, 6th Ed. Philadelphia: Mosby, 2012.

4. The story of the marathon runner and his wife is drawn from a copy of an unsigned typescript called "Roads to fitness – August 29, 1991," given to me by J. McBride.

5. Davis C et al. Wilderness Medical society practice guidelines for the prevention and treatment of lightning injuries: 2014 update. *Wilderness & Environmental Medicine* 25 (1): S86-S95, 2014.

Solar radiation and Eye Protection

Effects of UV radiation on the eye

1. Cullen AP: Additive Effects of Ultraviolet Radiation. *Am J Optom Physio Optics* 57:808-814, 1980

2. Brillant LB, et al: Associations among Cataract Prevalence, Sunlight Hours and Altitude in the Himalayas. *Am J Epid* 118:250-264, 1983

3. Rigel DS, Rigel EG, Rigel AC: Effects of Altitude and Latitude on Ambient UVB Radiation. *J Am Acad Dematol.* 40(1):114-6, 1999

4. Taylor HR, et al: Effect of Ultraviolet Radiation on Cataract Formation. *New England J Med* 319: 1429-1433, 1988

5. Pitts DG: The Human Ultraviolet Action Spectrum. *Am J Optom Physiol Optics* 51:946-960, 1974

6. Pitts DG, Cullen AP, Hacker PD: Ocular Effects of Ultraviolet Radiation from 295 to 365 nm. *Invest Ophthal Vis Sci* 16:932-939, 1977

7. Rosenthal FS, Satrum M, Taylor HR: The Ocular Dose of Ultraviolet Radiation to Outdoor Workers. *Invest Ophthal Vis Sci* 29:649-656, 1988

8. Tannoudji D, Sahel J, Picaud S: Phototoxic Action Spectrum on a Retinal Pigment Epithelium Model of Age-Related Macular Degeneration Exposed to Sunlight Normalized Conditions. *PlosOne* 8 (2013), DOI:10.1371/journal.pone.0071398

9. Sliney DH: Physical Factors in Cataractogenesis: Ambient Radiation and Temperature. *Invest Ophthal Vis Sci* 27:781-790, 1986

10. Polycarbonate lens update. *Optical World* 13(80):21-22, 1984

11. Scotto J, Fears TR, Gori GB: Ultraviolet Exposure Patterns. *Env Res* 12:228-237, 1986

12. Jinna S, Adams BB: Ultraviolet Radiation and the Athlete: Risk, Sun Safety, and Barriers to Implementation of Protective Strategies. *Sports Med* 43(7):531-537, 2013

Lenses for sun protection

1. Kors K, Peters HB: *Absorption Characteristics of Selected Commercially Available Ophthalmic Lenses.* Am J Optom Arch Am Acad of Optom 49(9):727-735, 1972

2. Fannin TE, Grosvenor TP: *Clinical Optics*, 179-230. Stoneham, MA: Butterworth., 1987

3. Mahjoob M, Heydarian S, Koochi S: Effect of Yellow Filter on Visual Acuity and Contrast

Sensitivity under Glare Condition among Different Age Groups. *Int Ophthalmol* 36:509-514, 2016

4. Harwood L: The Effects of Combining Optical Coating and Photochromic Lenses. *Am J Optom Arch Am Acad Optom* 48(8):659-661, 1971

5. Young, JM: How Polarized Lenses Really Work. *Eye Care Business* 3(5):42-46, 1988

6. Nyman JS, London R: *Problems in Optometry.* Ocular Emergencies 1(1), Oct-Dec 1989

7. Luria SM: Preferred Density of Sunglasses. *Am J Optom & Phys Opt* 61(6):397-402, 1984

8. Dain SJ: Sports Eyewear Protective Standards. *Clin Exp Optom* 99:4-23, 2016

9. American National Standard: *Sunglasses and fashion eyewear.* Publication #Z80.3-1986. N.Y., American National Standards Institute, Inc. 1986

10. Young RW: Sunglasses for Visual Health. *Eye Care Business* 3(5):48-53, 1988

11. Denison J: Tinting Optical Plastic Lenses Made from CR-39 Monomer: Part 3. *Optical Index* 55(10):59-64, 1980

12. Technical Information on Xperio UV. Essilor of America, Inc., 2016

13. Technical information. Corning Photochromic Ophthalmic Lenses, OPO-181. Corning, NY: Corning Corp., 1985

14. TransitionsPRO.com: Transitions Optical, Inc., 2015

Other topics

1. Fraunfelder FT: *Drug Induced Ocular Side Effects and Drug Interactions,* 271-272, 331-332. Philadelphia, Lea and Febiger, 1976

2. Watanabe K, Kaido M, Ishida R, et al: The Effect of Soft Contact Lens Wear on Functional Visual Acuity and Higher Order Aberrations. *Contact Lens & Anterior Eye* 37:203-208, 2014

3. Hoskins AK, Philip S, Dain SJ, Mackey DA: Spectacle-related Eye Injuries, Spectacle-impact Performance and Eye Protection. *Clin Exp Optom* 98:203-209, 2015

Sunburn and Skin Protection

1. Anti-photoaging and photoprotective compounds derived from marine organisms. *Mar Drugs* 8(4): 1189-1202, 2010. Published online: http://www.ncbi.nlm.nih.gov/pmc/articles/PMC 2866482/

2. Environmental Working Group: *Guide to sunscreens.* http://www.ewg.org/2015sunscreen/

3. Stege H et al. Enzyme plus light therapy to repair DNA damage in ultraviolet B irradiated human skin. Proc Natl Acad Sci USA 97(4): 1790-1795, Feb 15, 2000. Available online: http://www.ncbi.nlm.nih.gov/pmc/articles/PMC26 514/

4. Krakowski AC, Kaplan LA. Exposure to radiation from the sun. In: Auerbach P, ed. *Wilderness Medicine*, 6th Ed. Philadelphia: Mosby, 2012.

Contaminated water & disinfection

1. Gerba CP, Johnson D, Hasan MN. Efficacy of iodine water purification tablets against Cryptosporidium oosphere cysts and Giardia cysts. *Wilderness & Environmental Medicine* 8(2):96-100, May 1997.

2. Backer HD. Field water disinfection. In: Auerbach P, ed. *Wilderness Medicine*, 6th Ed. Philadelphia: Mosby, 2012.

3. Adachi JA, Backer HD, Dupont HL. Infectious diarrhea from wilderness and foreign travel. In: Auerbach P, ed. *Wilderness Medicine*, 6th Ed. Philadelphia: Mosby, 2012.

4. Gerba CP, Naranjo JE. Microbiological water purification without the use of chemical disinfection. *Wilderness & Environmental Medicine* 11(1):12-16, Spring 2000.

Mosquitoes, Ticks and Disease

Books

1. Sherman IW. *The Elusive Malaria Vaccine: Miracle or Mirage?* Washington D.C.: American Society for Microbiology, 2009.

2. Desowitz, RS. *The Malaria Capers.* New York: W.W. Norton & Company, Inc., 1991.

3. McNeill WH. *Plagues and Peoples.* New York: Anchor Books, 1998.

4. Drummond R. *Ticks: And what you can do about them*, Wilderness Press, 2440 Bancroft Way, Berkeley, CA 94704.

Diseases

1. Kanzaria HK, Hsia RY. Mosquitoes and mosquito-borne diseases. In: Auerbach P, ed. *Wilderness Medicine*, 6th Ed. Philadelphia: Mosby, 2012.

2. Erickson TB, Marquez A. Arthropod envenomation and parasitism. In: Auerbach P, ed. *Wilderness Medicine*, 6th Ed. Philadelphia: Mosby, 2012.

3. Patel SS. Malaria. In: Auerbach P, ed. *Wilderness Medicine*, 6th Ed. Philadelphia: Mosby, 2012.
4. William T et al. Increasing Incidence of *Plasmodium knowlesi* Malaria following Control of *P. falciparum* and *P. vivax* Malaria in Sabah, Malaysia. *PLoS Negl Trop Dis.* 2013 Jan; 7(1): e2026. http://www.ncbi.nlm.nih.gov/pmc/articles/PMC35 54533/.
5. Traub SJ, Cummins GA. Tick-borne diseases. In: Auerbach P, ed. *Wilderness Medicine*, 6th Ed. Philadelphia: Mosby, 2012.

Repellents

1. Stanczyck NM, Brookfield JFY, Field LM, Logan JG. Aedes Aegypti mosquitoes exhibit decreased repellency by DEET following previous exposure. PLOS One 8(2), February 2013. http://journals.plos.org/plosone/article?id=10.1371/journal.pone.0054438
2. Effectiveness of a repellant containing DEET and EBAAP foe preventing tick bites. *Wilderness & Environmental Medicine* 13(1):12-20, Spring 2002.
3. Fradin MS, Carroll SP. Protection from blood-feeding arthropods. In: Auerbach P, ed. *Wilderness Medicine*, 6th Ed. Philadelphia: Mosby, 2012.

Tick removal

1. Stewart RL, Burgdorfer W, Needham GR. Evaluation of three commercial tick-removal tools. *Wilderness & Environmental Medicine* 9(3):137-142, Fall 1998.
2. Celenza A, Rogers IR. The "knot method" of tick removal. *Wilderness & Environmental Medicine* 13(2):179-180, 2002.

Spiders, Bees and Wasps

1. Yang S et al. A bimodal activation mechanism underlies scorpion toxin-induced pain. *Science Advances* 3(8), 2 August 2017.
2. Wingert W. Black widow spider envenomation. *Wilderness Medicine Letter* 12(4):12, Fall 1995.
3. Abroug f, Nouira S, El Atrous S, et al. A canine study of immunotherapy in scorpion envenomation. *Intensive Care Med* 2003.

4. Maynor ML. Hyperbaric oxygen to treat brown recluse spider bites. *Wilderness Medicine Letter* 13(4):12-13, Fall 1996.
5. Minton SA, Bechtel HB, Erickson TB. North American arthropod envenomation and parasitism. In: Auerbach PS, ed. *Wilderness Medicine*,4th Ed. St. Louis: Mosby, 2001.
6. Boyer LV, Binford GJ, Degan JA. Spider bites. In: Auerbach P, ed. *Wilderness Medicine*, 6th Ed. Philadelphia: Mosby, 2012.
7. Suchard JR. Scorpion envenomation. In: Auerbach P, ed. *Wilderness Medicine*, 6th Ed. Philadelphia: Mosby, 2012.

Venomous Snakes

Books

1. Klauber LM. *Rattlesnakes: Their Habits, Life Histories, & Influence on Mankind*, Abridged Edition. Berkeley: University of California Press, 1982.
2. Russell FE. *Snake Venom Poisoning*. Great Neck, J.B. Lippencott Company, 1983.

Snakebite effects

1. Norris RL, Bush S, Smith JC. Bites by venomous reptiles in Canada, the United States, and Mexico. In: Auerbach P, ed. *Wilderness Medicine*, 6th Ed. Philadelphia: Mosby, 2012.
2. Warrell DA. Envenoming and injuries by venomous and nonvenomous reptiles worldwide. In: Auerbach PS, ed. *Wilderness Medicine*, 6th Ed. Philadelphia: Mosby, 2012.

Snakebite treatment

1. Kanaan NC et al. Wilderness Medical Society practice guidelines for the treatment of pit viper envenomations in the United States and Canada. *Wilderness and Environmental Medicine* 26:472-487, 2015.
2. NOTE: The recommendation in the American Heart Association and American Red Cross Guidelines for First Aid (2010, 2015) to use constricting bands for North American pit viper envenomation has been REJECTED by North American snakebite experts, including the authors of the only article cited in the AHA Guidelines to support their recommendation.

Antivenom

1. Horowitz RS, Dart RC. Antivenins and immunobiologicals: immunotherapeutics of envenomation. In: Auerbach PS, ed. *Wilderness Medicine,*4th Ed. St. Louis: Mosby, 2001.
2. Norris RL, Dery R, Johnson C, et al. Regional vs. systemic antivenom administration in the treatment of snake venom poisoning in a rabbit model: A pilot study. *Wilderness & Environmental Medicine* 14(4): 231-235, 2003.
3. LoVeccio F, Klemens J, Roundy EBA, Klemens A. Serum sickness following administration of antivenin (Crotalidae) polyvalent in 181 cases of presumed rattlesnake envenomation. *Wilderness & Environmental Medicine* 14(4): 220-221, 2003.

What NOT to do

1. Davis D, Branch K, Egan NB, Russell FE, Gerrish K, Auerbach PS. The effect of electrical current on snake venom toxicity. *Journal of Wilderness Medicine* 3(1):48-53, February 1992.
2. Bush SP, Hegewald GK, Green SM, Cardwell MD, Hayes WK. Effects of a negative pressure traction device (Extractor) on local tissue injury after artificial rattlesnake envenomation in a porcine model. *Wilderness and Environmental Medicine* 11(3):180-188, Fall 2000.
3. Alberts MB, Shalit M, LoGalbo F. Suction for venomous snakebite: A study of "mock venom" extraction in a human model. *Annals of Emergency Medicine* 43:181-186, 2004.
4. Welch EB, Gales BJ. Use of stun guns for venomous bites and stings: a review. *Wilderness & Environmental Medicine* 12(2):111-117, Summer 2001.

Hazardous Mammals

Book

Herrero S. *Bear Attacks: Their Causes and Avoidance.* Lyons & Burford, 1985.

Articles & chapters: Attacks

1. Freer L, French SP. Bear behavior and attacks. In: Auerbach P, ed. *Wilderness Medicine*, 6th Ed. Philadelphia: Mosby, 2012.
2. Floyd T. Bear-inflicted human injury and fatality. *Wilderness & Environmental Medicine* 10(2):75-87, Summer 1999.
3. Bradford JE, Freer L. Bites and injuries inflicted by wild and domestic animals. In: Auerbach P, ed. *Wilderness Medicine*, 6th Ed. Philadelphia: Mosby, 2012.
4. Conrad LC. Wild animal attacks in the United States. *Wilderness Medicine Letter* 13(2):1,607; Spring 1996

Infections

1. Neumann K. Hantavirus infections in the Southwestern United States. *Wilderness Medicine Letter* 11(2):1,9; Spring 1994
2. Wilkerson JA. Rabies. In: Auerbach P, ed. *Wilderness Medicine*, 6th Ed. Philadelphia: Mosby, 2012.

Hazardous Marine Animals

Book

Auerbach PS. *Medicine for the Outdoors.* Boston: Little, Brown & Co., 1991.

Articles & chapters

1. Breault, JL. Candiru: Amazonian parasitic catfish. *Journal of Wilderness Medicine* 2(4):304-312, November 1991.
2. Kizer KW. Aquatic infections: from the benign to the life-threatening. *Emergency Medicine* July 15, 1991:77-90.
3. Kimball AB, Arambula KZ, et al. Efficacy of a jellyfish sting inhibitor in preventing jellyfish stings in normal volunteers. *Wilderness & Environmental Medicine* 15(2):102-108, 2004.
4. Auerbach PS. Envenomation by aquatic vertebrates. In: Auerbach P, ed. *Wilderness Medicine*, 6th Ed. Philadelphia: Mosby, 2012.
5. Auerbach PS. Envenomation by aquatic invertebrates. In: Auerbach P, ed. *Wilderness Medicine*, 6th Ed. Philadelphia: Mosby, 2012.
6. Auerbach PS, Burgess GH. Injuries from nonvenomous aquatic animals. In: Auerbach P, ed. *Wilderness Medicine*, 6th Ed. Philadelphia: Mosby, 2012.

7. Lakkis NA, Maalouf GJ, Mahmassani DM. Jellyfish stings: A practical approach. *Wilderness & Environmental Medicine* 26(3): 422-429, 2015.
8. Kizer KW. When a stingray strikes: treating common marine envenomations. *The Physician and Sportsmedicine* 18(8):93-109, August 1990.

Hazardous Plants

Book

Auerbach PS. *Medicine for the Outdoors*: A Guide to Emergency Medical Procedures and First Aid, rev. ed. Boston: Little, Brown & Co., 1991.

Chapter

Schofner JD, Kimball AB. Plant-induced dermatitis. In: Auerbach P, ed. *Wilderness Medicine*, 6th Ed. Philadelphia: Mosby, 2012.

EMS in the Wilderness

Books

1. Forgey WW, ed. *Wilderness Medical Society Practice Guidelines for Wilderness Emergency Care*, 2nd Ed. Guilford: The Globe Pequot Press, 2001.
2. National Association for Search and Rescue. *Fundamentals of Search and Rescue*, 2nd Edition. NASAR July 2018.
3. Setnicka TJ. *Wilderness Search and Rescue*. Appalachian Mountain Club, 1980.

Articles & chapters

1. Shimanski C. Helicopter evacuation of the injured patient. *Wilderness Medicine Letter* 17(3):1-7; 17(4):1-7, Summer & Fall 2000.
2. Allen RC, Cooper JL. Helicopter rescue and aeromedical transport. In: Auerbach P, ed. *Wilderness Medicine*, 6th Ed. Philadelphia: Mosby, 2012.
3. Cooper DC, LaValla PH, Stoffel RC. Search and rescue. In: Auerbach P, ed. *Wilderness Medicine*, 6th Ed. Philadelphia: Mosby, 2012.
4. Hubbell FR. Wilderness emergency medical services and response systems. In: Auerbach P, ed. *Wilderness Medicine*, 6th Ed. Philadelphia: Mosby, 2012.

Respiratory Illness

Books

1. Auerbach PS. *Medicine for the Outdoors: A Guide to Emergency Medical Procedures and First Aid*, rev. ed. Boston: Little, Brown & Co., 1991.
2. Moser KM, Spragg RC. *Respiratory Emergencies*, 2nd Ed. St. Louis: The C.V. Mosby Company, 1982.
3. Lehrer S. Understanding Lung Sounds. Philadelphia: W.B. Saunders Co., 1984.
4. Dormandy T. *The White Death: A History of Tuberculosis*. New York: New York University Press, 2000.
5. Forgey WW. *Wilderness Medicine*, 4th Ed. Merrillville: ICS Books, 1994.

Articles & chapters

1. Slovis CM. 5-step asthma approach. *JEMS* 28(12):65-72, Dec. 2003.
2. For the hygiene hypothesis on why asthma is so prevalent in developed countries, see: Okada H, Kuhn C, Feillet H, Bach JF. The 'hygiene hypothesis' for autoimmune and allergic diseases: An update. *Clin Exp Immunol*. Apr 2010; 160(1): 1-9. Accessible at: www.ncbi.nlm.nih.gov/pmc/articles/PMC2841828/

Web site

Physiopedia: Auscultation. www.physio-pedia.com/Auscultation.

Gastrointestinal Illness

Books

1. Youmans GP, Paterson PY, Sommers HM, ed. *The Biologic and Clinical Basis of Infectious Disease*. Philadelphia: W.B. Saunders Company, 1986.
2. Auerbach PS. *Medicine for the Outdoors: A Guide to Emergency Medical Procedures and First Aid*, rev. ed. Boston: Little, Brown & Co., 1991.

Articles & chapters

1. Backer HD. Field water disinfection. In: Auerbach P, ed. Wilderness Medicine, 6th Ed. Philadelphia: Mosby, 2012.
2. Adachi JA, Backer HD, DuPont HL. Infectious diarrhea from wilderness and foreign travel. In: Auerbach P, ed. Wilderness Medicine, 6th Ed. Philadelphia: Mosby, 2012.

Diabetes and Seizures

Books

1. Auerbach PS. *Medicine for the Outdoors: A Guide to Emergency Medical Procedures and First Aid*, rev. ed. Boston: Little, Brown & Co., 1991.

2. Forgey WW. *Wilderness Medicine*, 4th Ed. Merrillville: ICS Books, 1994.

Articles & chapters

1. Bhaskarabhatla KV, Birres R. Physical activity and Type II diabetes. *Physician and Sportsmedicine* 32(1), January 2004.

2. Krolak S. Searching for seeds in the southwest. *Calypso Log* 21(3):20-21, June 1994.

Pregnancy and wilderness activity

1. Anderson S. Women in the wilderness. In: Auerbach P, ed. *Wilderness Medicine*, 6th Ed. Philadelphia: Mosby, 2012.

CPR and oxygen in the Wilderness

1. *2015 American Heart Association Guidelines for Cardiopulmonary Resuscitation and Emergency Cardiovascular Care Science*. Available at: http://circ.ahajournals.org/content/122/18_suppl_3.toc
2. Flesche CW et al. The ability of health professionals to check the carotid pulse. *Circulation* 90 (Suppl. 1):288, 1994.
3. Valenzuela TD, et al. Case and survival definitions in out-of-hospital cardiac arrest: effect on survival rate calculation. *JAMA* 267(2): 272-274, Jan. 8, 1992.
4. Eberle B. et al. Checking the carotid pulse check: diagnostic accuracy of first responders in patients with diagnostic accuracy of first responders inpatients with and without a pulse. Resuscitation 33:107-116, 1996.
5. Navarro, Kenneth. Getting with the 2015 Guidelines: The science behind the scenes. Presentation at The Wine Country Field Care Symposium, 2015.
6. Sasson C, Rogers MAM, Dahl J, Kellerman AL. Predictors of survival from out-of-hospital cardiac arrest: A systematic review and meta-analysis. Circ Cardiovasc Qual Outcomes 2010;3;63-81; originally published online November 10, 2009. Available at: http://circoutcomes.ahajournals.org/content/3/1/63.full.
7. Koenig WJ, Ostrow LS. Prehospital cardiac care. *J Emerg. Med. Serv.* 21(5):42-52, May 1996.
8. Bahr J et al. Skills of lay people in checking the carotid pulse. *Resuscitation* 35:23-26, 1997.
9. Kaye W et al. The problem of poor retention of CPR skills may lie with the instructor. *Resuscitation* 21:61-87, 1991.
10. Moser DK, Coleman S. Recommendations for improving cardiopulmonary resuscitation skills retention. *Heart and Lung* 21(4):372-380, July/August 1992.

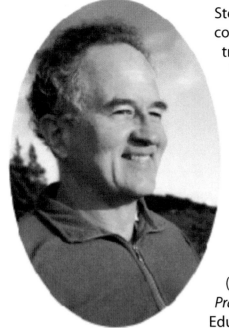

Steve Donelan, NREMT, has been designing, developing and teaching courses in wilderness and prehospital emergency care for over 30 years, and training instructors almost as long. Earlier versions of his courses (Basic Wilderness First Aid, Wilderness First Aid, Wilderness First Responder, and Wilderness EMT Upgrade) have been available through other organizations, but they are now supported by the National Association for Search and Rescue. Steve has a BA in Philosophy and Greek from the University of California, Berkeley, and did years of graduate studies in the history of science. He has published over 60 articles on emergency care and how to teach it, as well as several textbooks. He has been an instructor of the National Ski Patrol's Outdoor Emergency Care course since the beginning of the program, and is a peer reviewer of the OEC textbook. He is also the section editor and columnist on education for *Wilderness and Environmental Medicine* (journal of the Wilderness Medical Society), a peer reviewer of their *Practice Guidelines for Wilderness Emergency Care*, and a recipient of their Education Award.

Steve can be contacted about teaching and instructor training through his web site:

www.wildernessemergencycare.com.

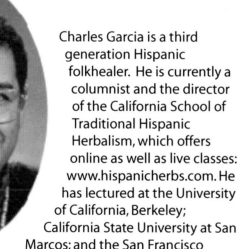

Charles Garcia is a third generation Hispanic folkhealer. He is currently a columnist and the director of the California School of Traditional Hispanic Herbalism, which offers online as well as live classes: www.hispanicherbs.com. He has lectured at the University of California, Berkeley; California State University at San Marcos; and the San Francisco Healthcare Consortium. His other vocation is talking down potential suicides, and he hasnt lost one yet. His novel, Forever Faire: A Post Apocalyptic Fantasy is available on Amazon for download. Charles is married with two daughters, one granddaughter, and a cat.

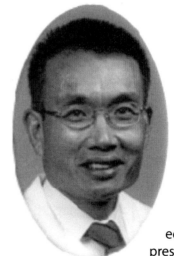

Stephen R. Chun, O.D., F.A.A.O. is Clinical Professor of Optometry at the University of California, Berkeley, and founding partner of the Berkeley Optometric Group. Since 1996, he has directed a U.C. Berkeley program to develop optometry in China at Beijing University. He is interested in optometry education and has served as president and licensure examination chair of the California Board of Optometry. In 1993, he was honored as California Optometrist of the Year, and in 1994 as Optometry Alumnus of the Year at U.C. Berkeley.

Made in the USA
Middletown, DE
09 March 2020